Guide to

Peripheral and Cerebrovascular Intervention

By the same editor:
Essential Concepts in Cardiovascular Intervention
Handbook of Acute Coronary Syndromes

Published by Remedica Publishing
32–38 Osnaburgh Street, London, NW1 3ND, UK
Civic Opera Building, 20 North Wacker Drive, Suite 1642, Chicago, IL 60606, USA

Email: books@remedica.com
www.remedica.com
Tel: +44 20 7388 7677
Fax: +44 20 7388 7457

Publisher: Andrew Ward
In-house editor: Cath Harris

ISBN 1 901346 61 7
British Library Cataloguing-in-Publication Data
A catalogue record for this book is available from the British Library.

Guide to

Peripheral and Cerebrovascular Intervention

Deepak L Bhatt, Editor

Editor

Deepak L Bhatt, MD, FACC, FSCAI, FESC
Director, Interventional Cardiovascular Fellowship
Associate Director, Cardiovascular Medicine Fellowship
Staff, Cardiac, Peripheral, and Cerebrovascular Intervention
Department of Cardiovascular Medicine
Cleveland Clinic Foundation
9500 Euclid Avenue, Desk F25
Cleveland, OH 44195
USA

Authors

Alex Abou-Chebl, MD
Interventional Neurology Section
of Stroke and Neurological
Critical Care
Department of Neurology, S91
Cleveland Clinic Foundation
9500 Euclid Avenue
Cleveland, OH 44195, USA

Christopher T Bajzer
Associate Director, Vascular Intervention
Department of Cardiovascular Medicine
Cleveland Clinic Foundation
9500 Euclid Avenue, Desk F25
Cleveland, OH 44195, USA

Charles T Burke, MD
Assistant Professor of Radiology
University of North Carolina at Chapel Hill
Chapel Hill, NC 27599-7212, USA

Ivan P Casserly, MD
Department of Cardiovascular Medicine
Cleveland Clinic Foundation
9500 Euclid Avenue, Desk F25
Cleveland, OH 44195, USA

Albert W Chan, MD
Associate Director, Catheterization Laboratory
Department of Cardiology
Ochsner Clinic Foundation
1514 Jefferson Highway
New Orleans, LA 70121, USA

Yung-Wei Chi, DO
Ochsner Heart and Vascular Institute
Department of Cardiology
Ochsner Clinic Foundation
1514 Jefferson Highway
New Orleans, LA 70121, USA

Leslie Cho, MD
Director, Carotid Intervention
Assistant Professor of Medicine
Stritch School of Medicine
Loyola University Medical Center
2160 S. First Avenue, Building 110 #6215
Maywood, IL 60153, USA

Frank J Criado, MD
Director, Center for Vascular Intervention
Chief, Division of Vascular Surgery
Union Memorial Hospital/MedStar Health
3333 N. Calvert Street, Suite 570
Baltimore, MD 21218, USA

Gregory S Domer, MD
Division of Vascular Surgery and
Center for Vascular Intervention
Union Memorial Hospital/MedStar Health
3333 N. Calvert Street, Suite 570
Baltimore, MD 21218, USA

J Emilio Exaire, MD
Department of Cardiovascular Medicine
Cleveland Clinic Foundation
9500 Euclid Avenue, Desk F25
Cleveland, OH 44195, USA

Brendan P Girschek, BS
Division of Vascular Surgery and
Center for Vascular Intervention
Union Memorial Hospital/MedStar Health
3333 N. Calvert Street, Suite 570
Baltimore, MD 21218, USA

Samir R Kapadia, MD
Interventional Cardiologist
Department of Cardiovascular Medicine
Cleveland Clinic Foundation
9500 Euclid Avenue, Desk F25
Cleveland, OH 44195, USA

Steven P Marso, MD
Assistant Professor
University of Missouri-Kansas City
St Luke's Hospital
Mid America Heart Institute
4401 Wornall
Kansas City, MO 64111, USA

Debabrata Mukherjee, MD, MS, FACC
Director, Peripheral Vascular
Interventions, Cardiology
Assistant Professor, Department
of Internal Medicine
University of Michigan Health System
University Hospital, TC B1 228
1500 E. Medical Center Drive
Ann Arbor, MI 48109-0311, USA

Marco Roffi, MD
Andreas Grüntzig Cardiovascular
Catheterization Laboratories
Cardiology
University Hospital
Raemistrasse 100
8091 Zurich, Switzerland

Jacqueline Saw, MD
Department of Cardiovascular Medicine
Cleveland Clinic Foundation
9500 Euclid Avenue, Desk F25
Cleveland, OH 44195, USA

Guido Schnyder, MD
Centre Cardio Vasculaire
La Riviera
Vevey, Switzerland

Walter A Tan, MD, MS
Director, Vascular Medicine Program
Assistant Professor of Medicine (Cardiology)
Assistant Professor of Radiology
University of North Carolina at Chapel Hill
Chapel Hill, NC 27599-7075, USA

Michael H Wholey, MD, MBA
Associate Professor
Cardiovascular and Interventional Radiology
University of Texas Health Science Center
at San Antonio
San Antonio, TX 78284, USA

Jay S Yadav, MD
Director, Vascular Intervention
Department of Cardiovascular Medicine
Cleveland Clinic Foundation
9500 Euclid Avenue, Desk F25
Cleveland, OH 44195, USA

Preface

We are at the dawn of a new era in the treatment of vascular disease. The time of the scalpel is fading and endovascular intervention is becoming the dominant mode of treatment for peripheral and cerebrovascular diseases.

In keeping with the rapid expansion of knowledge in the field of endovascular intervention, this book brings together experts from various backgrounds to provide the essential content for the reader to perform complex endovascular interventions.

I am grateful to the authors for providing such excellent technical treatises, describing intricate procedures that are in a state of evolution, while at the same time providing the scientific data to justify their positions. I am appreciative of the efforts by Remedica to provide the highest quality reproductions of angiographic images, a prerequisite for any truly useful book pertaining to vascular disease. It is my wish that readers of assorted backgrounds at various stages in their adoption of endovascular techniques will find this book informative, exciting, and also enjoyable, as we enter the brave new world of endovascular intervention.

Deepak L Bhatt

To my wife Shanthala, my sons Vinayak and Arjun,
and my parents, for their unwavering love and support
through this and many other of life's endeavors

Contents

1 Anatomical considerations

Christopher T Bajzer

Introduction

A detailed knowledge and understanding of normal vascular anatomy and the common variants are essential to perform quality angiography and plan endovascular intervention.

Thoracic aorta and the great vessels

The thoracic aorta includes the aortic root, ascending aorta, aortic arch, and a portion of the descending aorta. There is variability in the aortic arch and the origin of the vessels off the aortic arch, which are usually termed the great vessels. The variability in the anatomy of the great vessels is both congenital and acquired. After the origin of the coronary arteries, the great vessels arise off the aortic arch and include:

- the innominate artery (also known as the brachiocephalic artery)

- the left common carotid artery (CCA)

- the left subclavian artery

The angiographic appearance of the origin of the great vessels off the aortic arch is classified as to whether the great vessels arise more from the ascending or the descending portion of the aortic arch. A reference dimension is defined as the diameter of either the left or right CCA. An imaginary horizontal line is drawn tangentially to the top of the aortic arch. Parallel imaginary lines are drawn inferiorly to this index line, spaced by the reference dimension set by the diameter of the CCA (see **Figure 1**).

- If the origins of all the great vessels arise within the arc segment of the aortic arch subtended by the first parallel reference line, it is termed a type I arch.

- If the origins of all the great vessels are included in the arc segment of the aortic arch subtended by the second index line, it is termed a type II arch.

- If the origins of all of the great vessels are included in the arc segment of the aortic arch subtended by the third index line, it is termed a type III arch.

Different arch types occur due to congenital variations as well as acquired variations due to unfolding of the aorta related to various pathologic processes, including long-standing hypertension.

Variations in the origins of the great vessels are often encountered. The innominate artery usually gives rise to the right CCA and right subclavian artery. When the left CCA also originates off the innominate it is termed a "bovine origin" of the left CCA (see **Figure 2**). The term bovine is used because this is the most common anatomy encountered in the bovine species. This variation in the origin of the great vessels is encountered in approximately 7%–20% of individuals.

Another commonly encountered variation is a separate origin of the left vertebral artery off the aortic arch. In this instance, the left vertebral artery is usually identified between the origins of the left CCA and the left subclavian artery. This is encountered in approximately 0.5%–6%

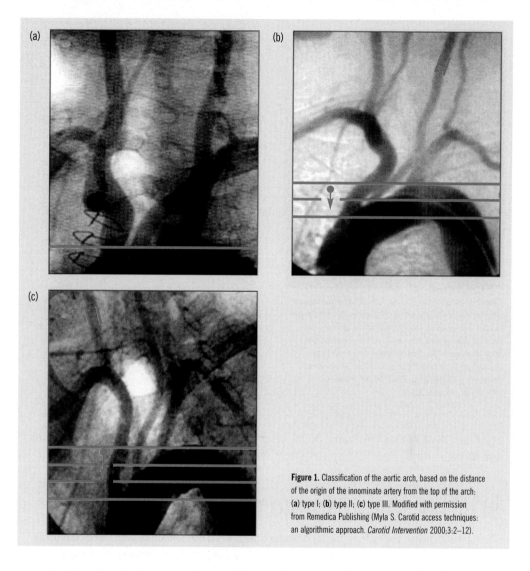

(a)

(b)

(c)

Figure 1. Classification of the aortic arch, based on the distance of the origin of the innominate artery from the top of the arch: (a) type I; (b) type II; (c) type III. Modified with permission from Remedica Publishing (Myla S. Carotid access techniques: an algorithmic approach. *Carotid Intervention* 2000;3:2–12).

of individuals. A less frequently encountered congenital anomaly is a separate origin of the right subclavian artery with a retroesophageal course (0.2%–0.4% of individuals). A further, uncommon, variation in arch anatomy is a persistent right aortic arch; this is sometimes termed the avian arch because it is the most commonly encountered anatomy in birds. A double aortic arch is extremely uncommon and has been termed an amphibian arch (not surprisingly, it is the most common anatomy encountered in amphibians).

Optimal views

Arch aortography is optimal with the patient's head turned towards the right and their chin elevated. The camera's field of view is centered so that it includes the top of the arch and the extent of the carotid arteries to the level of the mandible. Filters minimize areas of over-exposure. Digital subtraction acquisition is utilized with the patient instructed to "Hold your breath, don't

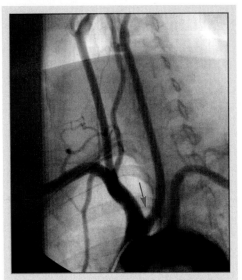

Figure 2. An arch aortogram performed in the 30° left anterior oblique projection with the patient's head turned towards the right and their chin elevated. This run was un-subtracted to show bony landmarks and placement of wedge filters. A bovine origin of the left common carotid artery (arrow) can be seen. The left vertebral artery is only faintly visualized and the right vertebral artery is dominant. There is good visualization of the carotid bifurcations, including both bulbs of the internal carotid arteries.

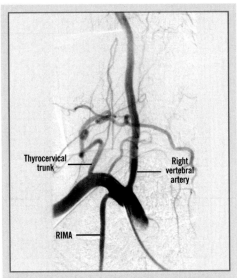

Figure 3. Right subclavian angiography performed in a posteroanterior projection using digital subtraction. This shows the origin and course of the right vertebral artery, as well as of the right internal mammary artery (RIMA) and the thyrocervical trunk.

move, and don't swallow." A total of 30 mL of contrast is utilized at a rate of 15 mL/min with no rate of rise.

Arterial supply to the upper extremities

The right subclavian arises from the innominate artery, while the left subclavian most commonly arises directly off the aortic arch. The subclavian artery gives rise to the internal mammary and vertebral arteries, as well as to the high thoracic artery and thyrocervical trunk (see **Figure 3**). The subclavian artery is terminally demarcated by the first rib. As the subclavian artery courses over the first rib it becomes the axillary artery. The first segment of the axillary artery gives rise to the thoracoacromial trunk and the highest thoracic artery. The distal segment of the axillary artery gives rise to the lateral thoracic artery and the subscapular artery, which in turn gives rise to the circumflex scapular and the thoracodorsal artery (see **Figure 4**). The axillary artery then gives rise to the posterior and anterior circumflex humeral arteries before becoming the brachial artery (see **Figure 5**), which courses over the anterior aspect of the shaft of the humerus. Before this anterior course, the brachial artery gives rise to a radial collateral branch that courses posteriorly and laterally to the humerus itself. The radial collateral then courses anteriorly to the lateral epicondyle and usually rejoins the radial artery at the level of the antecubital fossa. On occasion, the radial collateral will give rise to a branch termed the middle collateral artery, which courses posteriorly to the lateral epicondyle of the humerus and often rejoins the interosseus artery.

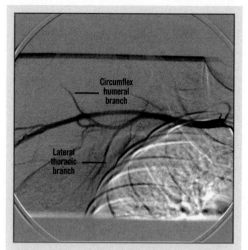

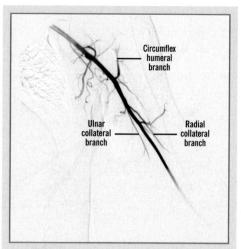

Figure 4. The right axillary artery with continuation into the brachial artery in a posteroanterior projection using digital subtraction. The lateral thoracic and circumflex humeral branches can be seen. Note the presence of a motion artifact that degrades the image quality due to the patient's inability to hold their breath.

Figure 5. The left axillary artery with continuation into the brachial artery in a posteroanterior projection using digital subtraction. Note the origin of the circumflex humeral branches and the radial collateral branch, as well as the ulnar collateral branch.

After giving rise to the radial collateral artery, the brachial artery will first give rise to the superior ulnar collateral and then to the inferior ulnar collateral. These arteries course posteriorly and anteriorly to the medial epicondyle of the humerus, respectively. They rejoin the ulnar artery as the posterior ulnar recurrent artery and the anterior recurrent artery. The brachial artery bifurcates just below the trochlea of the humerus, dividing into the radial artery (which courses laterally) and the ulnar artery (which courses medially) (see **Figure 6**). The interosseous artery commonly arises from the ulnar artery, but has been observed to arise from the radial artery, or as a true trifurcation of the brachial artery. The interosseous artery often divides into an anterior and posterior interosseous artery, which either terminate at the level of the metacarpal bones or rejoin the ulnar or radial arteries via a carpal arch (see **Figure 7**).

At the level of the carpal bones, the radial artery divides into superficial and deep branches, which join the superficial and deep branches of the ulnar artery, forming the superficial and deep palmar arches. Commonly, a continuation of the ulnar artery forms a superficial palmar arch and a continuation of the radial artery forms a deep palmar arch, although there is considerable variability. Palmar mediocarpal branches then arise from both the superficial and deep palmar arch and join together at the base of the interdigital spaces. At this level, the proper digital arteries arise directly. The proper digital arteries for the thumb and second and fifth digits often arise from the deep and superficial palmar arches (see **Figure 8**).

Optimal views

An upper extremity angiogram is optimally obtained with piecemeal stepped static digital subtraction images. The patient's arm is fixed in an anatomic position, palm upwards and fingers separated. At least six stepped views are obtained with the catheter sequentially moved from more proximal to more distal positioning for optimal opacification of the small vessels.

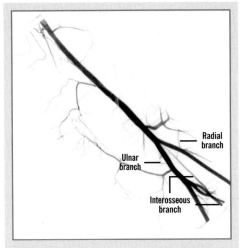

Figure 6. The left brachial artery branching at the antecubital fossa in a posteroanterior projection. The brachial artery can be seen to divide into the ulnar and radial branches. Note the origin of the interosseous artery off the ulnar artery. In this case, an interosseous branch forms as an almost true trifurcation of the brachial artery.

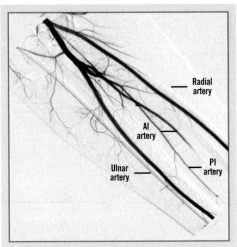

Figure 7. The radial and ulnar arteries, and the anterior (AI) and posterior (PI) interosseous arteries, coursing into the forearm using digital subtraction.

The initial image has a field of view from the origin of the subclavian to the axillary artery, with the catheter positioned at the beginning of the subclavian artery. With the catheter advanced into the axillary artery, two stepped views of the upper arm are performed: first to encompass the shoulder to the mid biceps and second the mid biceps to the antecubital fossa.

The catheter is then advanced to the distal brachial artery prior to its bifurcation. Two stepped views of the forearm are obtained. The first encompasses the antecubital fossa to the mid forearm, with careful visualization of the forearm vessel bifurcations. Some slight oblique angulation can be utilized to optimally view these bifurcations. The next stepped view is from the mid forearm to the base of the wrist or metacarpal bones. Finally, a magnified view of the hand is performed, including the distal phalanges of all five fingers. On occasion, over-exposure is encountered with magnified views of the hand. If filtering is inadequate to allow image acquisition, the automatic exposure software can be assisted by placing a bag of saline over the x-ray source.

External carotid artery

Both the right and left carotid arteries divide into the internal (ICA) and external (ECA) carotid arteries at the level of the angle of the mandible (see **Figure 9**). There is considerable variability in the branching of the ECA. From an inferior to anterior and posterior course, commonly encountered branches of the ECA include:

• superior thyroidal artery

• ascending pharyngeal artery

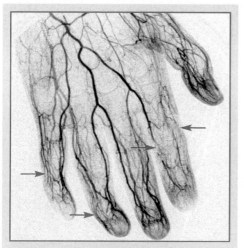

Figure 8. A magnified view of the left hand in the anatomic position using digital subtraction. The mediocarpal branches predominantly arise from the ulnar artery and then divide into proper digital arteries. Note the absence of a well-developed superficial and/or deep palmar arch. There are "skip lesions" (arrows) in the digital arteries; evidence for a collateral arterial supply is most prominent in the index finger and thumb.

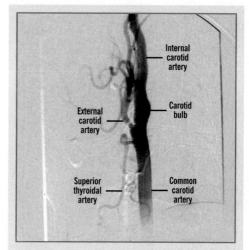

Figure 9. Carotid artery bifurcation in an ipsilateral oblique angulation using digital subtraction. The carotid bulb has a fairly normal appearance at the origin of the left internal carotid artery. There is a near-separate origin of the superior thyroidal artery off the common carotid artery, and the external carotid artery exhibits early branching.

- lingual artery

- facial artery

- maxillary artery

- superficial temporal artery

- posterior auricular artery

- occipital artery

The variability in the branching of the ECA was demonstrated in one study in which 80% of ECAs had a separate origin of the superior thyroidal, lingual, and facial arteries. In 20% of ECAs, both the lingual and facial arteries arose from a common trunk originating low in the ECA.

Optimal views

Carotid angiography is optimal with the patient's head immobilized in the anatomic position and the chin slightly elevated. The innominate bifurcation is optimally viewed with the camera in a right anterior oblique position. Again, the patient is instructed not to breathe, move, or swallow when digital acquisition images are obtained. Selective carotid angiography is performed with the field of view focused on the carotid bifurcation; this is optimally viewed with an ipsilateral oblique in addition to a cross-table 90° lateral. On occasion, the geometry and anatomy of the carotid bifurcation varies, and a contralateral oblique or posteroanterior (PA) projection will optimally "open" the bifurcation.

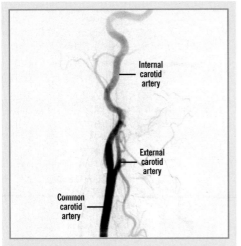

Figure 10. Carotid bifurcation and ipsilateral oblique angulation using digital subtraction. The tortuosity of the cervical internal carotid artery is clearly visualized.

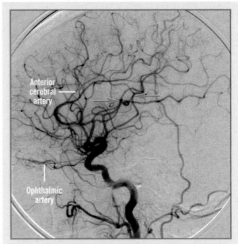

Figure 11. Intracranial run-off of a carotid injection demonstrating the course of the anterior cerebral artery towards and then around the top of the corpus callosum. Branches of the middle cerebral artery are identified by the hairpin turns (arrows) of the branches of the middle cerebral artery and the sulcus of the insula. The ophthalmic artery is well visualized.

Internal carotid artery

The ICA can be divided into four or five anatomic segments. The first is the cervical segment, which originates at the common carotid bifurcation and terminates at the base of the skull (see **Figure 10**). There are usually no branches off the cervical segment of the ICA. The carotid bulb is in the most proximal portion of the ICA and ranges from 1.1 to 1.4 times the diameter of the distal cervical ICA. The second segment is the petrous portion of the ICA, which traverses the temporal bone and begins at the skull base to the foramen lacerum. Again, this segment of the ICA usually has no branches.

The third segment is the cavernous segment. This segment begins at the foramen lacerum, traverses the venous sinuses, and terminates at the anterior clinoid process. One or two branch vessels can be seen originating from the cavernous segment; these include the meningohypophyseal artery and the inferolateral trunk artery.

The final segment is the cerebral segment, which occurs within the cranial subarachnoid space. This segment is sometimes divided into clinoidal and supraclinoidal subsegments. The clinoidal portion is extremely short, and traverses the dural ring and then enters the subarachnoid space. The supraclinoidal ICA begins at the dural ring and terminates at the ICA bifurcation. Branches off the cerebral segment or supraclinoidal subsegment of the ICA include the ophthalmic and hypophyseal branches and the posterior communicating artery (see **Figure 11**).

Optimal views

Acquisition of intracranial images is performed with the field of view encompassing the entire skull. With the patient's head fixed in the anatomic position (if necessary, using adhesive tape on the forehead or a soft foam head support), the camera is positioned as needed in a right or left oblique angulation in order to have the camera's line of sight parallel to the falx cerebri. Cranial or caudal angulation is then adjusted to align the petrous ridge in the inferior aspect of the orbits. Digital acquisition images are obtained with the patient instructed not to breathe, move, or swallow. Imaging is continued until venous drainage is complete. A cross-table 90° lateral view is also obtained. The field of view again encompasses the entire skull.

Oblique angulation is performed until the sella turcica is clearly in view and the petrous ridges (or tympanic membranes) are clearly aligned. Again, digital acquisition images are obtained with the patient instructed not to breathe, move, or swallow, and imaging continues until venous drainage is complete. To optimally view the anterior cerebral artery (ACA), the camera is positioned in an ipsilateral oblique with cranial or caudal angulation – this places the segment within a field of view with minimal bony density to avoid subtraction artifact. This is often performed with the intent to place the segment within the orbit. Likewise, focal views of the middle cerebral artery (MCA) can be performed with a slight contralateral oblique or ipsilateral oblique view with cranial or caudal angulation added in order to minimize overlapping bony densities and focus on the segment of interest.

Anterior cerebral artery

The ACA is anatomically divided into five segments. The first segment (A1) begins at the origin of the ACA (the carotid bifurcation) and is demarcated by where the artery turns superiorly between the frontal and temporal lobes. The A1 segment can give rise to the medial striate artery and the anterior communicating artery, which connects to the contralateral ACA (see **Figure 12**). As the ACA enters the interhemispheric fissure, it ascends superiorly on the medial surface of the hemisphere and then continues posteriorly on the superior surface of the corpus callosum.

The A2–A5 segments are demarcated as the ACA gives rise to side branches – such as the orbital artery, the frontal polar artery, and the callosal marginal artery – and then terminates as the pericallosal artery (see **Figure 11**). Variations or anomalies of the ACA occur in about 25% of brains. These include unpaired arteries and instances where branches are given off to the contralateral hemisphere.

Middle cerebral artery

The MCA often appears as a continuation of the ICA beyond the origin of the ACA. The MCA is angiographically subdivided into four segments. The M1 segment, also called the horizontal segment, originates at the carotid bifurcation and terminates as the middle cerebral artery, and its branches turn superiorly into the area between the temporal lobe and the insula. The M2 segment (the insular segment) originates as the artery enters between the temporal lobe and the insula and ascends along the insular cleft before making a hairpin turn at the sulcus of the insula. The M3 segment (the opercular segment) begins at the apex of the hairpin turn in the sulcus of the insula and terminates as the branches reach the lateral convexity of the hemisphere. The M4 segment (the cortical segment) is visible on the lateral convexity of the hemisphere as the artery arises between the frontal, parietal, and temporal lobes (see **Figure 12**).

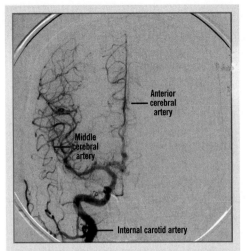

Figure 12. Cerebral run-off of an injection of the right carotid artery in a posteroanterior projection. The course and bifurcations of the middle and anterior cerebral arteries can be seen. Note the visualization of the contralateral anterior cerebral artery via right to left flow in the anterior cerebral artery, which is not clearly delineated.

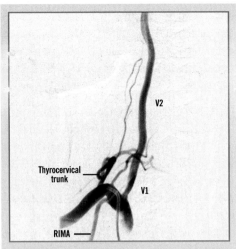

Figure 13. The right subclavian artery with visualization of the vertebral artery origin and the V1 and V2 segments. The right internal mammary artery (RIMA) can also be seen, as can the thyrocervical trunk with an ascending cervical branch.

The MCA is the most complex of the three cerebral arteries and divides into a number of large branches. In the insular region, anything from five to eight branches of the MCA lie within the Sylvian triangle. The apex of the Sylvian triangle is angiographically determined by the most posterior branch of the MCA to emerge onto the lateral convexity. The lowest branches of the MCA form the inferior margin of the Sylvian triangle. The superior margin is formed by the apices of the hairpin turns that define the M2 and M3 segments (see **Figure 11**). The Sylvian triangle is angiographically helpful in that mass lesions can be easily detected as a displacement or distortion of the triangle.

The terminal branches of the MCA fan out over the lateral convexity of each hemisphere. The branches to the frontal, anterior temporal, and anterior parietal regions are small in comparison with those to the posterior parietal, posterior temporal, and terminal occipital regions, but they are more numerous. Branches of the MCA include the lenticulostriate arteries and the anterior choroidal artery, which arise from the M1 segment. The posterior communicating artery can also arise from the M1 segment. The cortical branches of the MCA include the anterior temporal artery, pre-rolandic artery, rolandic artery, anterior parietal artery, posterior parietal artery, and posterior temporal artery.

Vertebral artery

The vertebral artery usually arises from the subclavian artery and is angiographically divided into five segments. The first segment (V1) begins at the origin of the subclavian artery and extends to the point where the artery enters the transverse foramen of the sixth cervical vertebra. The V2 segment begins where the artery enters the sixth cervical vertebra and ascends through all the

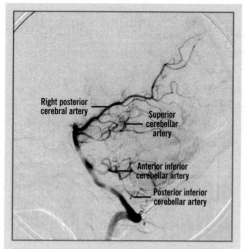

Figure 14. Intracranial run-off of an injection of the vertebral artery in a cross-table lateral projection using digital subtraction. This shows a solitary posterior inferior cerebellar artery; two superimposed anterior inferior cerebellar arteries; two superimposed superior cerebellar arteries; and a solitary posterior cerebral artery with obvious branching. The blush of the cerebellum is faintly visualized.

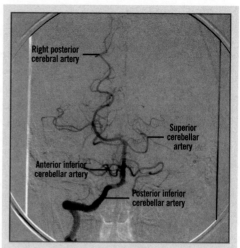

Figure 15. Intracerebral run-off of an injection of the right vertebral artery in the posteroanterior cranial view. There is faint visualization of a solitary posterior inferior cerebellar artery; both anterior inferior cerebellar arteries; both superior cerebellar arteries; and only a right posterior cerebral artery. The left posterior cerebral artery is supplied by the left carotid artery via a fetal posterior cerebral artery circulation. Note the slight motion artifact manifest by visualization of the nasal bones.

foramina transversaria of the cervical vertebrae to the second cervical vertebra or the Atlas (see **Figure 13**). The V3 segment traverses the transverse foramen of C2 and terminates as the artery pierces the posterior atlanto-occipital membrane. The V4 segment is demarcated by the atlanto-occipital membrane and where the artery finally enters the foramen magnum at the base of the skull. The V5 segment traverses the foramen magnum and courses along the anterior lateral surface of the medulla oblongata, before it finally unites with the opposite vertebral artery at the inferior border of the pons to form the basilar artery. V5 commonly gives rise to the ipsilateral posterior inferior cerebellar artery (PICA) (see **Figure 14**).

Basilar artery

The basilar artery is formed when the right and left vertebral arteries join at the inferior margin of the pons, and terminates as it divides into the right and left posterior cerebral arteries (PCAs). Branches of the basilar artery include the anterior inferior cerebellar arteries (AICAs) and the superior cerebellar artery (SCA). There are also smaller labyrinthine arteries, as well as numerous peri-median and pontine branches (see **Figures 14** and **15**).

The PCA is angiographically divided into three segments. The first segment begins at the origin of the PCA to the origin of the posterior communicating artery. The second segment begins at the origin of the posterior communicating artery and terminates at the posterior aspect of the midbrain. The third segment begins at the posterior segment of the brain and terminates in the main arteries of the posterior temporal, parietal, and occipital lobes. There is a great deal of variability in these named arteries (see **Figures 14** and **15**).

Optimal views

With the patient's head immobilized in the anatomic position, the field of view is centered on the inferior margin of the nasal passage or the superior margin of the maxilla. A steep cranial angulation in a PA projection optimally displays the branches of the distal vertebral and basilar arteries. A cross-table 90° lateral view is also performed. The field of view is centered on the posterior third of the skull in the area of the cerebellum. The occiput and sella turcica should be clearly in the field of view. Digital subtraction imaging is acquired with the patient instructed not to breathe, move, or swallow. Imaging continues until venous drainage is complete.

Common congenital anomalies of the intracranial circulation

A PCA that is predominately supplied by the ICA or an M1 segment that is smaller than the posterior communicating artery is termed a fetal PCA. On occasion, the PICA is absent and the territory that is usually perfused by this artery is instead perfused by a very large and wandering AICA. This is termed the AICA–PICA complex.

Cerebral vascular venous drainage

Delicate venous drainage from the cerebral hemispheres emerges from the brain to form small venous structures in the pia mater. These larger venous channels then form cerebral veins, which bridge the subarachnoid space and enter into endothelial-lined sinuses within the dura mater. Small veins from the scalp also communicate with the dural sinus via emissary veins that perforate the skull. The majority of the cerebral convexities ultimately drain into the mid-line structure in the dura mater (the superior sagittal sinus). The superior sagittal sinus courses posteriorly back towards the occiput, where it receives drainage from the straight sinus. The straight sinus itself receives drainage from the inferior sagittal sinus, which courses in the falx cerebri. The inferior margin of the superior sagittal sinus divides into a right and left transverse sinus in the tentorium cerebelli, which is again made up of dura mater. Each transverse sinus curves downward and backward as a sigmoid sinus, and is ultimately drained by each of the internal jugular veins. Venous drainage is often asymmetrical, with the superior sagittal sinus most commonly draining into the right transverse sinus, while the straight sinus usually drains into the left transverse sinus.

The cavernous sinus is an irregular network of venous channels on each side of the sphenoid sinus and sella turcica, extending from the superior orbital fissure to the petrous portion of the temporal bone. The cavernous sinus encloses a segment of the ICA. Each cavernous sinus is connected to the other by a basilar venous plexus. Each cavernous sinus drains posteriorly into the superior and inferior petrosal sinus, which enter the transverse sinus and the bulb of the internal jugular vein (see **Figures 16** and **17**).

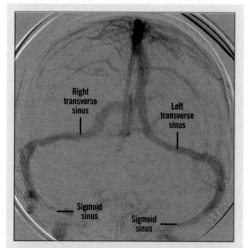

Figure 16. Venous drainage of the brain and skull in a posteroanterior projection. Venous channels course from the right and left cerebral convexities towards the mid-line to form the superior sagittal sinus, which drains into the right and left transverse sinuses. The inferior sagittal sinus drains into the straight sinus, which connects with the left transverse sinus. Each transverse sinus then drains into a sigmoid sinus, which ultimately empties into each of the jugular veins.

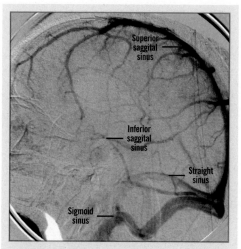

Figure 17. Venous drainage of the brain and skull. The superior sagittal sinus is abbreviated from the mid skull forward (arrow). This is due to either a thrombosis or a congenital anomaly. The superior sagittal sinus predominantly empties into the right transverse sinus; the inferior sagittal sinus drains into the straight sinus, which drains into the left transverse sinus. Both transverse sinuses drain into the sigmoid sinuses, and ultimately into the jugular veins.

There is considerable variability in the venous drainage of the brain and skull. There are also numerous interconnections between venous drainage systems. The superior anastomotic vein (vein of Trolard) connects to the superficial middle cerebral vein, which usually empties into the cavernous sinus common with the superior sagittal sinus. The inferior anastomotic vein (vein of Labbé) connects the superficial middle cerebral vein with the transverse sinus.

Abdominal aorta and mesenteric arteries

As the descending thoracic aorta crosses through the crus of the diaphragm it becomes the most proximal segment of the abdominal aorta (see **Figure 18**). The first and often largest visceral branch of the abdominal aorta is the celiac trunk. The celiac trunk quickly bifurcates or trifurcates into branches. The main branches are the common hepatic and splenic arteries, and, in the case of a trifurcation, the left gastric artery (see **Figure 19**). Otherwise, the left gastric artery will arise off the splenic artery. The splenic artery also gives rise to the left gastroepiploic artery, prior to terminating at the spleen. The common hepatic artery gives rise to the right gastric artery and then the gastroduodenal artery. The gastroduodenal artery divides into the superior pancreaticoduodenal artery and the right gastroepiploic artery. Each of the right and left gastroepiploic arteries may have anastomoses to the superior mesenteric artery (SMA) and often form the prime source for collateral circulation between these two main mesenteric arteries.

The SMA is immediately inferior to the origin of the celiac trunk (see **Figure 20**). One of the first several branches of the SMA can be a collateral connection to the right and/or left gastroepiploic arteries. The SMA gives rise to jejunal and ileo branches, which fan out towards the left side of the abdomen. At the level of the first jejunal branches, the SMA gives rise to the middle colic

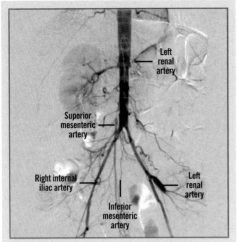

Figure 18. Abdominal aortogram in a posteroanterior projection in a patient with fibromuscular dysplasia. Note the absence of the hepatic and splenic branches of the celiac artery, which is occluded. The left renal artery is occluded at the site of a previously placed stent, which suffered the expected severe in-stent restenosis that occurs in fibromuscular dysplasia. The left kidney was autotransplanted to the left external iliac artery. There are severe stenoses in the branches of the superior mesenteric artery. The branches of the inferior mesenteric artery can be seen. Note the absence of a left internal iliac artery and the underdeveloped right internal iliac artery.

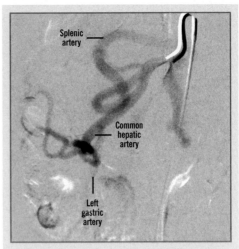

Figure 19. Selective injection of the celiac artery and a cross-table lateral projection using digital subtraction. The main branches of the celiac artery can be seen, including the common hepatic, splenic, and left gastric arteries.

artery, followed by the right colic artery and the ileocolic artery. At their periphery, the middle colic, right colic, and ileocolic arteries can form an interconnection that courses to the junction of the transverse colon and descending colon; this is termed the wandering artery of Drummond. Cecal branches are seen to arise from the ileocolic branch. The wandering artery of Drummond will anastomose with the left colic artery, which is a branch of the inferior mesenteric artery (IMA) and provides the primary source of collaterals between these two mesenteric arteries.

There are usually one or two sets of paired lumbar branches off the abdominal aorta before the origin of the right renal artery (see **Figure 21**) and then the left renal artery (see **Figure 22**). Branches to the adrenal gland can originate from either the aorta or the renal arteries. Accessory renal arteries are commonly encountered. An accessory renal artery supplies a portion of the superior or inferior pole of the kidney and is termed a polar artery. Right and left gonadal arteries originate from the infrarenal abdominal aorta, as do paired and unpaired lumbar branches. Just before the distal aortic bifurcation is the origin of the IMA (see **Figure 23**). The IMA gives rise to the left colic artery, as well as several sigmoid and then superior and inferior rectal branches. The middle sacral branch is sometimes identified at the level of the aortic bifurcation, especially in diseased states, where the sacral branch can provide significant collateral circulation. The distal abdominal aorta then bifurcates into the right and left common iliac arteries; each common iliac artery bifurcates into an external and internal iliac artery (see **Figure 24**). As the external iliac artery approaches the pelvic brim and the inguinal ligament, it is termed the common femoral artery. The internal iliac artery gives rise to the superior and inferior gluteal arteries, as well as the lateral sacral arteries. It then gives rise to the middle rectal artery and

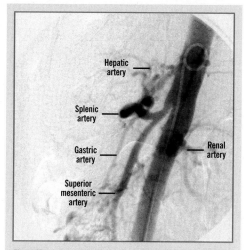

Figure 20. An abdominal aortogram in a cross-table lateral projection using digital subtraction. There is a congenitally anomalous common origin of the celiac artery with the hepatic, splenic, and gastric arteries, as well as the superior mesenteric artery. There is faint visualization of the right and left renal arteries coursing posteriorly to the posterior wall of the aorta.

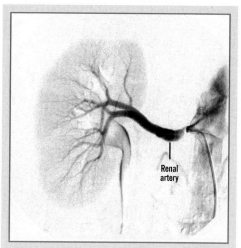

Figure 21. Selective injection of the right renal artery in a shallow right anterior oblique projection. There is severe stenosis of the renal artery near its ostium. Note the motion artifact of peristalsis of the renal pelvis and ureter.

hemorrhoidal arteries, and then to internal pudendal and vesicular arteries as well as an obturator artery. The true terminus of the internal iliac artery is the obliterated umbilical artery.

Optimal views

Abdominal aortography is performed using PA and cross-table 90° lateral views. On the PA projection, the field of view is from the level of the diaphragm to the top of the iliac wings; on the lateral projection, the field of view is the top of the diaphragm to the iliac wings, with visualization of the vertebral bodies and the anterior surface of the abdomen. Patients are instructed to hold their breath, preferably in exhalation, and not to move while digital acquisition images are obtained.

The first two views of the abdominal aorta are performed with a flush or pigtail catheter tip located at the first lumbar vertebra. The catheter is then withdrawn to a position just superior to the aortic bifurcation and two pelvic or iliac views are obtained in right and left anterior oblique projections. Power injection of contrast is utilized for the initial aortogram at a rate of 15–20 mL/s for a total of 30–40 mL of contrast. No rate of rise is necessary. For the pelvic aortogram, lower flow rates and volumes are used, usually in the order of 7 mL/s for a total of 14 mL or 2-second injection.

Arterial supply of the lower extremities

The arterial supply of the lower extremities begins with the iliofemoral system. The common iliac artery supplies the external iliac artery and then the common femoral artery. The common femoral artery gives rise to the superficial epigastric artery, the external pudendal artery, and the superficial circumflex artery, prior to bifurcating into the deep femoral artery (also known as the profunda femoris) and the superficial femoral artery (SFA) (see **Figure 25**). The profunda femoris

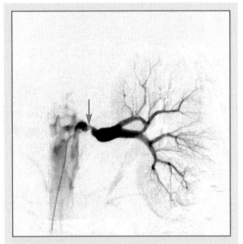

Figure 22. Selective injection of the left renal artery in a shallow left anterior oblique projection. There is high-grade stenosis in the proximal left renal artery (arrow) with poststenotic dilatation.

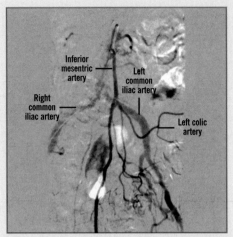

Figure 23. Selective injection of the inferior mesenteric artery. There is faint visualization of the distal abdominal aorta with its bifurcation, and right and left common iliac arteries, as well as internal and external iliac arteries on the left. The inferior mesenteric artery is seen to give rise to a left colic artery and several branches to the rectosigmoid.

gives rise to the medial and lateral circumflex femoral arteries, as well as to perforating arteries that provide the blood supply to the muscles of the thigh. A descending branch of the profunda femoris supplies a lateral geniculate artery, which can supply collaterals to the above-knee popliteal artery in the setting of a diseased or obstructed SFA.

The SFA courses inferiorly with few, if any, side branches, and then enters the adductor canal and courses posteriorly to the femur to form the popliteal artery (see **Figure 26**). A descending medial geniculate branch originates from the distal SFA just prior to its entering the adductor canal. In the setting of obstructive atherosclerotic disease, this branch often provides additional collateral circulation around the knee. The popliteal artery courses along the posterior surface of the femur and tibia. It divides into two just below the proximal anastomosis of the fibula to the tibia, giving rise to an anterior tibial artery and a tibial peroneal trunk (see **Figure 27**). The anterior tibial artery pierces the interosseus membrane between the tibia and the fibula and courses along the anterior surface of the interosseus membrane close to the tibia, where it changes at the mortis joint of the ankle and becomes the dorsalis pedis artery. Lateral and medial malleolar branches can form interconnections between the anterior and posterior tibial arteries and the peroneal artery as a form of collateral circulation in diseased states.

The tibial peroneal trunk courses along the posterior surface of the interosseus membrane and divides into a posterior tibial artery and a peroneal artery (see **Figure 28**). The peroneal artery (also known as the fibular artery) courses along the posterior surface of the interosseus membrane close to the fibula and terminates at the ankle, usually with lateral and medial calcaneal branches. There is a distal communicating branch between the peroneal artery and the distal posterior tibial artery at the level just above the lateral malleolus. This also forms a source of collateral circulation in diseased states. The posterior tibial artery courses along the posterior aspect of the tibia and forms the medial and lateral plantar arches. The plantar arch gives rise to metatarsal and then plantar digital arteries. Perforating branches from the plantar

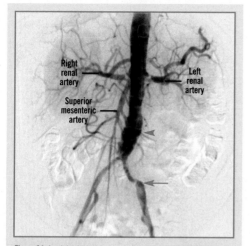

Figure 24. An abdominal aortogram performed in a posteroanterior projection using digital subtraction. There are high-grade stenoses at both the right and left renal arteries and ectasia of the infrarenal abdominal aorta prior to its bifurcation into the right and left common iliac arteries (arrowhead). Note how the overlap of the left internal and external iliac arteries gives the false appearance of an aneurysmal dilatation of the external iliac artery (arrow).

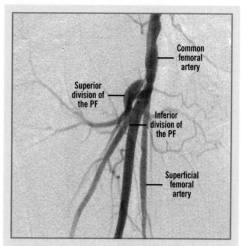

Figure 25. Bifurcation of the right common femoral artery into the profunda femoris (PF) and right superficial femoral artery. There is irregularity of the right common femoral artery consistent with atherosclerotic plaque. There is also a separate origin of the superior division of the profunda femoris, with high-grade stenosis prior to the main origin of the profunda femoris proper. Note the small caliber of the right superficial femoral artery, which, in this particular example, ultimately occludes in the mid thigh.

arch communicate with the superficial or dorsal arch, which is usually formed as a sweeping terminus of the dorsalis pedis artery, and also give rise to the dorsal metatarsal arteries and dorsal digital arteries coursing into the toes (see **Figure 29**).

Optimal views

Different strategies can be utilized to a obtain a lower extremity run-off study. Both legs can potentially be run-off simultaneously with imaging equipment with a large field of view. With the pigtail catheter just above the aortic bifurcation, stepped digital subtraction views can be obtained with injection of 90–100 mL of contrast at a rate of 10–15 mL/s. The patient is instructed not to move their legs or feet. Alternatively, the aortic bifurcation can be crossed over with a diagnostic catheter and guidewire for placement of a straight-tip flush catheter with sideholes in the contralateral external iliac artery. This facilitates unilateral lower extremity run-off using stepped digital subtraction imaging acquisition. Half of the contrast, or 45–50 mL, is utilized at a flow rate of 7–10 mL/s, with a reasonable rate of rise ranging from 0.5 to 1.0 seconds to ramp up the injection to the set flow rate. The flush catheter is then withdrawn to the ipsilateral iliac artery and the same procedure is repeated for a run-off of the remaining limb.

To obtain high-quality images, it is imperative that the patient does not move and that there is adequate filtering of overexposed areas. On occasion, it is important to utilize a guidewire and a straight flush catheter to position the catheter more distally in the leg for high magnification and digital subtraction images of the lower leg and/or foot. A sidehole straight-tip flush catheter can be safely placed in the popliteal artery and hand injections can be used to obtain high-magnified views of the distal lower extremity and foot. Placing the patient's leg in a "frog" position can facilitate a lateral view of the foot.

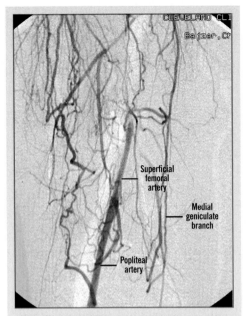

Figure 26. Reconstitution of the distal right superficial femoral artery and the above-knee popliteal artery via medial and lateral collateral branches from the right profunda femoris artery. Note the descending medial geniculate branches, which provide additional collateral circulation around the knee-joint proper.

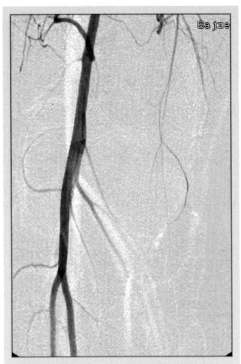

Figure 27. The below-knee popliteal artery branching into the anterior tibial artery and the tibial peroneal trunk in the posteroanterior projection using digital subtraction. A subtraction artifact consistent with venous drainage can be seen.

Venous drainage of the lower extremities

Venous drainage of the lower extremities is divided into the superficial and deep systems. There is significant variability in the venous drainage of the lower extremities, with more variability noted in the superficial as compared with the deep venous drainage. Perforating or anastomotic veins on the medial aspect of the foot form the greater saphenous vein, which courses somewhat anteriorly as it superiorly ascends the leg to the level of the groin. The lesser saphenous vein forms from a confluence of perforating or anastomotic veins from the lateral aspect of the foot and courses posteriorly in the calf, where it joins the popliteal vein in the popliteal fossa.

The deep venous system courses alongside the arterial system and includes the anterior tibial, posterior tibial, and the peroneal veins, which ultimately form the popliteal vein. It is joined by the lesser saphenous vein from the superficial system, ascends, and forms the superficial femoral vein and ultimately the common femoral vein. The common femoral vein is joined by the greater saphenous vein, which usually receives the external pudendal vein as well as the superficial epigastric vein, and the superficial circumflex iliac vein. The common femoral vein empties into the external iliac vein, which, when joined by the internal iliac vein, forms the common iliac vein. Both the right and left common iliac veins join to form the inferior vena cava. The lumbar veins, as well as the left and right renal veins, empty into the inferior vena cava. The hepatic veins empty into the inferior vena cava prior to entering the right atrium. The mesenteric veins follow

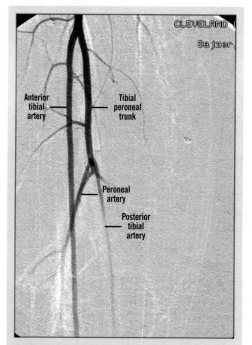

Figure 28. Below-knee trifurcation in a shallow ipsilateral oblique angulation using digital subtraction. Note the origin of the anterior tibial artery and tibial peroneal trunk, with ultimate division into the peroneal artery and posterior tibial arteries. Again, there is a subtraction artifact related to venous drainage.

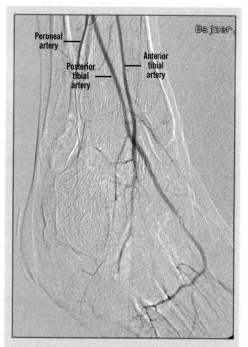

Figure 29. The right ankle and foot in a shallow right anterior oblique projection using digital subtraction. Note the motion artifact due to patient movement. The posterior tibial artery descends posterior to the medial malleolus, giving rise to the plantar arch and subsequently to the digital arteries. The peroneal artery terminates at the distal terminus of the interosseous membrane between the fibula and the tibia. The anterior tibial artery can be seen descending and forming the dorsalis pedis artery.

their named mesenteric arteries, which ultimately join the portal artery that courses into the liver. This venous drainage is described as the portal system. There are connections or anastomoses between the portal and systemic venous drainage systems located in the rectum, esophagus, and the umbilicus; these can be points of manifestation of dilated venous structures in the setting of portal hypertension.

Venous drainage of the upper extremities

The venous drainage of the upper extremities is again divided into a superficial and deep system. The dorsal digital veins are highly interconnected and form an array of superficial dorsal veins. These form a dorsal venous arch at the base of the back of the hand before the wrist. There are numerous perforating veins with connections to deeper venous structures and drainage. The cephalic vein courses from the dorsal venous arch, from the dorsal radial aspect of the forearm to the anterior radial aspect of the forearm. The basilic vein arises from either the dorsal or the palmar aspect of the hand and courses towards the palmar or anterior aspect of the forearm along the ulnar aspect of the forearm. An array of veins along the palmar or anterior surface of the forearm ultimately forms the median vein of the forearm. This vein flows into either the basilic vein or the median cubital vein in the antecubital fossa. The median cubital vein is the largest connecting vein between the cephalic and basilic veins within the antecubital fossa. The cephalic vein courses out of the arm on the radial or lateral aspect and then courses between the deltoid and the pectoralis major to ultimately join the subclavian vein. The basilic vein ultimately becomes the axillary vein at the lower border of the teres major muscle. The axillary vein becomes the subclavian vein at the first rib. The subclavian vein joins the internal jugular vein to become the brachiocephalic or innominate vein just behind the sternal end of the clavicle.

There is great variability in the venous structures of the arm. There are numerous interconnecting veins between the superficial and deep systems of the arm and there is great variability in the location of the numerous venous valves. Within the deep system, several brachial veins surrounding the brachial artery (the venae comitantes) ultimately unite and join the axillary artery near the middle of the axilla. The right brachiocephalic vein joins the left brachiocephalic vein and forms the superior vena cava. Intercostal veins on the right form an ascending posterior paraspinal vein that drains into the azygos vein, which drains into the superior vena cava prior to its insertion in the right atrium. On the left, a similar venous system of intercostal veins drains into a posterior paraspinal vein that ascends into the hemiazygos system, which commonly drains into the left brachiocephalic vein, but occasionally drains directly into the superior vena cava. Both the right and left intercostal veins also drain anteriorly into the internal thoracic veins, which ascend superiorly and drain into the left and right subclavian veins. The largest lymphatic drainage in the body, the thoracic duct, joins the subclavian vein just before the insertion of the left internal jugular vein forms the left brachiocephalic vein.

Suggested reading

• Mizeres NJ. *Human Anatomy: A Synoptic Approach*.
  New York: Elsevier Publishing, 1981.

• Anderson JE, editor. *Grant's Atlas of Anatomy*, 8th Edition.
  Baltimore: Williams and Wilkins Publishing, 1983.

• Carpenter MB. *Core Text of Neuro Anatomy*, 3rd Edition.
  Baltimore: Williams and Wilkins Publishing, 1985.

• Sadler TW, editor. *Langman's Medical Embryology*, 5th Edition.
  Baltimore: Williams and Wilkins Publishing, 1985.

2 Case selection

Leslie Cho

Introduction

Meticulous case selection sets the basis for a successful intervention. This chapter delineates the appropriate interventions for patients with peripheral vascular disease (PVD).

Risk factor modification

Aggressive risk factor modification is mandatory for all patients with PVD, regardless of the severity of their symptoms, since they frequently have coexisting coronary and cerebrovascular disease.

Smoking cessation

Smoking cessation has been shown to reduce the risk of myocardial infarction and death from vascular causes [1]. Therefore, all patients should be strongly encouraged to stop smoking. The most efficacious smoking cessation programs combine education, counseling, and pharmacologic therapies.

Lipid-lowering therapy

Multiple clinical trials have supported the use of 5-hydroxymethyl glutaryl-coenzyme A (statin) therapy for the reduction of myocardial infarction, stroke, and death in both primary and secondary prevention settings [2]. In PVD patients, the current recommendation is to achieve a serum low-density lipoprotein cholesterol level <100 mg/dL and serum triglyceride <150 mg/dL [1]. A high serum homocysteine level is an independent predictor for the development of PVD and increases the risk of death from cardiovascular events [3]. Even though the efficacy of homocysteine lowering in the prevention of cardiovascular events in patients with PVD has not been addressed in randomized trials, supplementing the diet with vitamin B and folic acid seems a reasonable approach.

Hypertension control

Several prospective studies have shown that hypertension control reduces cardiovascular events. In the HOPE (Heart Outcomes Prevention Evaluation) study, use of the angiotensin-converting enzyme (ACE) inhibitor ramipril was associated with a reduction in death from vascular causes, nonfatal myocardial infarction, and stroke compared with placebo, even in patients with PVD [4].

Diabetes control

Whether macrovascular complications are reduced with intensive control of blood glucose remains a source of debate; however, tight diabetes control was associated with a trend towards a reduction in myocardial infarction in one large trial [5]. Therefore, aggressive blood glucose control is recommended in all diabetics with PVD.

Antiplatelet therapy

All PVD patients should be on aspirin. A retrospective meta-analysis of 145 randomized trials of antiplatelet agents in patients at risk for vascular events demonstrated a 25% risk reduction in the combined endpoint of myocardial infarction, stroke, or vascular death with aspirin use [6]. In addition, aspirin has been shown to improve the vascular graft patency rate following coronary or peripheral bypass surgery or angioplasty [7]. Dipyridamole alone or in combination with aspirin does not reduce cardiovascular events in patients with PVD [8].

The CAPRIE (Clopidogrel Versus Aspirin in Patients at Risk of Ischemic Events) trial demonstrated a potential role for clopidogrel, an ADP receptor inhibitor, in patients with PVD [9]. In this study, cardiovascular events decreased from 4.9% in the aspirin group to 3.7% in the clopidogrel group with an adjusted risk reduction of 23.8% ($P=0.045$). The hypothesis that a combination of aspirin and clopidogrel is more efficacious than aspirin alone in patients at high risk for cardiovascular events is currently being tested in the CHARISMA (Clopidogrel for High Atherothrombotic Risk and Ischemic Stabilization, Management, and Avoidance) trial, which has enrolled over 15,000 patients.

Lower extremity disease

Smoking cessation

Smoking is the most significant independent predictor for the development of PVD and is associated with progression to disabling claudication and limb-threatening ischemia [1]. In a meta-analysis of published data, smoking cessation did not improve maximal treadmill walking distance in patients with symptomatic PVD [10]. However, patients who successfully stopped smoking had fewer myocardial infarctions and decreased mortality from vascular causes on follow-up [10]. Therefore, smoking cessation remains one of the mainstays of patient care in PVD.

Medical therapy

Lipid-lowering therapy

Over the last decade, statin trials have focused on cardiac morbidity and mortality, and only a few reports have addressed the impact of statins on PVD. In small studies, statin therapy has been associated with delayed progression and even regression of arterial occlusive disease and increased exercise time [11,12]. Two studies have evaluated the effects of lipid-lowering therapy on clinical endpoints in the leg. In a trial of ileal bypass surgery for the treatment of hyperlipidemia, 5-year follow-up showed a 15% absolute risk reduction in abnormal ankle–brachial index, claudication, or limb-threatening ischemia in the group treated with ileal bypass compared with controls [13]. In a subgroup of patients in 4S (Scandinavian Simvastatin Survival Study), the relative risk of new claudication or worsening of pre-existing claudication was reduced in patients treated with a statin compared with placebo [14].

Exercise therapy

In addition to aggressive risk factor modification, patients with moderate PVD and intermittent non-lifestyle-limiting claudication should receive exercise therapy. The importance of exercise therapy, the most consistently effective medical treatment for intermittent claudication, cannot be stressed enough [15]. All prospective studies of patients treated with at least 3 months of exercise therapy have demonstrated improvements in walking distance and pain relief [16]. Patient motivation is crucial, since exercise must be undertaken on a regular basis.

Vasodilators

Patients with moderate PVD and intermittent non-lifestyle-limiting claudication should receive a trial of vasodilator drugs, eg, cilostazol, a phosphodiesterase-III inhibitor. This compound has been shown to improve walking distance compared with pentoxifylline or placebo [17]. Disadvantages include that it is contraindicated in patients with a left ventricular ejection fraction <40% and that it can require 3–4 months of therapy to achieve full clinical response.

Pentoxifylline, a methylxanthine derivative, has been used to improve claudication and exercise capacity, but most contemporary studies have shown no benefit [1]. Pentoxifylline may have a role in rare patients with markedly reduced walking distances who do not respond to or cannot engage in exercise therapy. Vasodilator therapies may be indicated in patients with moderate intermittent claudication while undergoing an exercise program. Both cilostazol and pentoxifylline treat symptoms only and do not alter the disease course.

Indications for revascularization

Indications for revascularization for aortoiliac, femoropopliteal, and infrapopliteal disease include lifestyle-limiting claudication, ischemic rest pain, nonhealing ischemic ulcerations, critical limb ischemia, and gangrene. Percutaneous revascularization is best-suited for stenosis and for short focal occlusions, while long total occlusions are more suited to surgery. An algorithm for the treatment of patients with lower extremity PVD is shown in **Figure 1**.

Aortoiliac stenosis

Endovascular revascularization

Percutaneous transluminal angioplasty (PTA) is the procedure of choice for short (<10 cm) iliac stenosis (see **Table 1**). For short focal lesions, the procedural success rate of PTA is >90%. Chronic total occlusions have a lower success rate (50%) and, among those that are successful, the 2- to 4-year patency rate is 75% [18]. Overall, the reported patency rates for PTA are 75%–95% at 1 year, 60%–90% at 3 years, and 55%–85% at 5 years [18]. Factors associated with prolonged patency include a focal lesion, large vessel size, lesion in the common iliac artery, and a single lesion.

With stents, the 1-year patency rate is 90%, with an average 3-year patency rate of 75%; a meta-analysis found a 4-year patency rate of 77% [19]. There has been one randomized trial of iliac angioplasty with provisional stenting compared with planned stenting. At 2 years,

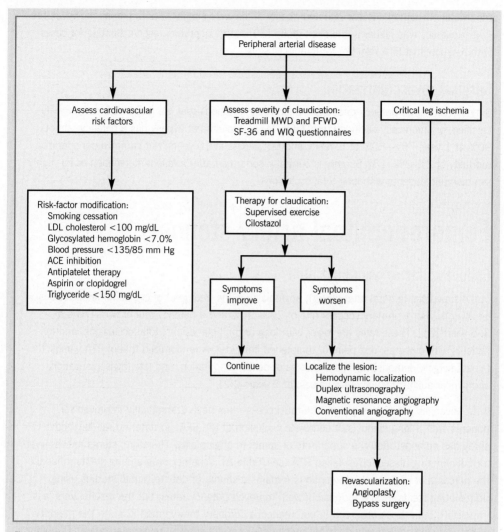

Figure 1. Algorithm for patients with lower extremity peripheral vascular disease. ACE: angiotensin-converting enzyme; LDL: low-density lipoprotein; MWD: maximum walking distance; PFWD: pain-free walking distance; SF-36: short-form-36 questionnaire; WIQ: walking impairment questionnaire. Reproduced with permission from the Massachusetts Medical Society (Hiatt WR. Drug therapy: Medical treatment of peripheral arterial disease and claudication *N Engl J Med* 2001;344:1608–21). Copyright © 2001 Massachusetts Medical Society. All rights reserved.

PTA	Surgery
Stenosis <10 cm	Stenosis >10 cm
Chronic occlusion <5 cm	Chronic occlusion >5 cm
	Heavily calcified lesions
	Lesions associated with aortic aneurysm

Table 1. Iliac revascularization: indications for percutaneous transluminal angioplasty (PTA) and surgery.

the overall procedural success rate and quality of life were similar in both groups; however, the 4-year patency was higher in the stent group [20]. Some operators reserve stenting for cases with a suboptimal PTA result or for total occlusions.

Surgical revascularization

Surgery has higher patency rates than angioplasty in lesions that are long (>10 cm), heavily calcified, or chronically occluded (see **Table 1**). Aortobifemoral bypass has a patency rate of 90% at 1 year, 75%–80% at 5 years, and 60%–70% at 10 years, but carries a perioperative mortality of 2%–3% [18]. Surgery is currently performed after a failed intervention or for highly symptomatic patients with long total occlusions.

Femoropopliteal artery stenosis

Endovascular revascularization

In the superficial femoral artery (SFA), angioplasty is the treatment of choice for short lesions (<10 cm), with a primary success rate of 70%–90% and a patency rate of 50%–70% at 3–5 years [21]. These rates are lower with long or multiple lesions, total occlusions, and in patients with diabetes, rest pain, or threatened limb loss. A randomized trial of PTA versus bypass surgery demonstrated similar rates of death, amputation, and late revascularization, and similar ankle–brachial index values, at 3 years [22].

With advances in equipment, procedural success rates have dramatically improved for patients with a long stenosis or complete occlusion of the SFA. To date, no randomized study has demonstrated the superiority of stents to angioplasty. Therefore, stents are reserved for flow-limiting dissection or failed PTA (see **Table 2**). Whether drug-eluting stents influence the outcome of peripheral interventions remains a source of debate. Initial studies using drug-eluting stents in SFA lesions showed improved patency rates, but the results were less impressive than those observed in percutaneous coronary intervention [23]. In the majority of cases, failed angioplasty does not preclude successful surgical revascularization. Therefore, utilizing endovascular intervention as the first line of therapy and then resorting to surgery at a later date seems a viable treatment option in patients with SFA disease.

Common femoral angioplasty is reserved for patients with severe fibrosis due to previous surgery. Currently, bare metal stents are not approved for use in the common femoral artery because of

PTA	Surgery
Discrete single lesions <10 cm	Lesion involving common femoral artery
Calcified stenosis <5 cm	Lesions >10 cm
	Heavily calcified lesion >5 cm
	Lesion involving superficial femoral artery origin
	Lesion involving popliteal artery

Table 2. Femoropopliteal artery revascularization: indications for percutaneous transluminal angioplasty (PTA) and surgery.

crush injury risk, though self-expanding nitinol stents have been used successfully. In addition, stenting of the common femoral artery limits further access for diagnostic angiograms and percutaneous intervention of the coronary arteries or other vascular beds. Profunda angioplasty is reserved for cases of limb-threatening ischemia with no surgical options. Since the SFA is occluded in these cases, this "last remaining vessel" percutaneous intervention is associated with increased risks.

Surgical revascularization

Surgery remains the treatment of choice for common femoral and profunda artery disease. In patients with above-knee vein-graft femoropopliteal bypass surgery, the 5-year cumulative patency is 78%, whereas a 5-year patency rate of 52% has been reported for Gore-Tex grafts [24,25]. Patients with diffuse disease or long occlusions (>10 cm) historically have better patency rates with surgery (see **Figure 2**), though this appears to be changing with advances in interventional techniques.

Infrapopliteal artery stenosis

Endovascular revascularization

Even though our ability to treat infrapopliteal disease has improved with technological advances, in particular the incorporation of coronary techniques, infrapopliteal angioplasty has generally been reserved for cases of threatened limb loss. The procedural success rate for infrapopliteal PTA is 85% and 1–2 year patency ranges from 40% to 85% [26]. This low patency rate may be due to the small size of the vessels and the characteristics of the patient population. PTA may be an appropriate choice for discrete, focal stenosis; however, such lesions only represent 20% of cases. Unlike with SFA lesions, failed endovascular intervention can preclude surgical revascularization. Therefore, careful case selection is crucial (see **Figure 3**). Stents are reserved for severe dissection. It remains to be seen whether drug-eluting stents improve the restenosis rate in the infrapopliteal vessels, though it is highly likely (see **Figure 4**).

Surgical revascularization

Due to the historically poor patency rate with PTA, infrapopliteal artery disease is often treated with autogenous vein bypass. Reports using the *in situ* technique for distal vein-graft bypass procedures have shown improved patency rates [18].

Carotid stenosis

Medical therapy

Data from large randomized trials suggest that medical therapy (aspirin) is appropriate for symptomatic patients with carotid stenosis of <50% and for asymptomatic patients with carotid stenosis of <60% [27–29]. Currently, patients with carotid stenosis should undergo broad

(a)

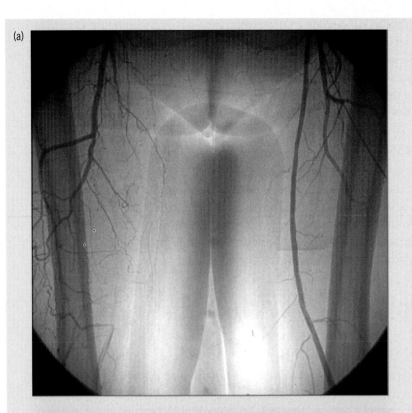

(b)

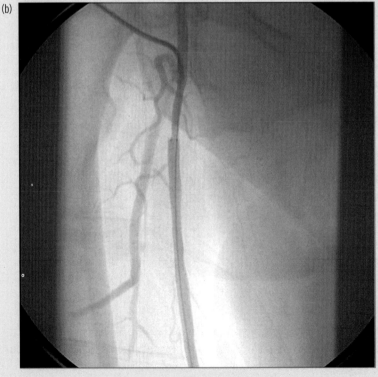

Figure 2. Longer than 10-cm chronic total occlusion of the right superficial femoral artery: (**a**) treated with balloon angioplasty and placement of a 10-cm nitinol self-expanding SMART stent (Cordis, Miami Lakes, FL, USA); (**b**) in a patient with lifestyle-limiting claudication who was told "nothing could be done". The stent was patent at 1-year follow-up. (Figure courtesy of Deepak L Bhatt, MD.)

(a)

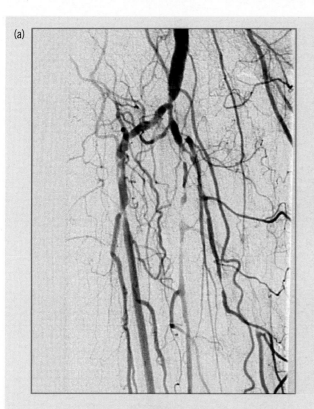

(b)

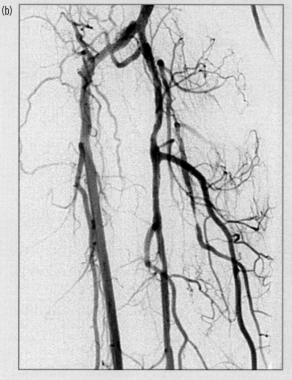

Figure 3. Severe stenosis of the right anterior tibial artery and chronic total occlusion of the peroneal artery: (**a**) in a patient with a nonhealing ulcer of the right foot. While classically this lesion morphology would be considered a contraindication for a percutaneous approach, incorporation of coronary angioplasty technology has now made infrapopliteal intervention much more feasible. Using coronary equipment, including hydrophilic 0.0014-inch wires, low-profile balloons, and the cutting balloon, both vessels were successfully treated with (**b**) a good angiographic result. (Figure courtesy of Deepak L Bhatt, MD.)

(a)

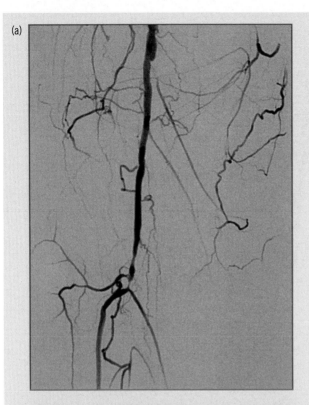

(b)

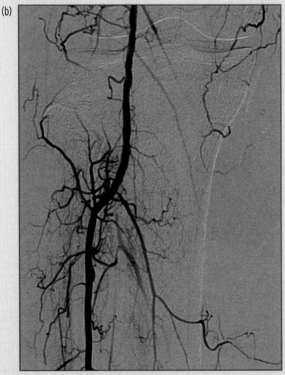

Figure 4. Severe stenosis of the distal right popliteal artery,
extending into the anterior tibial artery, (**a**) before and (**b**)
after placement of a Cypher drug-eluting coronary stent
(Cordis, Miami Lakes, FL, USA) in a woman with rest foot
pain. While the restenosis rate for such lesions has been
considered high after angioplasty alone, drug-eluting stents
are likely to reduce restenosis to acceptable rates.
(Figure courtesy of Deepak L Bhatt, MD.)

cardiovascular prevention, including statin therapy, and, if appropriate, beta-blocker or ACE-inhibitor therapy. Large-scale trials are addressing the use of clopidogrel, with or without aspirin, in the setting of cerebrovascular disease.

Indications for revascularization

The American Heart Association (AHA) Stroke Council has issued guidelines for carotid endarterectomy (CEA) [30]. According to the guidelines, which are based on large trials, CEA is the treatment of choice for symptomatic patients with carotid stenosis of >70% and asymptomatic patients with carotid stenosis of >60%. Symptomatic patients with carotid stenosis of 50%–69% may benefit from CEA [30].

Endovascular revascularization

Percutaneous carotid intervention offers several advantages over surgery. It eliminates the potential risk of general anesthesia and the local surgical complications of endarterectomy, such as neck hematoma, infection, cervical strain, and cranial nerve damage. Also, patients at high risk for surgery may be treated, such as those with previous ipsilateral CEA, previous radiation therapy to the neck or previous neck surgery, contralateral carotid occlusion, lesions above the mandible or below the clavicle, neurological instability, and coexistent coronary or pulmonary disease. CAVATAS (Carotid and Vertebral Artery Transluminal Angioplasty Study) compared carotid angioplasty with CEA in 504 symptomatic patients: at 30 days, the two groups had a similar rate of death or stroke (10% in the angioplasty group vs 10% in the surgery group). In addition, the ipsilateral stroke rate was comparable between the groups at 3 years [31].

Interest in carotid intervention has grown rapidly due to the invention of emboli protection devices. The multicenter SAPPHIRE (Stenting and Angioplasty with Protection in Patients at High Risk for Endarterectomy) trial compared CEA and carotid stenting with filter emboli protection in patients at high risk for surgery. The trial enrolled 723 patients (307 randomized patients, 409 stent registry patients, seven surgery registry patients). The 30-day rate of death, stroke, or myocardial infarction was 5.8% among patients randomized to carotid stenting and 12.6% among those who underwent surgery ($P=0.047$) [32]. A nonstatistically significant benefit was observed across the individual endpoints. Patients who were considered to be at too high risk for surgery and therefore entered a carotid stent registry also had a favorable 30-day death, stroke, or myocardial infarction rate of 7.8%. At 1 year, the results of SAPPHIRE continued to support the superiority of carotid stenting.

A large study is underway to evaluate carotid stenting versus CEA in low-risk symptomatic patients. Since CEA has been proven to be safe and efficacious, the AHA has recommended that carotid stenting be limited to well-designed, well-controlled studies performed by skilled interventionalists [33]. However, in the light of emerging data, carotid stenting appears to be a viable therapeutic option in the hands of the trained interventionalist for patients at high surgical risk (see **Table 3**). A consensus conference of cardiologists, vascular surgeons, and interventional radiologists has recommended that carotid stenting be performed in experienced centers in patients with CEA restenosis, previous radical neck dissection or cervical irradiation, high bifurcation or ostial carotid lesion, or in symptomatic or asymptomatic high surgical risk patients [34].

Clinical risk factors	Lesion characteristics
Age >80 years	Contralateral carotid occlusion
Congestive heart failure (New York Heart Association class III/IV) and/or known severe left ventricular dysfunction (ejection fraction <30%)	Contralateral laryngeal nerve palsy
	Radiation therapy to neck
Open heart surgery needed within 6 weeks	Previous carotid endarterectomy with recurrent stenosis
Recent myocardial infarction (>24 hours and <4 weeks)	High cervical internal carotid/below the clavicle common carotid lesions
Unstable angina (Canadian Cardiovascular Society class III/IV)	Severe tandem lesions
Severe pulmonary disease	

Table 3. Indications for carotid stenting.

There are currently five relative contraindications to carotid stenting. These are: lesions with intraluminal thrombus; complex bifurcation lesions that are long or severely angulated; heavily calcified lesions; patients with extensive aortic plaque, severe tortuosity, or a calcified aortic arch (these patients are at high risk for embolization during catheter manipulation); and patients with neurologic instability or who have had a very recent stroke.

Surgical revascularization

The risks and benefits of CEA are well defined. In NASCET (North American Symptomatic Carotid Endarterectomy Trial), which randomized symptomatic patients to CEA versus medical therapy, the surgical group had a death or stroke rate of 5.8% at 30 days [27,29]. At 3 years, the death or stroke rate was 12.3% in the CEA group compared with 21.9% in the medical group. Similarly, ACAS (Asymptomatic Carotid Atherosclerosis Study), which randomized asymptomatic patients to CEA versus medical therapy, found a 2.3% death or stroke rate at 30 days [28]. At 5 years, the stroke rate was 5.1% in the CEA group compared with 11.0% in the medical group. Myocardial infarctions were not included in the primary endpoints in these trials. These trials enrolled much lower-risk patients than the carotid stent studies.

Subclavian artery stenosis

Indications for revascularization

Subclavian steal syndrome results from significant subclavian stenosis and may cause coronary ischemia in patients with an internal mammary bypass graft, symptoms of vertebrobasilar insufficiency, or upper extremity claudication.

Endovascular revascularization

Although no randomized trials have compared surgery with PTA for subclavian disease, PTA is considered the first-line therapy due to a superior safety profile. Studies of subclavian PTA have reported a procedural success rate of 97%. A multicenter trial of subclavian artery PTA and stenting found an overall procedural success rate of 98.5%, with a major complication rate of 1%.

The primary patency rate (the patency rate of the vessel without additional intervention) with stents was 89% at 2 years and the secondary patency rate (the patency rate of the vessel with additional intervention, such as angioplasty or lysis) was 98.5% [35]. Restenosis rates were 5%–10%; restenosis in the subclavian artery can be treated by stenting or balloon angioplasty. Complications with stenting or PTA of the subclavian artery include vascular access bleeding and stent embolization. Treatment for occlusive subclavian disease is more controversial since PTA is associated with a low procedural success rate (50%–75%) and a slightly increased risk of embolization of the thrombus or atheroma into the cerebral, upper extremity, or coronary circulations.

Surgical revascularization

Surgical intervention for subclavian stenosis – carotid to subclavian artery bypass – is associated with high procedural success rates, but also with high procedural morbidity and mortality. A surgical registry recorded 2% mortality with a 3% stroke rate during the postoperative period, with a patency rate of 85% at 4 years [36–38]. Complications specific to open repair are phrenic nerve palsy, Horner's syndrome, thoracic duct fistula, and chylothorax. Surgical revascularization is now reserved for patients with long subclavian occlusions that cannot be treated percutaneously.

Renal artery stenosis

The two most common causes of renal artery stenosis (RAS) are atherosclerosis and fibromuscular dysplasia (FMD). Much controversy surrounds the indications for renal artery revascularization. Patients with irreversible renal dysfunction, hemodynamically insignificant stenosis, and <6-cm kidney size generally do not benefit from renal artery intervention. Diffuse intrarenal stenosis and poor cortical blood flow do not benefit from revascularization.

Indications for revascularization

PTA is the treatment of choice in patients with FMD who have refractory hypertension and RAS. In patients with refractory hypertension and atherosclerotic RAS, PTA will not cure hypertension but will decrease the patient's medication requirement and may preserve renal function [39]. Renal artery stenting may improve blood pressure control in patients with refractory hypertension, unstable angina or heart failure, and RAS [40].

Endovascular revascularization

Even though no randomized trials have compared surgery with PTA for the treatment of RAS, PTA is considered the first-line therapy due to a superior safety profile. PTA is the treatment of choice for FMD associated with renovascular hypertension that is refractory to medical therapy. Studies have shown that PTA cures >75% of patients with refractory hypertension and FMD [39]. In contrast, patients with refractory hypertension and atherosclerotic RAS are rarely cured by any form of revascularization therapy, even though medication requirements may decrease [39]. PTA for atherosclerotic disease has been associated with a high restenosis rate. Aorto-ostial renal artery lesions are unsuitable for PTA due to high elastic recoil and dissection. Stents are preferred for ostial lesions. Procedural success rates for renal stenting are 90%–100% and restenosis rates

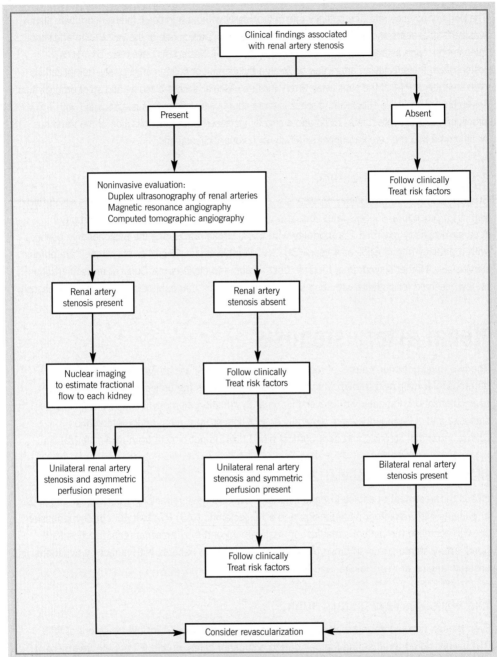

Figure 5. Renal artery stenosis algorithm. Reproduced with permission from the Massachusetts Medical Society (Safian RD, Textor SC. Renal-artery stenosis. *N Engl J Med* 2001;344:431–42). Copyright © 2001 Massachusetts Medical Society. All rights reserved.

at 1 year are ≤10% [41]. Patients with ulcerative lesions in the abdominal aorta are at increased risk for cholesterol emboli during catheter manipulation. Also, patients with renal artery aneurysm may be at higher risk for rupture or perforation during renal intervention. Drug-eluting stents and emboli protection devices are being evaluated for the treatment of RAS.

Surgical revascularization

Surgery is infrequently employed for RAS. Perioperative mortality rates range from 2.1% to 6.1% for extra-anatomical bypass and from 1% to 4.7% for renal endarterectomy [42]. Other complications of the procedure include myocardial infarction, stroke, hemorrhage, and cholesterol embolization. At 5 years, the secondary patency rate has been reported to be 75% [42]. An algorithm for the treatment of RAS is given in **Figure 5**.

Conclusion

Careful case selection is the most important factor in the success of any endovascular intervention. It is crucial that all patients undergo aggressive risk factor modification. Continued advances in peripheral interventional equipments and therapies will further expand the range of patients who may benefit from endovascular procedures.

References

1. Hiatt WR. Medical treatment of peripheral arterial disease and claudication. *N Engl J Med* 2001;344:1608–21.
2. LaRosa JC, He J, Vupputuri S. Effect of statins on risk of coronary disease: a meta-analysis of randomized controlled trials. *JAMA* 1999;282:2340–6.
3. Graham IM, Daly LE, Refsum HM, et al. Plasma homocysteine as a risk factor for vascular disease. The European Concerted Action Project. *JAMA* 1997;277:1775–81.
4. Yusuf S, Sleight P, Pogue J, et al. Effects of an angiotensin-converting-enzyme inhibitor, ramipril, on cardiovascular events in high-risk patients. The Heart Outcomes Prevention Evaluation Study Investigators. *N Engl J Med* 2000;342:145–53.
5. UK Prospective Diabetes Study (UKPDS) Group. Intensive blood-glucose control with sulphonylureas or insulin compared with conventional treatment and risk of complications in patients with type 2 diabetes (UKPDS 33). *Lancet* 1998;352:837–53.
6. Antithrombotic Trialists' Collaboration. Collaborative meta-analysis of randomised trials of antiplatelet therapy for prevention of death, myocardial infarction, and stroke in high risk patients. *Br Med J* 2002;324:71–86.
7. Antiplatelet Trialists' Collaboration. Collaborative overview of randomised trials of antiplatelet therapy – II: Maintenance of vascular graft or arterial patency by antiplatelet therapy. *Br Med J* 1994;308:159–68.
8. Antiplatelet Trialists' Collaboration. Collaborative overview of randomised trials of antiplatelet therapy – I: Prevention of death, myocardial infarction, and stroke by prolonged antiplatelet therapy in various categories of patients. *Br Med J* 1994;308:81–106.
9. CAPRIE Steering Committee. A randomised, blinded, trial of clopidogrel versus aspirin in patients at risk of ischaemic events (CAPRIE). *Lancet* 1996;348:1329–39.
10. Girolami B, Bernardi E, Prins MH, et al. Treatment of intermittent claudication with physical training, smoking cessation, pentoxifylline, or nafronyl: a meta-analysis. *Arch Intern Med* 1999;159:337–45.
11. Corti R, Fuster V, Fayad ZA, et al. Lipid lowering by simvastatin induces regression of human atherosclerotic lesions: two years' follow-up by high-resolution noninvasive magnetic resonance imaging. *Circulation* 2002;106:2884–7.
12. McDermott MM, Guralnik JM, Greenland P, et al. Statin use and leg functioning in patients with and without lower-extremity peripheral arterial disease. *Circulation* 2003;107:757–61.
13. Buchwald H, Bourdages HR, Campos CT, et al. Impact of cholesterol reduction on peripheral arterial disease in the Program on the Surgical Control of the Hyperlipidemias (POSCH). *Surgery* 1996;120:672–9.
14. Pedersen TR, Kjekshus J, Pyorala K, et al. Effect of simvastatin on ischemic signs and symptoms in the Scandinavian Simvastatin Survival Study (4S). *Am J Cardiol* 1998;81:333–5.
15. Nehler MR, Hiatt WR. Exercise therapy for claudication. *Ann Vasc Surg* 1999;13:109–14.
16. Stewart KJ, Hiatt WR, Regensteiner JG, et al. Exercise training for claudication. *N Engl J Med* 2002;347:1941–51.
17. Dawson DL, Cutler BS, Hiatt WR, et al. A comparison of cilostazol and pentoxifylline for treating intermittent claudication. *Am J Med* 2000;109:523–30.
18. Ouriel K. Peripheral arterial disease. *Lancet* 2001;358:1257–64.

19. Bosch JL, Hunink MG. Meta-analysis of the results of percutaneous transluminal angioplasty and stent placement for aortoiliac occlusive disease. *Radiology* 1997;204:87–96.

20. Richter G, Noeldge G, Roeren T, et al. First long term results of a randomized multicenter trial: iliac balloon expandable stent placement versus regular percutaneous transluminal angioplasty. In: Lierman D, editor. *State of the Art and Future Developments*, 1st edn. Morin Heights, Canada: Polyscience, 1995.

21. Weitz JI, Byrne J, Clagett GP, et al. Diagnosis and treatment of chronic arterial insufficiency of the lower extremities: a critical review. *Circulation* 1996;94:3026–49.

22. Wilson SE, Wolf GL, Cross AP. Percutaneous transluminal angioplasty versus operation for peripheral arteriosclerosis. Report of a prospective randomized trial in a selected group of patients. *J Vasc Surg* 1989;9:1–9.

23. Duda SH, Pusich B, Richter G, et al. Sirolimus-eluting stents for the treatment of obstructive superficial femoral artery disease: six-month results. *Circulation* 2002;106:1505–9.

24. Abbott WM, Green RM, Matsumoto T, et al. Prosthetic above-knee femoropopliteal bypass grafting: results of a multicenter randomized prospective trial. Above-Knee Femoropopliteal Study Group. *J Vasc Surg* 1997;25:19–28.

25. Verhelst R, Bruneau M, Nicolas AL, et al. Popliteal-to-distal bypass grafts for limb salvage. *Ann Vasc Surg* 1997;11:505–9.

26. Matsi PJ, Manninen HI, Suhonen MT, et al. Chronic critical lower-limb ischemia: prospective trial of angioplasty with 1–36 months follow-up. *Radiology* 1993;188:381–7.

27. North American Symptomatic Carotid Endarterectomy Trial Collaborators. Beneficial effect of carotid endarterectomy in symptomatic patients with high-grade carotid stenosis. *N Engl J Med* 1991;325:445–53.

28. Executive Committee for the Asymptomatic Carotid Atherosclerosis Study. Endarterectomy for asymptomatic carotid artery stenosis. *JAMA* 1995;273:1421–8.

29. Barnett HJ, Taylor DW, Eliasziw M, et al. Benefit of carotid endarterectomy in patients with symptomatic moderate or severe stenosis. North American Symptomatic Carotid Endarterectomy Trial Collaborators. *N Engl J Med* 1998;339:1415–25.

30. Biller J, Feinberg WM, Castaldo JE, et al. Guidelines for carotid endarterectomy: a statement for healthcare professionals from a Special Writing Group of the Stroke Council, American Heart Association. *Circulation* 1998;97:501–9.

31. Endovascular versus surgical treatment in patients with carotid stenosis in the Carotid and Vertebral Artery Transluminal Angioplasty Study (CAVATAS): a randomised trial. *Lancet* 2001;357:1729–37.

32. Yadav J. Stenting and Angioplasty with Protection in Patients at High Risk for Endarterecomy. Presented at the 75th Scientific Sessions of the American Heart Association. Chicago, 2002.

33. Bettmann MA, Katzen BT, Whisnant J, et al. Carotid stenting and angioplasty: a statement for healthcare professionals from the Councils on Cardiovascular Radiology, Stroke, Cardio-Thoracic and Vascular Surgery, Epidemiology, and Prevention, and Clinical Cardiology, American Heart Association. *Circulation* 1998;97:121–3.

34. Veith FJ, Amor M, Ohki T, et al. Current status of carotid bifurcation angioplasty and stenting based on a consensus of opinion leaders. *J Vasc Surg* 2001;33(2 Suppl.):S111–6.

35. Jain S, Zhang S, Khosla S. Subclavian and innominate arteries stenting: acute and long term results. *J Am Coll Cardiol* 1998;31:63A (Abstr.).

36. Gershony G, Basta L, Hagan AD. Correction of subclavian artery stenosis by percutaneous angioplasty. *Cathet Cardiovasc Diagn* 1990;21:165–9.

37. Dorros G, Lewin RF, Jamnadas P, et al. Peripheral transluminal angioplasty of the subclavian and innominate arteries utilizing the brachial approach: acute outcome and follow-up. *Cathet Cardiovasc Diagn* 1990;19:71–6.

38. Beebe HG, Stark R, Johnson ML, et al. Choices of operation for subclavian-vertebral arterial disease. *Am J Surg* 1980;139:616–23.

39. Safian RD, Textor SC. Renal-artery stenosis. *N Engl J Med* 2001;344:431–42.

40. Khosla S, White CJ, Collins TJ, et al. Effects of renal artery stent implantation in patients with renovascular hypertension presenting with unstable angina or congestive heart failure. *Am J Cardiol* 1997;80:363–6.

41. van de Ven PJ, Kaatee R, Beutler JJ, et al. Arterial stenting and balloon angioplasty in ostial atherosclerotic renovascular disease: a randomised trial. *Lancet* 1999;353:282–6.

42. Torsello G, Sachs M, Kniemeyer H, et al. Results of surgical treatment for atherosclerotic renovascular occlusive disease. *Eur J Vasc Surg* 1990;4:477–82.

3 Equipment

Steven P Marso

Introduction

Percutaneous peripheral intervention is now a common therapy for the alleviation of lifestyle-limiting claudication, limb salvage, and to re-establish flow following acute arterial occlusion. Numerous techniques and devices have been developed to facilitate reperfusion. These have resulted in an improved rate of successful completion of these procedures and a broadening of patients deemed eligible for peripheral percutaneous interventions. This section highlights many of the devices currently available for use.

Peripheral balloon angioplasty

Balloon angioplasty of the peripheral arteries is the most common technique, and numerous balloons are available (see **Table 1**, p. 43). The recent trend in peripheral dilatation balloons has been to decrease the crossing profile and decrease maximum guidewire compatibility. Many companies have also introduced rapid-exchange balloons into the peripheral device marketplace.

The PolarCath system (see **Figure 1**), developed by CryoVascular Systems (Los Gatos, CA, USA) and distributed by Boston Scientific (Natick, MA, USA), appears to offer a promising new approach that differs from conventional balloon angioplasty. The PolarCath system achieves balloon inflation with pressurized nitrous oxide gas instead of conventional saline or contrast, thus providing rapid cold dilatation of the diseased artery. This results in a temperature decrease to −10°C. The device consists of a disposable, hand-held controlled inflation unit, a balloon dilatation catheter with dual, coaxial balloons, and a cartridge of nitrous oxide. Balloon dilatation is performed in a standardized inflation protocol. The balloon is inflated to 8 atm with a dwell time of 25 seconds. The balloons are sized from 4 to 7 mm in diameter, with lengths of 20, 40, and 60 mm, and both an 80 and a 120 mm shaft length. The PVD-CHILL study is currently investigating this technology for use in both the peripheral and coronary arterial circulations. The 9-month clinical patency rate for the first 102 patients was 85%. Ankle–brachial indices were improved in 75% of patients, and claudication symptoms were improved in 64% of patients.

Peripheral stents

There has been a marked increase in the number of balloon-expandable stents available for use in the peripheral arteries. Balloon-expandable stents are frequently used in the abdominal aorta, renal arteries, common and proximal external iliac arteries, and, occasionally, the superficial femoral artery. Commonly used balloon-expandable stents are shown in **Table 2** (p. 45).

Many of the frequently used self-expanding stents are shown in **Table 3** (p. 46). These stents are most often deployed in the superficial femoral artery and, to a lesser extent, in the distal iliac and common femoral arteries. Visibility and precise placement limitations permit less frequent use of these stents in the proximal iliac artery. This is a rapidly changing field, with many companies investing resources into stent development for peripheral applications. Thus, the available stents

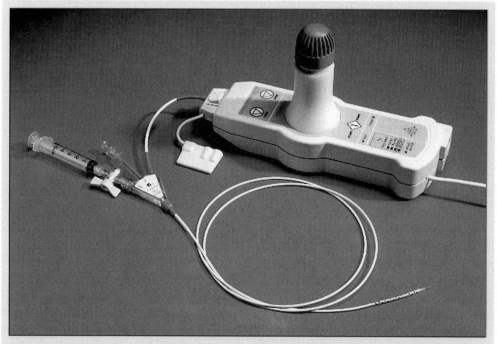

Figure 1. The PolarCath system (Boston Scientific, Natick, MA, USA).

are likely to change frequently. There was an initial interest in developing over-the-wire platforms with decreasing maximal guidewire compatibility. However, the recently released SMART Control (Cordis, Miami Lakes, FL, USA) and Aurora (Medtronic Vascular, Minneapolis, MN, USA) stents were released in a 0.035-inch platform. The Dynalink (Guidant, Indianapolis, IN, USA) is available in both 0.018- and 0.035-inch platforms.

Carotid artery stents

Table 4 (p. 47) depicts many of the stents under investigation or in development for use in the carotid arteries. Many of these stents are specially designed for use in proximal internal carotid artery lesions. These stents have a tapered design in order to accommodate the size discrepancy between the distal common carotid artery and the proximal internal carotid artery.

Emboli protection devices

Embolic protection is being utilized with increasing frequency in peripheral artery interventional procedures, and is common in carotid artery interventions. There is growing interest in embolic protection for high-risk renal artery intervention, including for patients with bulky atherosclerotic disease and elevated creatinine levels. Many options are evolving for embolic protection; a select list of filters is shown in **Table 5** (p. 47). The Medtronic GuardWire is an occlusion balloon

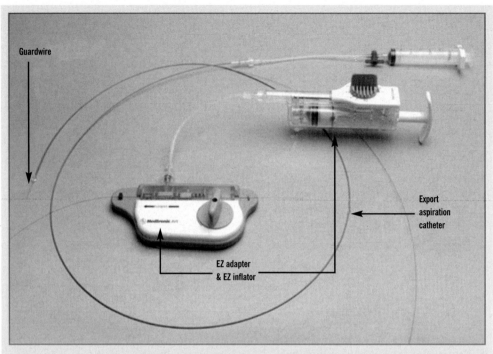

Guardwire

Export aspiration catheter

EZ adapter & EZ inflator

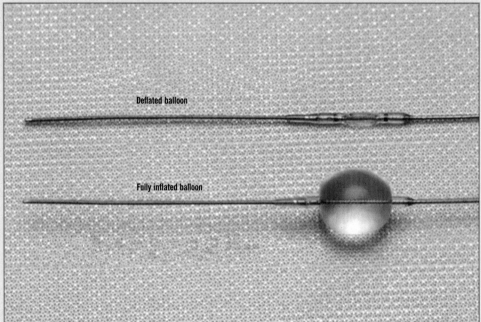

Deflated balloon

Fully inflated balloon

Figure 2. The GuardWire (Medtronic Vascular, Minneapolis, MN, USA).

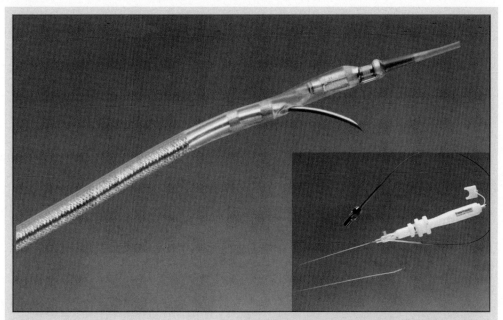

Figure 3. The CrossPoint TransAccess Catheter (Medtronic Vascular, Minneapolis, MN, USA).

device that is frequently used for coronary intervention (see **Figure 2**). The occlusion balloon is inflatable to either 3–6 or 2.5–5.0 mm and is available in 200- and 300-cm wires. After balloon occlusion, an export catheter is used to remove debris from the artery. The crossing profile for the export catheter is 0.068 inches.

Peripheral wires, catheters, and sheaths

Given the breadth of procedures, complexity, variability in anatomy, and vascular approach in the periphery, there are a plethora of available wires, introducer sheaths, and delivery, diagnostic, and interventional guiding catheters. Many of the available devices are shown in **Tables 6** and **7** (see p. 48 and 49).

Two unique devices are available for crossing total occlusions in lower extremity arteries. The CrossPoint TransAccess catheter (Medtronic) allows for controlled re-entry into the distal vessel following purposeful subintimal entry of the proximal occlusion using intravascular ultrasound (IVUS) guidance (see **Figure 3**). The device is placed proximal to the occlusion using a contralateral approach. It is compatible with a 7-Fr sheath, and has an internal diameter of 0.087 inches and a shaft length of 120 cm. The 6.2-Fr catheter tracks over a 0.014-inch guidewire, and a 24-G needle at the near tip of the catheter allows the delivery of a 0.014-inch wire into the distal artery. Ultrasound facilitates the entry of the needle into the true arterial lumen. An integrated 64-element phased-array 20-MHz IVUS transducer at the tip of the catheter enables use with the Jomed/Endosonics IVUS console. IVUS imaging is used to direct the needle towards the true lumen. A 0.014-inch needle is advanced through the CrossPoint needle in order to gain access to the true distal lumen.

(a)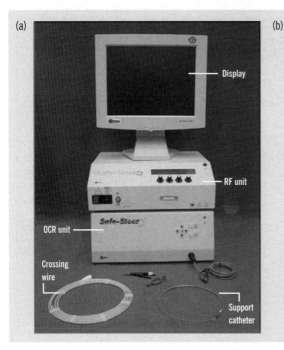

Display

RF unit

Safe-Steer

OCR unit

Crossing wire

Support catheter

(b)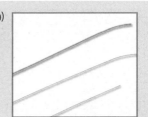

Figure 4. The Safe-Cross system (IntraLuminal Therapeutics, Carlsbad, CA, USA). (**a**) The Safe-Cross console and display. (**b**) The Safe-Cross crossing wire. The crossing wire has multiple tip configurations (straight and angled) and multiple sizes for coronary and peripheral applications.

The Safe-Cross Total Occlusion RF Crossing Wire (IntraLuminal Therapeutics, Carlsbad, CA, USA) is a forward-looking guidance device that uses optical coherence reflectometry for guidance and radiofrequency energy for microablation of the lesion (see **Figure 4**). The guidance works through a fiberoptic strand that is located in the center of the guidewire and looks out the distal tip of the wire. By analyzing the reflection of near infrared light from the tissue adjacent to the guidewire tip, the proximity to the arterial wall can be determined and displayed to the operator. If the guidewire is within the lumen of the artery and not near the artery wall, the radiofrequency energy can be used for microablation at the distal tip of the guidewire, such that the operator can create small voids and fissures in the occlusion to facilitate advancement of the guidewire. This guidewire system recently received market clearance from the Food and Drug Administration for use in coronary, iliac, and superficial femoral arteries.

Conclusion

Medical device availability is rapidly changing for peripheral interventions. This has created a need for continuing and consistent education regarding new devices. This will allow a broadening of initiatives for peripheral interventions, which will benefit the patient in terms of improved successful completion rates and a widening of patient criteria for these procedures.

Balloon name	Maximum guidewire size (inches)	Balloon diameter (mm)	Balloon length (mm)	Shaft length (cm)	Sheath fit	Company
AGIL/TRAC	0.035	4–14	2, 4, 6, 8, 10	55, 80, 135	5 Fr (4–6 mm) 6 Fr (7–10 mm) 7 Fr (12, 14 mm)	Guidant
AGIL/TRAC OTW	0.018	4–10, 12	20, 30, 40, 60	80, 135	5 Fr (4–8 mm) 6 Fr (9–10 mm) 7 Fr (12 mm)	Guidant
Aviator	0.014	4–7 (with 0.5-mm sizing)	10, 15, 17, 20, 25, 30, 40	75, 135	6 Fr (4–6.5 mm) 7 Fr (7 mm)	Cordis
Blue Max 20 (NC)	0.035	4–10	2–4, 8, 10	40, 75, 120	6 Fr (4–6 mm) 7 Fr (7–8 mm) 8 Fr (9–10 mm)	Boston Scientific
Gazelle Monorail (CC)	0.018	2–6 (with 0.5-mm sizing)	2	90, 135	4 Fr	Boston Scientific
Maxi LD	0.035	14, 15, 16, 18, 20, 22, 25	20, 40, 60, 80	65, 80, 110	8 Fr (14–18 mm) 9 Fr (20 mm) 11 Fr (22–25 mm)	Cordis
Opta Pro	0.035	3–12	8–9, 40, 60, 80, 100	65, 80, 110, 135	5 Fr (3–8 mm) 6 Fr (8–10 mm) 7 Fr (12 mm)	Cordis
Powerflex Extreme	0.035	4–10	20, 40, 60	40, 65, 80, 120	6 Fr (4–7 mm) 7 Fr (8–10 mm)	Cordis
Powerflex P3	0.035	4–12	10, 15, 20, 30, 40, 60, 80, 100	40, 65, 80, 110, 135	5 Fr (4–6 mm) 6 Fr (7–8 mm) 7 Fr (9–12 mm)	Cordis
Savy	0.018	2–6 (with 0.5-mm sizing)	20, 30, 40, 60, 100	80, 120, 150	4 Fr (2–5 mm) 5 Fr (6 mm)	Cordis

Table 1. Peripheral balloons. C: compliant; CC: controlled compliant; NC: noncompliant.

Balloon name	Maximum guidewire size (inches)	Balloon diameter (mm)	Balloon length (mm)	Shaft length (cm)	Sheath fit	Company
Slalom High	0.018	3.0–8.0	15, 20, 40	80, 120, 135	5 Fr (3–6 mm)	Cordis
Symmetry (NC)	0.018	1.5–6 (with 0.5-mm sizing)	2, 4, 10	std-90, 135, stiff-90, 135, 150	4 Fr (1.5–4×40 mm) 5 Fr (4–6×100 mm)	Boston Scientific
Synergy (C)	0.035	3–12	1.5, 2–4, 6, 8, 10	50, 75, 90, 135, 150	5 Fr (3.6×40 mm) 6 Fr (6–8×40–80 mm) 7 Fr (8–12×60 mm)	Boston Scientific
Talon (NC)	0.018	4–7	1.5, 2, 4	90, 130	5 Fr (4–6 mm) 6 Fr (7 mm)	Boston Scientific
Ultra-Soft SV Monorail (CC)	0.018	4–7 (with 0.5-mm sizing)	1.5, 2	90, 150	4 Fr (4–5 mm) 5 Fr (5.5–7 mm)	Boston Scientific
Ultra-Thin (NC) Diamond	0.035	3–12	1.5, 2–4, 6, 10	40, 75, 120, 135, 150	5 Fr (3–6 mm) 6 Fr (7–8 mm) 7 Fr (9–12 mm)	Boston Scientific
Ultra-Thin SDS (NC)	0.035	4–10	1.5, 2–4, 6, 8	50, 75, 90, 135	5 Fr (4–7×40 mm) 6 Fr (7–8×60 mm) 7 Fr (9–10 mm)	Boston Scientific
VIA/TRAC Rx	0.014 (with 0.5-mm sizing)	4–7	15, 20, 30, 40	80, 135	4 Fr (4–4.5 mm) 5 Fr (5–7 mm)	Guidant
XXL (NC)	0.035	12, 14, 16, 18	2, 4, 6 cm	55, 75, 80, 120, 135	7 Fr (12, 14 mm) 8 Fr (16, 18 mm)	Boston Scientific

Table 1. *Continued*

Device name	Maximum guidewire size (inches)	Stent diameter (mm)	Stent length (mm)	Shaft length (cm)	Sheath size	Material	Company
Bridge Assurant	0.035	6–10	20, 30, 40, 60	80, 130	6 Fr	Stainless steel	Medtronic Vascular
Bridge Extra Support	0.035	5–7	10, 17	75, 120	7 Fr	Stainless steel	Medtronic Vascular
Racer	0.018	4–7	12, 18	80, 130	5 Fr (4–6 mm) 6 Fr (7 mm)	Cobalt	Medtronic Vascular
Express LD	0.035	5–10	17, 27, 37, 57 (5–8 mm) 25, 37, 57 (9–10 mm)	75, 135	6 Fr (6–8×37 mm) 7 Fr (8×57 mm-10)	Stainless steel	Boston Scientific
GENESIS XD	Stent alone	8–10	19, 25, 29, 39, 59	N/A	N/A	Stainless steel	Cordis
LifeStent LP SDS	0.018	4–7	18, 36, 56	75, 120	5 Fr, 6 Fr	Stainless steel	Edwards Lifesciences
LifeStent SDS	0.035	6–10	18, 26, 36, 56	75, 120	6 Fr, 7 Fr	Stainless steel	Edwards Lifesciences
Omnilink	0.018, 0.035	5–10 4–10	18, 28, 38, 58 12, 16, 18, 28, 38,58	80, 135 80, 135	5 Fr (4–7 mm) 6 Fr (8–10 mm) 7 Fr (7–9 mm) 8 Fr (10 mm)	Stainless steel	Guidant
Palmaz	Unmounted	4–8	10, 15, 20, 29, 39	Unmounted	6 Fr, 7 Fr	Stainless steel	Cordis Endovascular
Palmaz XL	Stent alone	10–12	30, 40, 50	N/A	N/A	Stainless steel	Cordis
ParaMount	0.035	5–8	16, 26, 36	75	6 Fr, 7 Fr	Stainless steel	ev3
ParaMount Mini GPS	0.014, 0.018	5, 6, 7	14, 18, 21	80	5 Fr, 6 Fr	Stainless steel	ev3
ParaMount XS	0.035	5–8	12, 17	75	6 Fr	Stainless Steel	ev3
Racer	0.014, 0.018	4–7	12, 18	80, 130	5 Fr, 6 Fr	Cobalt	Medtronic Vascular
RX HERCULINK PLUS	0.014	4–7	12, 15, 18	80, 135	5 Fr, 6 Fr	Stainless steel	Guidant
Symphony	0.035	6–14	20, 40, 60	75, 110	7 Fr	Nitinol	Boston Scientific

Table 2. Balloon-expandable stents. N/A: not available.

Device name	Maximum guidewire size (inches)	Stent diameter (mm)	Stent length (mm)	Shaft length (cm)	Sheath size	Material	Company
Absolute	0.035	5–10	20, 40, 60, 80, 100	80, 135	6 Fr	Nitinol	Guidant
Aurora	0.035	6–10	20, 40, 60, 80	75, 120	6–7 Fr	Nitinol	Medtronic
Conformexx	0.035	6–6	20–40, 60, 80, 100, 120	135	6 Fr	Nitinol	Bard
Dynalink	0.018, 0.035	5–10	28, 38, 56, 80, 100	80, 120	6 Fr	Nitinol	Guidant
Luminexx	0.035	6–10, 12	20–60, 80, 100, 120	80, 135	6 Fr	Nitinol	Bard
Monorail Wallstent	0.014	6, 8, 10	21, 22, 24, 29, 31, 36, 37	135	5 Fr (6, 8 mm) 6 Fr (10 mm)	Elgiloy	Boston Scientific
Precise	0.018 0.018	5–7 8–10	20–40 20–40	135 135	5.5 Fr 6 Fr	Nitinol	Cordis
Precise Rx	0.014 0.014	5–7 8–10	20–40 20–40	135 135	5 Fr 6 Fr	Nitinol	Cordis
Protégé	0.018 0.035 0.035	6–9 6–10, 12 6–8	20–40, 60, 80 20–40, 60, 80 150	135 80, 120 120	6 Fr 7 Fr 7 Fr	Nitinol	ev3
Smart Control	0.035 0.035	6–10 12, 14	20–40, 60, 80, 100 30, 40, 60, 80	80, 120 80, 120	6 Fr 7 Fr	Nitinol	Cordis
Wallgraft	0.035	6–14	20, 30, 50, 70	90	9 Fr (6–8 mm) 10 Fr (9–10 mm) 11 Fr (12 mm) 12 Fr (14 mm)	Elgiloy	Boston Scientific
Wallstent	0.035	5–24	18, 20, 23, 24, 34, 35, 36, 38, 39, 40, 42, 45, 46, 47, 49, 52, 55, 59, 60, 61, 66, 67, 69, 80, 90, 94	75, 135	6 Fr (thru 10 mm)	Elgiloy	Boston Scientific
Zilver	0.035	6–10	20, 40, 60, 80, 100	80	7 Fr	Nitinol	Cook

Table 3. Self-expanding stents.

Device name	Tapered stents		Straight stents		Company
	Diameter (proximal/distal) (mm)	Length (mm)	Diameter (mm)	Length (mm)	
Carotid Wallstent	N/A	N/A	6, 8, 10	20–40	Boston Scientific
Exponent	N/A	N/A	6–10	20, 30, 40	Medtronic
Mednova Xact	10/8, 9/7, 8/6	30, 40	7–10	20, 30	Abbott Vascular
NexStent	Self-tapering; all diameters 4–9	30	4–9	30	EndoTex
Precise	10/7, 9/7, 8/6	30	5–10	20–40	Cordis
Precise RX	10/7, 9/7, 8/6	30	5–10	20–40	Cordis
Protégé	10/7, 8/6	30, 40	6, 8–10	20, 30, 40, 60, 80	ev3
RX Acculink	10/7, 8/6	30, 40	5–10	20, 30, 40	Guidant

Table 4. Carotid stents.

Name	Type	Position
AngioGuard	RX Filter	Distal
AngioGuard XP	Filter	Distal
EmboShield	Filter	Distal
FilterWire EX	Filter	Distal
Filterwire EZ	Filter	Distal
GuardWire	Occlusion	Distal
Interceptor	Filter	Distal
PAES	Continuous flow reversal	Proximal
RX Acunet	Filter	Distal
Spider	Filter	Distal

Table 5. Embolic protection devices.

Wire name	Diameter (inches)	Length (cm)	Tip shape	Material	Company
Amplatz Super Stiff	0.035, 0.038	75, 145, 180, 260	Straight/J	Tip lengths: 1, 3.5, 6 cm	Boston Scientific
Glidewire					
Standard	0.032, 0.035	120, 150, 180, 260	Straight/angled	Hydrophilic-coated	Boston Scientific
Stiff Shaft	0.035, 0.038	80, 150, 180, 260	Straight/angled	Hydrophilic-coated	Boston Scientific
Long Taper	0.035, 0.038	150	Straight/angled	Hydrophilic-coated	Boston Scientific
Stiff Shaft/ Long Taper	0.035, 0.038	150, 260	Straight/angled	Hydrophilic-coated	Boston Scientific
J-tip	0.035, 0.038	150	3-mm J	Hydrophilic-coated	Boston Scientific
Small Vessel	0.018, 0.025	150, 180, 260	Straight/angled	Hydrophilic-coated	Boston Scientific
Tapered Gold	0.016, 0.018–0.013	180	45°/70°	Hydrophilic-coated	Boston Scientific
Shapeable	0.018, 0.035, 0.038	150/180	Shapeable	Hydrophilic-coated	Boston Scientific
Magic Torque	0.035	180, 260	Shapeable	10 cm (Glidex); 11–50 cm (PTFE)	Boston Scientific
Meier Wire	0.035	185, 260, 300	J/C	Extra-stiff wire	Boston Scientific
Platinum Plus Glidex hydrophilic coating	0.014 ST 0.018 LT 0.018 LT 0.025 ST	180 60, 180, 260 145, 180, 260 180, 260	3-cm floppy tip 3-cm floppy tip 8-cm floppy tip 3-cm floppy tip	11-cm platinum shapeable tip 3 cm 11-cm platinum shapeable tip 3 cm 15 cm platinum shapeable tip 3 cm 14 cm platinum shapeable tip 3 cm	Boston Scientific
Spartacore	0.014	130, 190, 300	Straight	Stainless steel with MICROGLIDE	Guidant
MEMCORE Firm	0.014	130	Straight	Stainless steel with Hydrocoat	Guidant
Steelcore	0.018	190, 300	Straight	Stainless steel with MICROGLIDE	Guidant
Supracore	0.035	145, 190, 300	Straight	Stainless steel with MICROGLIDE	Guidant
Thruway b	0.018	130, 190, 300	Straight/J	Stainless steel core with platinum coil tip	Boston Scientific
Trooper Patriot ext. wire	0.018	130, 190, 300	Straight/J	Teflon coating	Boston Scientific
Storq	0.035	180, 300	Straight /J	Stainless steel	Cordis
V-18	0.018	–	8-, 12-cm taper	ICE hydrophilic coating/distal end 2-cm shape tip. Scitanium core	Boston Scientific
SV-5	–	180, 300	5-cm taper	Stainless steel	Cordis
SV-8	–	180, 300	8-cm taper	Stainless steel	Cordis
SV-14	0.018	180, 300	14-cm taper	Stainless steel	Cordis
Jindo	0.022, 0.035	145, 180, 300	Taper	Stainless steel	Cordis
Amplatz Super Stiff	0.035, 0.038	150	Straight	Stainless steel	Cordis

Table 6. Peripheral wires. LT: long taper; PTFE: polytetrafluoroethylene; ST: short taper.

Name	Size (Fr)	Length (cm)	Shape/function	Construction	Company
Avanti	4–10	5.5, 11, 23	Straight	Braided nylon	Cordis
Brite Tip Sheaths	4–11	5.5, 11, 23, 35, 45, 55, 90	Shapeable. Provides contralateral access for interventional procedures	Co-extruded polyethylene	Cordis
Flexor Introducer	5.5–8.0	40–45	Numerous	SS coil	Cook
Glidecath	4, 5	65, 100	Numerous	Selective, hydrophilic-coated	Boston Scientific
Imager II	4, 5	65, 90, 100	Numerous	Flush and selective	Boston Scientific
Launcher Guide	6–8	47, 55	Numerous	Vest-Tech nylon and encapsulated flatwire braid	Medtronic
Mach I	6–8	55, 90	Numerous	Tungsten and SS braid, PTFE inner lumen RO tip marker	Boston Scientific
Pinnacle Destination Guide	6–7	45, 90	Straight, Hockey, MP, RDC, LIMA	SS spiral	Boston Scientific
Pinnacle Sheath	4–11	10, 25	Straight	RO marker on 6, 7, 8 Fr	Boston Scientific
Royal Flush	4–5	65–110	Numerous: high-flow aortic injection	Nylon	Cook
Shuttle SL	6–8	80, 90	Straight, shapeable	SS coil with hydrophilic coating	Cook
Torcon NB	4–5	65–100	Numerous: visceral and cerebral applications	SS, braided nylon	Cook
Veripath Guide	6–8	50	Numerous	SS braid, nylon, PTFE	Guidant
Z^2 Guide	7, 8	47, 55	Numerous	Encapsulated flat wire braid with Pebax outer and inner jacket	Medtronic

Table 7. Guiding catheters/sheaths. LIMA: left internal mammary artery; MP: multipurpose; Pebax: polyetherbloxamide; PTFE: polytetrafluoroethylene; RDC: renal double curve; SS: stainless steel; RO: radiopaque.

4 Adjunctive pharmacology

Marco Roffi and Guido Schnyder

Introduction

As with percutaneous coronary intervention (PCI), the use of antithrombotic therapy in the setting of peripheral arterial angioplasty and stenting (percutaneous transluminal angioplasty [PTA]) relies on a balance between the reduction of ischemic complications and the bleeding risk. The endovascular treatment of peripheral and cerebrovascular disease has many similarities to PCI, namely: the basic equipment, the nature of the atherosclerotic disease, and the complications that may occur, both in the short-term (eg, dissection, abrupt vessel closure, thrombosis, embolization) and in the long-term (eg, restenosis, late occlusion).

Due to the variety of vascular beds involved in peripheral intervention, the consequence of a particular complication (eg, distal embolization) may range from catastrophic (eg, during carotid stenting) to a merely angiographic finding without clinical consequences. Therefore, the safety and efficacy of adjunctive pharmacologic treatment should be assessed for each vascular bed. With respect to access-site-related complications, similarities between PCI and PTA include a femoral approach and similar sheath size. The higher likelihood of atherosclerotic disease of the common femoral artery may be a source of increased local complications in patients undergoing PTA, although no comparative studies have been performed.

The evidence available on adjunctive pharmacologic treatment for PTA is far less solid than for PCI. One reason for this is the lack of surrogate markers of clinical outcome, such as creatine kinase-MB or troponin, which allow a more precise assessment of drug efficacy. Furthermore, the extrapolation of data from PCI trials to the peripheral vasculature is problematic due to incomparable endpoints. While PCI trials have focused on death, myocardial infarction, or the need for revascularization, peripheral vascular disease (PVD) intervention studies have mainly addressed patency rates and limb salvage.

Platelet activation, adhesion, and aggregation are pivotal mechanisms of thrombus formation and vessel occlusion in both the coronary and peripheral vasculature. Although the importance of adequate antithrombotic therapy for successful PTA is evident, the optimal regimen still needs to be determined. This chapter focuses on adjunctive antithrombotic therapy at the time of endovascular intervention. In addition, the value of secondary prevention in PVD patients is addressed.

Adjunctive antithrombotic therapy for endovascular procedures

Aspirin

Aspirin is the most widely used and studied platelet inhibitor for both coronary and peripheral vascular interventions. This agent irreversibly inhibits the production of cyclo-oxygenase-1 and thromboxane A_2. The most compelling data on the efficacy of antiplatelet agents among patients undergoing PTA are derived from a meta-analysis of the Antiplatelet Trialists' Collaboration, which

---

Summary of evidence

Patients undergoing endovascular intervention are at high risk for subsequent myocardial infarction and stroke.

Continuing the antiplatelet therapy at the time of vascular intervention may reduce the risk of periprocedural myocardial infarction.

Evidence extrapolated from percutaneous coronary interventions suggests that antiplatelet agents increase bleeding complications at the access site.

There is no evidence that antiplatelet agents reduce restenosis.

Recommendations

All patients with symptomatic peripheral arterial disease or who have undergone endovascular intervention should be considered for long-term antiplatelet therapy, unless contraindicated.

Aspirin should be continued periprocedure. In patients not on aspirin, a 300–325 mg aspirin loading dose should be given at least 2 hours prior to the procedure.

Table 1. Summary of evidence and recommendations for antiplatelet therapy in endovascular interventions according to the Peripheral Arterial Disease Antiplatelet Consensus Group. Adapted with permission from Elsevier Science (Antiplatelet therapy in peripheral arterial disease. Consensus statement. *Eur J Vasc Endovasc Surg* 2003;26:1–16).

showed a 47% reduction in occlusion rates among patients treated with platelet inhibitors (mostly aspirin) [1]. Therefore, all patients undergoing PTA should receive a 300–325 mg loading dose of aspirin at least 2 hours prior to the procedure (if not on chronic aspirin therapy) [2]. From a safety perspective, no large-scale prospective study has addressed the impact of antiplatelet therapy on PTA-related bleeding complications. **Table 1** summarizes the evidence for antiplatelet therapy in peripheral interventions.

Ticlopidine and clopidogrel

Ticlopidine and clopidogrel inhibit platelets by blocking the ADP receptor. Therefore, aspirin and ADP antagonists may have an additive effect in terms of both efficacy and bleeding complications. Due to its better safety profile and probable equal efficacy, clopidogrel has replaced ticlopidine for virtually all indications [3].

The combination of aspirin and ADP antagonists has been a major breakthrough in PCI and has led to a dramatic decrease in the subacute stent thrombosis rate [4]. In the peripheral circulation, stent thrombosis is less frequent due to higher flow and larger vessel size. Nevertheless, and despite the lack of prospective data, it is widely accepted that, following an endovascular procedure, patients should receive aspirin lifelong and clopidogrel for at least 1 month if a stent has been placed. Similarly, lifelong aspirin and at least 1 month of clopidogrel is recommended following carotid stenting [5]. Based on a recent randomized study, 1-year treatment with aspirin and clopidogrel should be considered the standard of care post-PCI [6]. Preliminary findings suggest that prolonged dual antiplatelet therapy significantly reduces cardiovascular events following PTA [7].

Platelet glycoprotein IIb/IIIa receptor antagonists

The glycoprotein (GP)IIb/IIIa receptor is the platelet binding site for fibrinogen. Occupancy of the receptor leads to blockage of fibrinogen cross-linking among platelets and consequent profound inhibition of platelet aggregation. Large-scale randomized clinical trials have established the efficacy of GPIIb/IIIa receptor antagonists in PCI, demonstrating a reduction in periprocedural myocardial infarctions and improved long-term survival [8]. Conversely, few data are available on the safety and efficacy of these agents as adjunctive treatment for cerebrovascular or peripheral interventions. Due to different safety and efficacy issues, the two fields are discussed separately below.

Carotid stenting

Distal embolization during carotid stenting may have catastrophic consequences. Therefore, it is mandatory that patients have adequate platelet inhibition at the time of the procedure. Standard therapy includes pretreatment with aspirin and clopidogrel, while the use of adjunctive GPIIb/IIIa receptor antagonists remains controversial. Although these agents have the potential to reduce distal embolization, they may increase intracranial bleeding. In a study of 151 consecutive patients undergoing unprotected carotid stenting, abciximab as an adjuvant to unfractionated heparin (UFH) was safe and possibly more efficacious than UFH alone in preventing ischemic events [9]. A small randomized report (N=70) also showed a lower rate of ischemic events in an abciximab-treated group compared with a heparin-treated group, though at the cost of two intracranial hemorrhages [10]. Conversely, a retrospective analysis of 550 carotid stenting patients (216 on GPIIb/IIIa receptor antagonists) showed that the rate of stroke or neurological death was higher among patients on GPIIb/IIIa receptor antagonists compared with those on UFH alone (6.0% vs 2.4%, $P=0.043$) [11]. Following the introduction of routine mechanical distal protection during carotid stenting, the advantage of potent intravenous platelet inhibition has decreased, while the potential for intracranial bleeding persists. Therefore, GPIIb/IIIa receptor antagonists cannot currently be recommended as a routine adjunctive treatment for carotid stenting.

Lower extremity interventions

Percutaneous catheter-based thrombolysis, discussed later in the chapter, is an established treatment of arterial thromboembolic disease and graft occlusion. Two trials have addressed the use of abciximab in conjunction with fibrinolytic therapy for lower limb thrombosis. A total of 84 patients with acute lower extremity arterial occlusion were randomized to aspirin or abciximab in the standard coronary dose along with intra-arterial recombinant tissue plasminogen activator (rt-PA) [12]. Patients receiving abciximab required a significantly shorter duration of lysis than those treated with aspirin (75 minutes vs 110 minutes, $P<0.001$). Moreover, abciximab significantly reduced the rates of rehospitalization, reintervention, and amputation.

The PROMPT (Platelet Receptor Antibodies in Order to Manage Peripheral Artery Thrombosis) trial prospectively evaluated the combination of abciximab and urokinase in the same setting [13]. Patients were randomized in a 2:5 ratio to receive urokinase and placebo (n=20) or urokinase and abciximab (n=50) in addition to aspirin and low-dose UFH. The amputation-free survival at 3 months was 96% in the combination group and 80% in the placebo group ($P=0.04$). At 90 days, the rates of survival without surgery or major amputation were 90% and 75%, respectively ($P=0.053$). There was no significant difference in the patency rates of the occluded vessels (66% vs 70%, respectively). Four major bleeding episodes (8%) were detected in the combination group; all related to the puncture site.

Data on the use of GPIIb/IIIa receptor antagonists during endovascular interventions are limited [14]. Because of cost issues and the potential for bleeding complications, the use of these agents should be reserved for procedures that carry a high risk of thrombosis or embolization. GPIIb/IIIa receptor antagonists may be considered for infrapopliteal angioplasty, particularly in the presence of single-vessel run-off, or long superficial femoral artery stenoses or occlusions. In total occlusions, it is recommended that these agents are administered after recanalization and documentation of intraluminal wire position in order to prevent extensive bleeding secondary to vessel wall perforation.

No data are available to determine whether one GPIIb/IIIa receptor antagonist is superior to another in peripheral intervention. According to coronary experience, abciximab may be preferable in the presence of a large thrombus burden [15]. Advantages of the small molecules tirofiban and eptifibatide include lower costs and shorter half-lives. The latter property may be crucial if urgent vascular surgery is needed or in case of bleeding complications. However, in life-threatening bleeding episodes abciximab-associated platelet inhibition can be antagonized by the administration of platelets, while the platelet inhibitory effect of small-molecule GPIIb/IIIa receptor antagonists cannot be opposed.

Periprocedural anticoagulation

Since the beginning of coronary and peripheral intervention, UFH has been the anticoagulant of choice. Although its effect is largely unpredictable due to poor and markedly variable bioavailability, this limitation is of minor importance in the angiography suite since the level of anticoagulation is easily monitored via the activated clotting time. The impact of other potential disadvantages of UFH described in the coronary circulation, such as a proaggregatory effect [16] and the inability to inactivate clot-bound thrombin, is unknown (see **Table 2**) [17]. With respect to safety, a series examining outcomes following heparin-based PTA found a major bleeding rate of 4.6% among 213 consecutive patients [18].

Whether UFH remains the anticoagulant of choice, in both the coronary and peripheral vasculature, is a source of debate [19]. Potential alternatives include low molecular weight heparins (LMWHs) and the direct thrombin inhibitor bivalirudin. From a cost perspective, UFH is far less expensive than its competitors. Nevertheless, LMWH has several advantages compared with UFH (see **Table 2**), including a predictable anticoagulant effect with no need for monitoring. Furthermore, LMWH has a higher ratio of factor Xa to thrombin inhibition, leading to inhibition of both thrombin generation and thrombin activity.

In the coronary circulation, most data on LMWH are based on acute coronary syndromes or acute myocardial infarction. In the setting of PCI, small studies have shown LMWH to be safe and efficacious alone or in combination with GPIIb/IIIa receptor antagonists [20]. Large-scale trials of UFH versus enoxaparin are underway [21]. To our knowledge, the use of LMWH in PTA has not been prospectively addressed.

Unfractionated heparin	Low molecular weight heparin	Direct thrombin inhibitor
Inhibits thrombin and factor Xa	Mainly inhibits factor Xa	Inhibits thrombin
Does not inactivate clot-bound thrombin	Does not inactivate clot-bound thrombin	Inactivates clot-bound thrombin
Anticoagulation fairly unpredictable	Anticoagulation more predictable	Anticoagulation more predictable
Elimination: reticuloendothelial system	Elimination: renal	Elimination: renal
Monitoring required	Generally, no monitoring is required	Monitoring required
Can be completely neutralized	Can be partially neutralized	Cannot be neutralized

Table 2. Pharmacologic properties of anticoagulants. Adapted with permission from the International Society on Thrombosis and Haemostasis (Verstraete M. Direct thrombin inhibitors: appraisal of the antithrombotic/hemorrhagic balance. *Thromb Haemost* 1997;78:357–63).

Recently, the direct thrombin inhibitor bivalirudin has gained attention as an anticoagulant during PCI and PTA. The advantages of direct thrombin inhibitors over UFH include a more specific and potent inhibition of thrombin, acting independently from antithrombin and other endogenous factors (see **Table 2**). Unlike UFH, direct thrombin inhibitors are able to inhibit clot-bound thrombin and produce a more stable level of anticoagulation over time. However, bivalirudin is more expensive than LMWH. In a large-scale, randomized PCI trial, the strategy of bivalirudin with bail-out GPIIb/IIIa inhibition was shown to be noninferior to UFH plus planned GPIIb/IIIa receptor antagonists and was associated with fewer bleeding complications [22].

Preliminary data on bivalirudin as an anticoagulant for PTA appear promising. A single-center experience reported only two major bleeding complications (4.2%) among 48 consecutive patients undergoing lower extremity intervention [23]. Similarly, a retrospective analysis of 180 iliac and 75 renal revascularization procedures described a major or minor bleeding rate of 3.9% [24]. A multicenter registry of bivalirudin in peripheral intervention called APPROVE is ongoing. Randomized trials comparing the safety and efficacy of bivalirudin, LMWH, and UFH in the setting of PTA are warranted.

Thrombolytic therapy

Thrombolytic therapy for peripheral vascular occlusions started as a systemic intravenous modality, but soon thereafter intra-arterial administration of lytic agents at the thrombus site gained popularity. The first agent studied was streptokinase. Subsequently, urokinase and rt-PA have been progressively used as agents of choice. The rate of successful reperfusion associated with intra-arterial thrombolysis (50%–85%) appears to be superior to that with intravenous application. In a small, randomized comparison (N=60) between intra-arterial rt-PA, intravenous rt-PA, and intra-arterial streptokinase, the use of intra-arterial rt-PA was associated with improved patency and a lower incidence of hemorrhagic complications [25]. Another study randomized 32 patients to intra-arterial administration of rt-PA or urokinase; there was faster reperfusion in the rt-PA arm and comparable bleeding complications [26].

The major drawback to intra-arterial thrombolysis is the prolonged intra-arterial catheter placement, a source of patient discomfort and bleeding complications. In an early review of thrombolytic series for lower extremity obstruction, the risk of hemorrhagic stroke was 1% and major and minor bleeding occurred in 5.1% and 14.8% of patients, respectively [27]. If a major bleeding event occurs at a noncompressible site, thrombolytic therapy and anticoagulants (eg, UFH) should be discontinued and coagulation factors should be substituted (eg, with fresh frozen plasma or cryoprecipitate). The use of agents to reverse the fibrinolytic state (eg, tranexamic acid or epsilon-aminocaproic acid) in life-threatening bleeding episodes remains controversial [28].

A larger, multicenter trial compared intra-arterial thrombolytic therapy with urokinase or rt-PA with surgery for recent onset, lower limb ischemia due to thrombotic native or bypass occlusion [29]. After 393 patients had been enrolled, the investigation was stopped prematurely due to better outcomes in the surgical group. Subsequent subgroup analyses detected a dichotomous response to therapy based on the time from onset of symptoms: in patients who had been symptomatic for over 2 weeks, surgical revascularization was superior; conversely, amputation rates were lower in the thrombolytic group among patients presenting within 2 weeks of symptom onset.

Few prospective randomized studies have compared different thrombolytic regimens. Therefore, no absolute recommendations can be given regarding drugs and doses. Commonly used thrombolytic regimens and contraindications to thrombolytic therapy are listed in **Tables 3** and **4**. Contemporary practice suggests that adding UFH to thrombolysis (either systemically or around the catheter through a proximal sheath) may reduce the risk of pericatheter thrombosis. Following thrombolytic therapy, oral anticoagulation should be continued until the underlying cause of occlusion is corrected. Although not prospectively investigated, long-term anticoagulation should be considered in the absence of a correctable cause of thrombosis.

Long-term antiplatelet therapy in PVD

PVD is a marker of generalized advanced atherosclerosis. Approximately half of the individuals with symptomatic disease have coronary disease [30]. In addition, PVD is associated with a 2- to 5-fold increase in cardiovascular mortality [31]. In this patient population, long-term antiplatelet therapy is associated with an approximately 25% reduction in subsequent vascular events [32,33].

Most data on the efficacy of antiplatelet therapy in secondary prevention among patients with PVD refer to aspirin. The CAPRIE (Clopidogrel versus Aspirin in Patients at Risk of Ischemic Events) trial is the largest head-to-head comparison of two antiplatelet regimens (aspirin and clopidogrel) in the long-term treatment of patients at high risk for cardiovascular events. Enrolling over 19,000 patients, this trial demonstrated an event reduction in the clopidogrel arm (relative risk reduction 9%, $P=0.043$) [34]. The greatest benefit of clopidogrel was observed among patients with PVD (relative risk reduction 24%, $P=0.0028$). The ongoing CHARISMA (Clopidogrel for High Atherothrombotic Risk and Ischemic Stabilization, Management, and Avoidance) trial, which has enrolled over 15,000 patients, will compare the safety and efficacy of the combination of aspirin and clopidogrel versus aspirin and placebo in the prevention of cardiovascular events among high-risk individuals [35].

Thrombolytic agent	Dose
Urokinase	240,000 IU/h for 2 hours, then 120,000 IU/h for 2 hours, then 60,000 IU/h until lysis complete; **or**
	240,000 IU/h for 4 hours, then 120,000 IU/h to a maximum of 48 hours
rt-PA	1 mg/h; **or**
	0.05 mg/kg/h

Table 3. Popular schemes for commonly used thrombolytic agents. rt-PA: recombinant tissue plasminogen activator.

Absolute contraindications
Established cerebrovascular events (including transient ischemic attack) within last 2 months
Active bleeding diathesis
Recent (<10 days) gastrointestinal bleeding
Neurosurgery (intracranial or spinal) within last 3 months
Intracranial trauma within last 3 months
Relative major contraindications
Cardiopulmonary resuscitation within last 10 days
Major nonvascular surgery or trauma within last 10 days
Uncontrolled hypertension (>180 mm Hg systolic or >110 mm Hg diastolic)
Puncture of noncompressible vessel
Intracranial tumor
Recent eye surgery
Minor contraindications
Hepatic failure, particularly with coagulopathy
Bacterial endocarditis
Pregnancy
Diabetic hemorrhagic retinopathy

Table 4. Contraindications to thrombolytic therapy according to the Working Party on Thrombolysis in the Management of Limb Ischemia. Reproduced with permission from Excerpta Medica (Working Party on Thrombolysis in the Management of Limb Ischemia. Thrombolysis in the management of lower limb peripheral arterial occlusion – a consensus document. *Am J Cardiol* 1998;81:207–18).

All patients with symptomatic PVD and those who have undergone PTA should receive long-term antiplatelet therapy. Based on efficacy and cost issues, aspirin is the first-line agent in a dose ranging from 75 to 325 mg/day. In patients who do not tolerate aspirin, clopidogrel is a valid alternative, and may even be more efficacious. Until further data become available, long-term dual antiplatelet therapy should be limited to selected patients who are deemed to be at particularly high risk for cardiovascular events.

Antiplatelet therapy and oral anticoagulation following peripheral arterial bypass surgery

As with PTA, the risks and benefits of antiplatelet therapy or anticoagulation following peripheral bypass surgery require careful evaluation. Compared with endovascular therapy, surgery is associated with an increased risk of cardiovascular events. More evidence is available on the impact of antithrombotic therapy following peripheral bypass surgery than post-PTA. An analysis of 10 randomized trials detected an overall 24% event reduction among patients undergoing lower limb bypass who were treated with antiplatelet agents compared with placebo [33]. A meta-analysis by the Antiplatelet Trialists' Collaboration demonstrated that, among around 2,000 patients undergoing peripheral bypass surgery, there was an approximately 40% reduction in graft occlusion in patients treated with antiplatelet agents (mostly aspirin) [1]. A placebo-controlled study similarly showed improved patency with ticlopidine [36]. The value of dual antiplatelet therapy in this setting is being investigated in the CASPAR (Clopidogrel and Acetylsalicylic Acid in Bypass Surgery for Peripheral Arterial Disease) trial.

Only one randomized study, which enrolled 130 patients and was neither blinded nor placebo-controlled, has addressed the efficacy of long-term oral anticoagulation on peripheral bypass graft patency [37]. In this study, patients treated with oral anticoagulation had a 55% lower occlusion rate than controls. The Dutch BOA (Bypass Oral Anticoagulants or Aspirin) study randomized 2,690 patients undergoing infrainguinal bypass to oral anticoagulation or aspirin [38]. Overall, no difference in patency was observed; however, anticoagulation was associated with a doubling of major bleeds. A randomized trial performed by the Veterans Administration on over 800 patients following lower extremity bypass surgery demonstrated that the combination of aspirin and warfarin had no benefit and was associated with more bleeding complications compared with aspirin alone [39].

Antirestenotic agents

Despite suggestive animal data, there is no evidence that antiplatelet therapy has any effect on restenosis, either in the coronary or peripheral vasculature. No systemic drug therapy has been proven to reduce restenosis after PTA. The value of homocysteine-lowering therapy, which has been associated with a significant reduction in restenosis [40] and improved outcomes [41] following PCI, has not been tested in the peripheral vasculature.

Preliminary reports on drug-eluting stents in the peripheral vasculature have been less compelling than those in the coronary vasculature [42]. Although this suggests that the technology may not have the same dramatic impact that has been observed in PCI, more studies are needed to assess its safety and efficacy in the peripheral vasculature.

Pentoxifylline and cilostazol for intermittent claudication

Pentoxifylline and cilostazol are the only two hemorheologic agents currently approved by the US Food and Drug Administration for the treatment of intermittent claudication. In patients with PVD, pentoxifylline has been reported to improve abnormal erythrocyte deformability, reduce blood viscosity, and decrease platelet reactivity and plasma hypercoagulability [43]. It is unclear whether these beneficial effects are derived from pentoxifylline's weak antithrombotic action or from other pharmacologic properties. Benefits in terms of improved treadmill walking distance have been demonstrated in several, but not all, randomized trials [44].

Cilostazol is a phosphodiesterase inhibitor with antiplatelet and vasodilating properties. Its mechanism of action as a treatment for intermittent claudication is not fully understood. This agent has been reported to increase walking distance and quality of life in a meta-analysis of randomized trials [45]. Importantly, cilostazol is contraindicated in patients with left ventricular ejection fraction <40%; echocardiography is recommended prior to beginning treatment.

Overall, the limited clinical efficacy of these hemorheologic agents may not justify the added expense for most patients. Nevertheless, these drugs may have a role in severely symptomatic patients for whom even a small increase in walking distance can have a major impact on their quality of life. Several other agents, including ketanserin, nifedipine, fish-oil supplementation, and chelation therapy, have failed to improve symptoms in intermittent claudication.

Secondary prevention

In addition to antiplatelet agents, several other drug classes appear to be effective in the secondary prevention of cardiovascular events among patients with PVD.

A meta-analysis of randomized trials described 698 patients with PVD. In this analysis, lipid-lowering agents were associated with a reduction in mortality [46].

The Heart Protection Study (HPS) demonstrated that statins produce substantial clinical benefit in a wide range of high-risk patients with coronary and vascular disease [47]. In addition, statins have recently been associated with improved walking distance in patients with claudication [48,49].

In the HOPE (Heart Outcomes Prevention Evaluation) study, the angiotensin-converting enzyme (ACE) inhibitor ramipril significantly reduced the rate of cardiovascular death, myocardial infarction, and stroke in patients with PVD [50].

Finally, the use of appropriate secondary preventative measures (eg, antiplatelet therapy, beta-blockers, statins, ACE inhibitors) has been shown to reduce major adverse cardiovascular events among patients undergoing PTA [51].

Conclusion

Antiplatelet therapy is one of the mainstays of successful PTA as well as of secondary prevention. In addition to lifelong aspirin, at least 1 month of clopidogrel is recommended for all patients undergoing stent-based PTA. The issue of whether long-term dual antiplatelet therapy is beneficial in post-PTA patients is currently being addressed in the CAMPER trial. The same strategy for secondary prevention in patients at high risk for cardiovascular events, and, among them, individuals with PVD, is being investigated in the CHARISMA trial.

With respect to periprocedural anticoagulation, UFH remains the most widely used agent. Ongoing studies are focusing on the administration of LMWH or direct thrombin inhibitors in this setting. Based on current knowledge, adjunctive GPIIb/IIIa receptor antagonists should be confined to patients at particularly high risk. From a surgical perspective, antiplatelet therapy enhances long-term patency after peripheral bypass surgery. In this setting, warfarin does not appear to be more beneficial than aspirin and is associated with more bleeding complications. In addition to antiplatelet agents, patients undergoing PTA or vascular surgery should enter a smoking cessation and exercise rehabilitation program, and should be given broad pharmacologic prevention therapy, including beta-blockers, ACE inhibitors, and statins.

References

1. Antiplatelet Trialists' Collaboration. Collaborative overview of randomised trials of antiplatelet therapy – II: Maintenance of vascular graft or arterial patency by antiplatelet therapy. *Br Med J* 1994;308:159–68.
2. Antiplatelet therapy in peripheral arterial disease. Consensus statement. *Eur J Vasc Endovasc Surg* 2003;26:1–16.
3. Bhatt DL, Bertrand ME, Berger PB, et al. Meta-analysis of randomized and registry comparisons of ticlopidine with clopidogrel after stenting. *J Am Coll Cardiol* 2002;39:9–14.
4. Cutlip DE, Baim DS, Ho KK, et al. Stent thrombosis in the modern era: a pooled analysis of multicenter coronary stent clinical trials. *Circulation* 2001;103:1967–71.
5. Bhatt DL, Kapadia SR, Bajzer CT, et al. Dual antiplatelet therapy with clopidogrel and aspirin after carotid artery stenting. *J Invasive Cardiol* 2001;13:767–71.
6. Steinhubl SR, Berger PB, Mann JT 3rd, et al. Early and sustained dual oral antiplatelet therapy following percutaneous coronary intervention: a randomized controlled trial. *JAMA* 2002;288:2411–20.
7. Mukherjee D, Dey S, Lingam P, et al. Predictors of clinical outcome in patients undergoing peripheral vascular interventions: insights from the University of Michigan Peripheral Vascular Disease Quality Improvement Initiative (PVD-QI2). *J Am Coll Cardiol* 2003;41:75A.
8. Kong DF, Hasselblad V, Harrington RA, et al. Meta-analysis of survival with platelet glycoprotein IIb/IIIa antagonists for percutaneous coronary interventions. *Am J Cardiol* 2003;92:651–5.
9. Kapadia SR, Bajzer CT, Ziada KM, et al. Initial experience of platelet glycoprotein IIb/IIIa inhibition with abciximab during carotid stenting: a safe and effective adjunctive therapy. *Stroke* 2001;32:2328–32.
10. Qureshi AI, Suri MF, Ali Z, et al. Carotid angioplasty and stent placement: a prospective analysis of perioperative complications and impact of intravenously administered abciximab. *Neurosurgery* 2002;50:466–73; discussion 473–5.
11. Wholey MH, Eles G, Toursakissian B, et al. Evaluation of glycoprotein IIb/IIIa inhibitors in carotid angioplasty and stenting. *J Endovasc Ther* 2003;10:33–41.
12. Schweizer J, Kirch W, Koch R, et al. Short- and long-term results of abciximab versus aspirin in conjunction with thrombolysis for patients with peripheral occlusive arterial disease and arterial thrombosis. *Angiology* 2000;51:913–23.
13. Duda SH, Tepe G, Luz O, et al. Peripheral artery occlusion: treatment with abciximab plus urokinase versus with urokinase alone – a randomized pilot trial (the PROMPT Study). Platelet Receptor Antibodies in Order to Manage Peripheral Artery Thrombosis. *Radiology* 2001;221:689–96.
14. Stavropoulos SW, Solomon JA, Soulen MC, et al. Use of abciximab during infrainguinal peripheral vascular interventions: initial experience. *Radiology* 2003;227:657–61.

15. Topol EJ, Moliterno DJ, Herrmann HC, et al. Comparison of two platelet glycoprotein IIb/IIIa inhibitors, tirofiban and abciximab, for the prevention of ischemic events with percutaneous coronary revascularization. *N Engl J Med* 2001;344:1888–94.

16. Xiao Z, Theroux P. Platelet activation with unfractionated heparin at therapeutic concentrations and comparisons with a low-molecular-weight heparin and with a direct thrombin inhibitor. *Circulation* 1998;97:251–6.

17. Weitz JI, Hudoba M, Massel D, et al. Clot-bound thrombin is protected from inhibition by heparin-antithrombin III but is susceptible to inactivation by antithrombin III-independent inhibitors. *J Clin Invest* 1990;86:385–91.

18. Shammas NW, Lemke JH, Dippel EJ, et al. In-hospital complications of peripheral vascular interventions using unfractionated heparin as the primary anticoagulant. *J Invasive Cardiol* 2003;15:242–6.

19. Bhatt DL. Heparin in peripheral vascular intervention – time for a change? *J Invasive Cardiol* 2003;15:249–50.

20. Bhatt DL, Lee BI, Casterella PJ, et al. Safety of concomitant therapy with eptifibatide and enoxaparin in patients undergoing percutaneous coronary intervention: results of the Coronary Revascularization Using Integrilin and Single Bolus Enoxaparin Study. *J Am Coll Cardiol* 2003;41:20–5.

21. Wong GC, Giugliano RP, Antman EM. Use of low-molecular-weight heparins in the management of acute coronary artery syndromes and percutaneous coronary intervention. *JAMA* 2003;289:331–42.

22. Lincoff AM, Bittl JA, Harrington RA, et al. Bivalirudin and provisional glycoprotein IIb/IIIa blockade compared with heparin and planned glycoprotein IIb/IIIa blockade during percutaneous coronary intervention: REPLACE-2 randomized trial. *JAMA* 2003;289:853–63.

23. Shammas NW, Lemke JH, Dippel EJ, et al. Bivalirudin in peripheral vascular interventions: a single center experience. *J Invasive Cardiol* 2003;15:401–4.

24. Allie DE, Lirtzman MD, Wyatt CH, et al. Bivalirudin as a foundation anticoagulant in peripheral vascular disease: a safe and feasible alternative for renal and iliac interventions. *J Invasive Cardiol* 2003;15:334–42.

25. Berridge DC, Gregson RH, Hopkinson BR, et al. Randomized trial of intra-arterial recombinant tissue plasminogen activator, intravenous recombinant tissue plasminogen activator and intra-arterial streptokinase in peripheral arterial thrombolysis. *Br J Surg* 1991;78:988–95.

26. Meyerovitz MF, Goldhaber SZ, Reagan K, et al. Recombinant tissue-type plasminogen activator versus urokinase in peripheral arterial and graft occlusions: a randomized trial. *Radiology* 1990;175:75–8.

27. Berridge DC, Makin GS, Hopkinson BR. Local low dose intra-arterial thrombolytic therapy: the risk of stroke or major haemorrhage. *Br J Surg* 1989;76:1230–3.

28. Working Party on Thrombolysis in the Management of Limb Ischemia. Thrombolysis in the management of lower limb peripheral arterial occlusion – a consensus document. *Am J Cardiol* 1998;81:207–18.

29. Results of a prospective randomized trial evaluating surgery versus thrombolysis for ischemia of the lower extremity. The STILE trial. *Ann Surg* 1994;220:251–66; discussion 266–8.

30. Aronow WS, Ahn C. Prevalence of coexistence of coronary artery disease, peripheral arterial disease, and atherothrombotic brain infarction in men and women ≥62 years of age. *Am J Cardiol* 1994;74:64–5.

31. Hiatt WR. Medical treatment of peripheral arterial disease and claudication. *N Engl J Med* 2001;344:1608–21.

32. Antithrombotic Trialists' Collaboration. Collaborative meta-analysis of randomised trials of antiplatelet therapy for prevention of death, myocardial infarction, and stroke in high risk patients. *Br Med J* 2002;324:71–86.

33. Robless P, Mikhailidis DP, Stansby G. Systematic review of antiplatelet therapy for the prevention of myocardial infarction, stroke or vascular death in patients with peripheral vascular disease. *Br J Surg* 2001;88:787–800.

34. CAPRIE Steering Committee. A randomised, blinded, trial of clopidogrel versus aspirin in patients at risk of ischaemic events (CAPRIE). *Lancet* 1996;348:1329–39.

35. Bhatt DL, Topol EJ. Scientific and therapeutic advances in antiplatelet therapy. *Nat Rev Drug Discov* 2003;2:15–28.

36. Becquemin JP. Effect of ticlopidine on the long-term patency of saphenous-vein bypass grafts in the legs. Etude de la Ticlopidine après Pontage Fémoro-Poplité and the Association Universitaire de Recherche en Chirurgie. *N Engl J Med* 1997;337:1726–31.

37. Kretschmer G, Herbst F, Prager M, et al. A decade of oral anticoagulant treatment to maintain autologous vein grafts for femoropopliteal atherosclerosis. *Arch Surg* 1992;127:1112–5.

38. Efficacy of oral anticoagulants compared with aspirin after infrainguinal bypass surgery (The Dutch Bypass Oral Anticoagulants or Aspirin Study): a randomised trial. *Lancet* 2000;355:346–51.

39. Johnson WC, Williford WO, Department of Veterans Affairs Cooperative Study #362. Benefits, morbidity, and mortality associated with long-term administration of oral anticoagulant therapy to patients with peripheral arterial bypass procedures: a prospective randomized study. *J Vasc Surg* 2002;35:413–21.

40. Schnyder G, Roffi M, Pin R, et al. Decreased rate of coronary restenosis after lowering of plasma homocysteine levels. *N Engl J Med* 2001;345:1593–600.

41. Schnyder G, Roffi M, Flammer Y, et al. Effect of homocysteine-lowering therapy with folic acid, vitamin B12, and vitamin B6 on clinical outcome after percutaneous coronary intervention: the Swiss Heart study: a randomized controlled trial. *JAMA* 2002;288:973–9.

42. Duda SH, Pusich B, Richter G, et al. Sirolimus-eluting stents for the treatment of obstructive superficial femoral artery disease: six-month results. *Circulation* 2002;106:1505–9.
43. Jackson MR, Clagett GP. Antithrombotic therapy in peripheral arterial occlusive disease. *Chest* 2001;119 (1 Suppl.): 283S–299S.
44. Hood SC, Moher D, Barber GG. Management of intermittent claudication with pentoxifylline: meta-analysis of randomized controlled trials. *CMAJ* 1996;155:1053–9.
45. Thompson PD, Zimet R, Forbes WP, et al. Meta-analysis of results from eight randomized, placebo-controlled trials on the effect of cilostazol on patients with intermittent claudication. *Am J Cardiol* 2002;90:1314–9.
46. Leng GC, Price JF, Jepson RG. Lipid-lowering for lower limb atherosclerosis. Cochrane Database Syst Rev 2000;CD000123.
47. Heart Protection Study Collaborative Group. MRC/BHF Heart Protection Study of cholesterol lowering with simvastatin in 20,536 high-risk individuals: a randomised placebo-controlled trial. *Lancet* 2002;360:7–22.
48. McDermott MM, Guralnik JM, Greenland P, et al. Statin use and leg functioning in patients with and without lower extremity peripheral arterial disease. *Circulation* 2003;107:757–61.
49. Mohler ER 3rd, Hiatt WR, Creager MA. Cholesterol reduction with atorvastatin improves walking distance in patients with peripheral arterial disease. *Circulation* 2003;108:1481–6.
50. Yusuf S, Sleight P, Pogue J, et al. Effects of an angiotensin-converting-enzyme inhibitor, ramipril, on cardiovascular events in high-risk patients. The Heart Outcomes Prevention Evaluation Study Investigators. *N Engl J Med* 2000;342:145–53.
51. Mukherjee D, Lingam P, Chetcuti S, et al. Missed opportunities to treat atherosclerosis in patients undergoing peripheral vascular interventions: insights from the University of Michigan Peripheral Vascular Disease Quality Improvement Initiative (PVD-QI2). *Circulation* 2002;106:1909–12.

5 Iliac and femoral artery intervention

Jacqueline Saw and Deepak L Bhatt

Introduction

Peripheral vascular disease (PVD) is prevalent in the western world, afflicting a staggering 8–12 million Americans and contributing to significant morbidity and mortality [1]. The prevalence of lower extremity arterial disease is ~17% for those between the ages of 55 and 74 years [2], with millions in America and Europe developing ischemic symptoms each year [3].

Atherosclerosis is the most common and important cause of lower extremity chronic arterial occlusive disease, although there are other infrequent causes (see **Table 1**). Patients typically present with intermittent claudication and subsequent slow deterioration over time to rest pain. Up to 20% of cases ultimately progress to critical leg ischemia (where limb viability is endangered) (see **Table 2** for symptom classifications) [4]. The atherosclerotic risk factors for the lower extremities are identical to those for other vascular beds, and include smoking, diabetes mellitus, hyperlipidemia, and hypertension.

Historically, the gold standard of therapy for severely symptomatic lower extremity PVD has been reconstructive vascular surgery. However, apart from the disadvantages of a long hospital stay and recovery time, the associated procedural morbidity (ie, myocardial infarction, wound infection) and mortality are not inconsequential with vascular surgery. Thus, percutaneous

Chronic causes
Atherosclerosis
Vasculitis (Buerger's disease, collagen vascular diseases, Takayasu's disease)
Radiation injury
Raynaud's disease or phenomenon
Trauma
Popliteal artery entrapment syndrome
Popliteal artery aneurysm (secondary thromboembolism)
Fibromuscular dysplasia
Iliac syndrome of the cyclist
Primary vascular tumors
Acute causes
Embolism (cardiac, paradoxical, proximal plaque, aneurysm)
Iatrogenic (catheterization, surgery)
Thrombosis (hypercoagulable states, graft thrombosis, plaque rupture)
Trauma
Dissection
Vasculitis
Extrinsic compression (eg, popliteal cysts)

Table 1. Causes of lower extremity arterial occlusive disease.

endovascular intervention (PEI) is an attractive alternative, offering a lower-risk, less invasive, and comparably effective option in selected patients when combined exercise and pharmacologic therapies have failed. Since the first PEI of femoropopliteal arterial PVD was performed by Dotter and Judkins in 1964 [5], percutaneous techniques and equipment have rapidly evolved, enabling the widespread application of percutaneous transluminal angioplasty (PTA) and stenting in numerous vascular beds.

Currently accepted indications for revascularization of the lower extremities include [6]:

• incapacitating claudication that interferes with work or lifestyle

• critical limb ischemia (rest pain, nonhealing ulcer, or gangrene)

• significant peripheral arterial disease in diabetics (high likelihood of progression to amputation)

• vasculogenic erectile dysfunction

The TransAtlantic Inter-Society Consensus (TASC) Working Group has developed a consensus document for the management of lower extremity PVD, aiming to optimize and maintain international standards [7]. Iliac and femoropopliteal lesions are each classified into four types: type A lesions are the most eligible for endovascular treatment (PEI), while type D lesions are most suitable for surgery (see **Tables 3** and **4**, **Figures 1** and **2**). There are inadequate data for firm treatment recommendations for type B and C lesions, although PEI is more commonly used. Even certain type D lesions are being approached percutaneously. In general, PEI of the iliac artery is associated with better procedural success and long-term patency than that of the femoral artery.

Fontaine classification of PAD		
Stage I	Asymptomatic	
Stage IIa	Mild claudication (>200 m)	
Stage IIb	Moderate to severe claudication (≤200 m)	
Stage III	Ischemic rest pain	
Stage IV	Tissue loss or ulceration	
Rutherford classification of PAD		
Grade 0	Category 0	Asymptomatic
Grade 1	Category 1	Mild claudication
Grade 1	Category 2	Moderate claudication
Grade 1	Category 3	Severe claudication
Grade 2	Category 4	Ischemic rest pain
Grade 3	Category 5	Mild tissue ulceration
Grade 3	Category 6	Tissue loss/gangrene

Table 2. Symptomatic classification of peripheral arterial disease. Adapted with permission from Elsevier (Management of peripheral arterial disease [PAD]. TransAtlantic Inter-Society Consensus [TASC]. *Eur J Vasc Endovasc Surg* 2000;19 [Suppl. A]:Si–xxviii, S1–250).

Lesion type	Description	Recommendation
Type A	Single stenosis <3 cm of CIA or EIA	PEI
Type B	Single stenosis 3–10 cm, not extending into CFA	PEI or surgery
	Total of two stenoses <5 cm in CIA and/or EIA, not extending into CFA	
	Unilateral CIA occlusion	
Type C	Bilateral stenosis 5–10 cm of CIA and/or EIA, not extending into CFA	PEI or surgery
	Unilateral EIA occlusion, not extending into CFA	
	Unilateral EIA stenosis extending into CFA	
	Bilateral CIA occlusion	
Type D	Diffuse, multiple unilateral stenoses involving CIA, EIA, and CFA (usually >10 cm)	Surgery
	Unilateral occlusion involving both CIA and EIA	
	Bilateral EIA occlusions	
	Diffuse disease in aorta and both iliac arteries	
	Iliac stenosis in patients with abdominal aortic aneurysm or lesion requiring aortic or iliac surgery	

Table 3. TransAtlantic Inter-Society Consensus morphologic classification of iliac artery lesions. CFA: common femoral artery; CIA: common iliac artery; EIA: external iliac artery; PEI: percutaneous endovascular intervention. Adapted with permission from Elsevier (Management of peripheral arterial disease [PAD]. TransAtlantic Inter-Society Consensus [TASC]. *Eur J Vasc Endovasc Surg* 2000;19[Suppl. A]:Si–xxviii, S1–250).

Lesion type	Description	Recommendation
Type A	Single stenosis <3 cm	PEI
Type B	Single stenosis 3–10 cm, not involving distal popliteal	PEI or surgery
	Heavily calcified stenoses up to 3 cm	
	Multiple lesions, each <3 cm (stenosis/occlusion)	
	Single or multiple lesions in the absence of continuous tibial run-off to improve inflow for distal surgical bypass	
Type C	Single stenosis or occlusion >5 cm	PEI or surgery
	Multiple stenoses or occlusions, each 3–5 cm, with or without heavy calcification	
Type D	Complete CFA or SFA occlusion, or complete popliteal and proximal trifurcation occlusions	Surgery

Table 4. TransAtlantic Inter-Society Consensus morphologic classification of femoropopliteal lesions. CFA: common femoral artery; PEI: percutaneous endovascular intervention; SFA: superficial femoral artery. Adapted with permission from Elsevier (Management of peripheral arterial disease [PAD]. TransAtlantic Inter-Society Consensus [TASC]. *Eur J Vasc Endovasc Surg* 2000;19[Suppl. A]:Si–xxviii, S1–250).

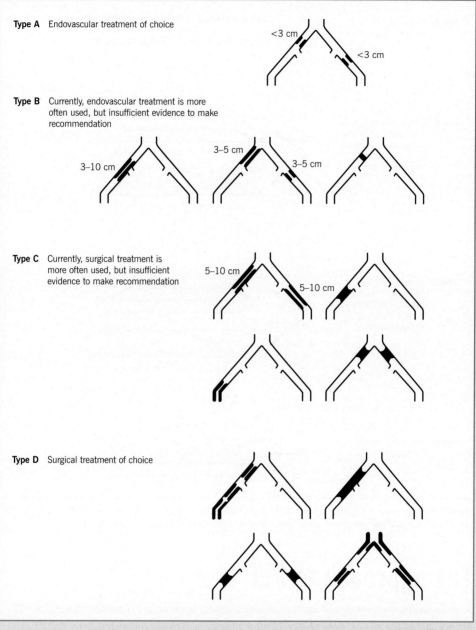

Figure 1. TransAtlantic Inter-Society Consensus classification of iliac lesions. Reproduced with permission from Elsevier (Management of peripheral arterial disease [PAD]. TransAtlantic Inter-Society Consensus [TASC]. *Eur J Vasc Endovasc Surg* 2000;19[Suppl. A]:Si–xxviii, S1–250).

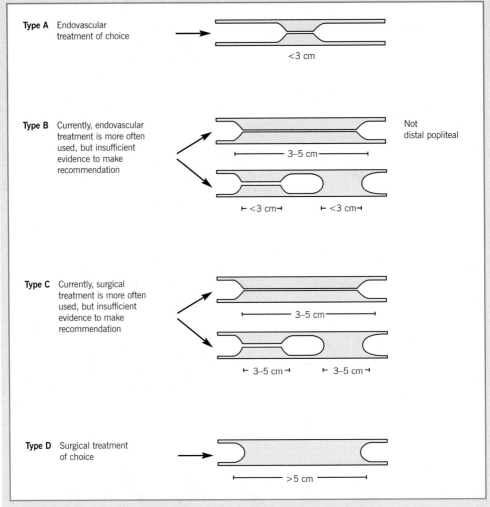

Type A Endovascular treatment of choice

<3 cm

Type B Currently, endovascular treatment is more often used, but insufficient evidence to make recommendation

Not distal popliteal

3–5 cm

<3 cm   <3 cm

Type C Currently, surgical treatment is more often used, but insufficient evidence to make recommendation

3–5 cm

3–5 cm   3–5 cm

Type D Surgical treatment of choice

>5 cm

Figure 2. TransAtlantic Inter-Society Consensus classification of femoropopliteal lesions. Reproduced with permission from Elsevier (Management of peripheral arterial disease [PAD]. TransAtlantic Inter-Society Consensus [TASC]. *Eur J Vasc Endovasc Surg* 2000;19[Suppl. A]:Si–xxviii, S1–250).

The approach to PEI

A comprehensive knowledge of lower extremity anatomy is necessary before embarking on PEI. Assessment of the clinical presentation of intermittent claudication and noninvasive testing of the severity of arterial disease are important to help decide upon the optimal treatment strategy. Full angiography to visualize the inflow, outflow, and run-off beds of the arterial tree is essential to provide anatomical details of disease and the presence of collateral circulation. Documentation of the arterial outflow is necessary, since clinical success and long-term patency are dependent on adequate outflow. Furthermore, full evaluation of the arterial tree is obligatory to identify whether multilevel revascularization is required, allowing preparation and strategizing of subsequent interventions.

Lower extremity anatomy

The abdominal aorta divides into the common iliac arteries at the L4–L5 level, which then divide near the lumbosacral junction into the internal and external iliac arteries (see **Figure 3**). The internal iliac artery is ~4 cm long and gives rise to an anterior trunk (branching off to the obturator, internal pudendal, inferior gluteal, and visceral arteries) and a posterior trunk (branching off to the iliolumbar, lateral sacral, and superior gluteal arteries). The external iliac artery (which is larger than the internal iliac artery) is the natural continuation of the common iliac artery, coursing directly to the groin behind the inguinal ligament, whereupon it becomes the common femoral artery (CFA). Just before or at the inguinal ligament, the distal external iliac artery gives rise medially to the inferior epigastric artery (which runs superiorly and communicates with the superior epigastric branch of the internal mammary artery) and laterally to the deep circumflex iliac artery (which ascends superiorly and anastomoses with the iliolumbar, superior gluteal, and ascending branch of the lateral circumflex femoral arteries). The CFA travels over the femoral head in the femoral sheath (the femoral vein runs medially while the femoral nerve runs laterally), branching off to the superficial epigastric, superficial circumflex iliac, and external pudendal arteries, before dividing into the superficial femoral arteries (SFA) and deep femoral arteries (DFA) near the bottom of the femoral head.

The DFA is the largest branch of the CFA, arising laterally and posteriorly, and giving rise to the lateral and medial circumflex femoral and perforating arteries (usually 3–4 pairs). The SFA travels along the anteromedial thigh, diving into the flexor muscle compartment, and ends when it passes through the adductor magnus (Hunter's) canal, where it becomes the popliteal artery. The popliteal artery runs deep to the popliteal vein behind the femur across the knee (see **Figure 4**), and continues as the tibioperoneal trunk after giving rise to the anterior tibial artery laterally. The anterior tibial artery pierces the interosseous membrane to run in front of the tibia towards the dorsum of the foot and become the dorsalis pedis artery. The tibioperoneal trunk branches into the posterior tibial artery (which travels posteromedially in the flexor compartment to the back of the medial malleolus) and peroneal artery (which runs between the anterior and posterior tibial arteries). Branches of the posterior tibial and dorsalis pedis arteries form the plantar arch, which then gives off the metatarsal arteries.

The presence of rare anatomical anomalies and collateral pathways may alter treatment decisions and these need to be recognized by the endovascular interventionalist. A persistent sciatic artery (~1/1000) may arise from the internal iliac artery, running through the greater sciatic foramen and joining the popliteal artery. It is associated with a hypoplastic or absent SFA. Benign variants of the tibial branches are common (~10%), such as high bifurcation of the popliteal artery (anterior tibial artery arising high) or actual trifurcation (common origin of the peroneal, anterior, and posterior tibial arteries). In the setting of aortoiliac femoral arterial occlusive disease, a complex collateral circulation can develop to supply distal vessels, primarily through branches of the lumbar, internal iliac, DFA, and popliteal arteries (see **Figure 5**).

Noninvasive imaging of lower extremity PVD

Clinical evaluation of PVD includes a comprehensive history and physical examination, concentrating on peripheral arterial pulses, presence of bruits, and skin ulcerations or gangrene.

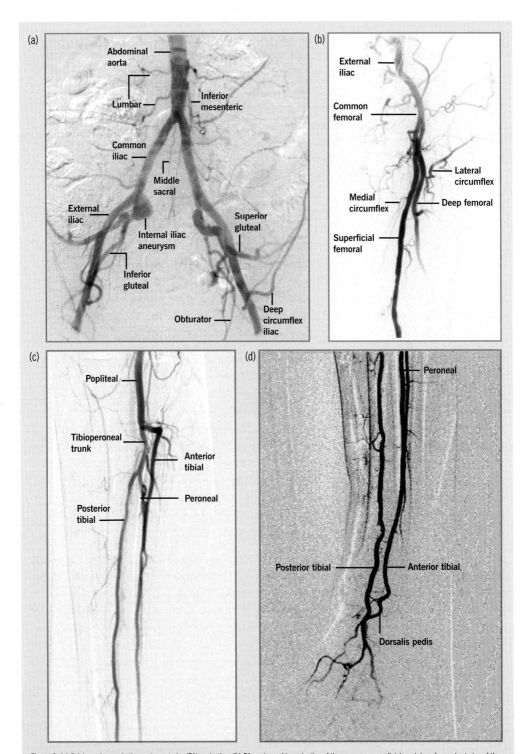

Figure 3. (**a**) Pelvic angiogram in the posteroanterior (PA) projection. (**b**) PA angiographic projection of the common, superficial, and deep femoral arteries of the left lower extremity. (**c**) PA angiographic projection of the popliteal and infrapopliteal arteries of the left lower extremity. (**d**) Infrapopliteal angiogram of the left lower extremity.

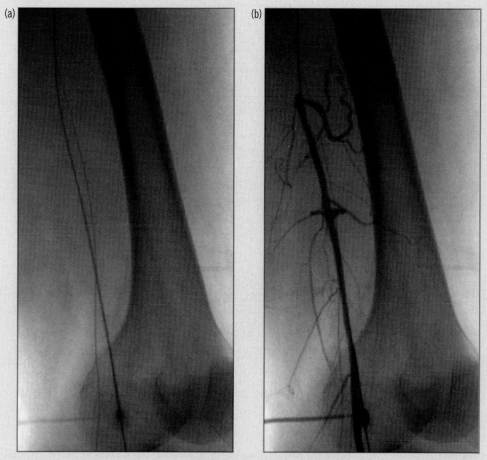

Figure 4. PA projection of the left knee, showing a retrograde arterial sheath and guidewire in the left popliteal artery, and a separate guidewire in the popliteal vein. The popliteal artery runs deep to the popliteal vein behind the femur across the knee. (**a**) Without contrast. (**b**) With contrast in the left popliteal artery.

ABI classification	Severity of PVD
≥0.9	Normal
0.70–0.89	Mild
0.50–0.69	Moderate
<0.5	Severe

Table 5. Classification of the ankle–brachial index (ABI). PVD: peripheral vascular disease.

Noninvasive imaging provides a more objective and quantifiable degree of peripheral arterial stenoses. The ankle–brachial index (ABI) is a simple, inexpensive measurement obtained using a blood pressure cuff and a Doppler probe. It is defined as the ratio of ankle systolic blood pressure (posterior tibial or dorsalis pedis artery) to the brachial systolic pressure (measuring both arms and using the higher level as the denominator) (see **Table 5**). If the resting level is normal then

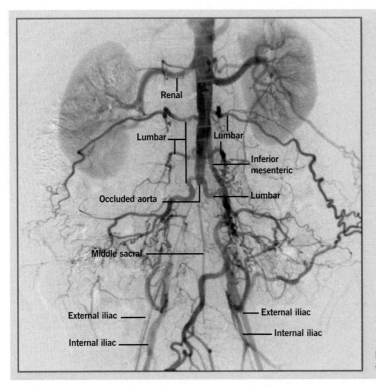

Figure 5. Collateral circulation with distal aortic occlusion.

the ABI should also be assessed after exercise, since the increase in blood flow heightens the pressure drop across a fixed stenosis. An ABI <0.9 was associated with 2.4-fold higher mortality in a Swedish study [8].

Segmental systolic pressures should also be obtained by placing the blood pressure cuff at different levels (upper and lower thigh, calf) to help determine the disease level (significant if the pressure drop is >15 mm Hg). Another useful test that is often performed to complement segmental pressures is the pulse volume recording (PVR), which utilizes air plethysmography to measure pulsatile arterial waveforms. Alternatively, Doppler velocity waveform analysis can be performed.

Abdominal, pelvic, and lower extremity arteriography

The retrograde femoral arterial route is most commonly used for a diagnostic abdominal and pelvic angiography, although a brachial approach can also be used. Either a 5- or 6-Fr pigtail catheter is placed at the level of T12, and the cineangiogram is taken in the posteroanterior (PA) projection visualizing the abdominal aorta (including the renal arteries), aortic bifurcation, and both iliac vessels. The contrast agent (nonionic iso-osmolar iodixanol, Visipaque [Amersham Health, Princeton, NJ, USA], is preferred to minimize pain in the lower extremities) is pressure injected at a rate of 10–15 cc/s for 20–30 cc. Oblique views of the pelvis should also be performed in patients with significant iliac and femoral disease (moving the pigtail catheter to the lower abdominal aorta L3–L4), positioning to include the aortic bifurcation and the femoral heads.

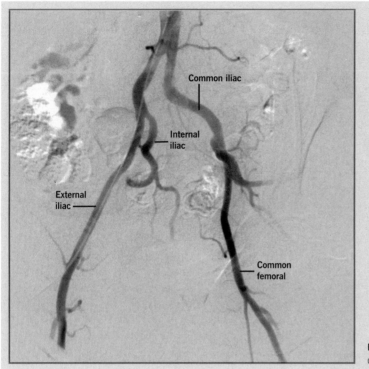

Figure 6. Pelvic left anterior oblique projection.

A 15°–30° left anterior oblique (LAO) projection enhances visualization of the right iliac and left femoral bifurcations (see **Figure 6**). A 15°–30° right anterior oblique (RAO) projection, in contrast, preferentially visualizes the left iliac and right femoral bifurcations (see **Figure 7**). These oblique views can be taken with a lower contrast volume (7 cc/s for 14 cc). Bilateral lower extremity run-offs can then be performed in the PA projection (with the pigtail catheter positioned near the aortic bifurcation) using the interactive digital subtraction bolus-chase method, or, if unavailable, serial descending digital subtraction filming to both feet (see **Figures 3b–d**). Alternatively, selective cineangiography run-offs can be performed separately in each leg using a catheter with side-holes (eg, multipurpose catheter) placed at the level of the external iliac artery or CFA.

Vascular access for lower extremity PEI

An important first step in performing PEI involves choosing and gaining arterial access. This depends on the lesion location, the presence of an arterial pulse at the preferred site, and the length of the equipment available (long wires, catheters, balloons, and stents). The recommended access routes are described in **Table 6**. In general, the ipsilateral retrograde femoral approach is ideal for common iliac and proximal to mid external iliac lesions. The contralateral retrograde femoral approach is preferred for lesions in the contralateral internal iliac, distal external iliac, CFA, DFA, SFA, and even popliteal arteries. Long occlusive SFA disease can be approached from both the ipsilateral antegrade femoral and retrograde popliteal routes (see **Figures 8** and **9**), which allow coaxial manipulation of wires and balloons. The ipsilateral antegrade femoral approach can also be used for DFA, popliteal, and infrapopliteal lesions.

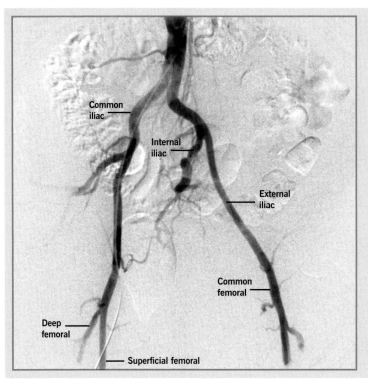

Figure 7. Pelvic right anterior oblique projection.

Lesion location	Preferred access site	Alternative access sites
Aortic bifurcation	Bilateral retrograde CFA	Bilateral brachial
Common iliac artery	Ipsilateral retrograde CFA	Brachial
Proximal and mid external iliac artery	Ipsilateral retrograde CFA	Contralateral retrograde CFA or brachial
Distal external iliac artery	Contralateral retrograde CFA	Brachial
CFA	Contralateral retrograde CFA	Brachial or popliteal
Proximal SFA	Contralateral retrograde CFA	Brachial or popliteal
Mid or distal SFA	Contralateral retrograde CFA	Ipsilateral antegrade CFA, brachial, or popliteal
Deep femoral artery	Contralateral retrograde CFA	Brachial
Popliteal artery	Contralateral retrograde CFA	Ipsilateral antegrade CFA or brachial

Table 6. Recommended arterial access sites, depending on lesion location. CFA: common femoral artery; SFA: superficial femoral artery.

Selection of the appropriate arterial sheath is also important to facilitate successful PEI with respect to providing adequate support and the correct luminal diameter for PTA/stent catheters. A 5- to 6-Fr sheath will accommodate a 0.035-inch wire and most balloon catheters. However, a 6- to 7-Fr sheath is often necessary for adequate contrast visualization when delivering a stent. Short sheaths can be used for the ipsilateral femoral, brachial, or popliteal approaches.

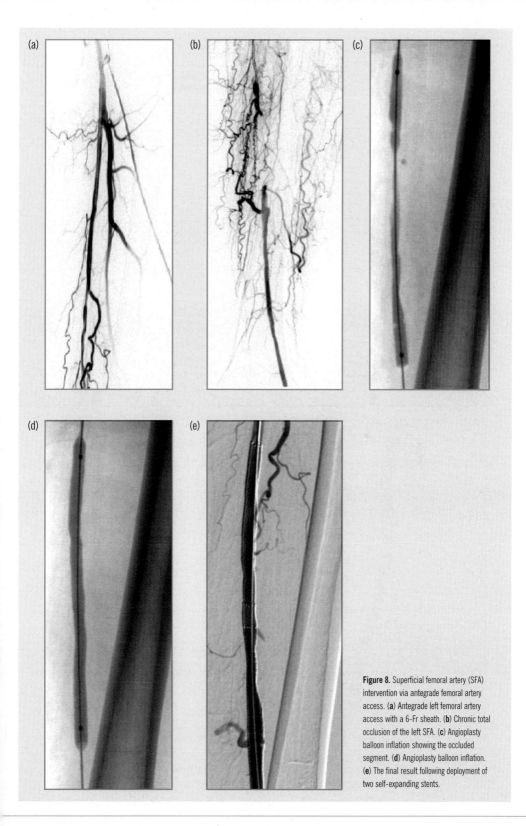

Figure 8. Superficial femoral artery (SFA) intervention via antegrade femoral artery access. (**a**) Antegrade left femoral artery access with a 6-Fr sheath. (**b**) Chronic total occlusion of the left SFA. (**c**) Angioplasty balloon inflation showing the occluded segment. (**d**) Angioplasty balloon inflation. (**e**) The final result following deployment of two self-expanding stents.

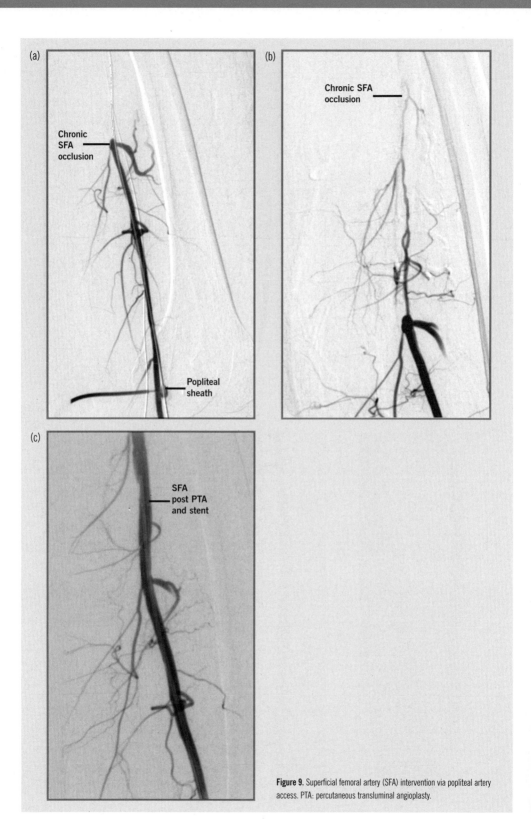

Figure 9. Superficial femoral artery (SFA) intervention via popliteal artery access. PTA: percutaneous transluminal angioplasty.

The contralateral retrograde femoral approach often requires a longer sheath to cross the aortic bifurcation (eg, Balkan [Cook, Bloomington, IN, USA] or Arrow [Arrow International, Reading, PA, USA] sheath), especially for occlusive disease that requires back-up support, or for PEI of more distal SFA or popliteal lesions. This is achieved by advancing a 0.035-inch guidewire to the aortic bifurcation, followed by using an angled catheter (eg, internal mammary artery, crossover, Cobra [Cardean, Cupertino, CA, USA], SOS [Angiodynamics, Queensbury, NY, USA], or Simmons Sidewinder catheter) to direct the wire down the contralateral iliac artery. The catheter is then advanced to about the CFA level, and a stiffer guidewire (eg, Stiff Amplatz wire) usually needs to be exchanged prior to advancing a Balkan sheath to the contralateral iliac artery.

Guidewire selection for PEI

Guidewires are selected based on the arterial diameter, the presence of occlusive disease or stenosis, and the PTA/stent equipment needed. Generally, PEI of iliac or femoral lesions requires the use of 0.035-inch guidewires (eg, Wholey wire [Mallinckrodt, Hazelwood, MO, USA], Magic Torque wire [Boston Scientific, Natick, MA, USA], Terumo Glidewire [Terumo Medical, Somerset, NJ, USA]) to cross the lesion. Hydrophilic wires (eg, stiff Terumo Glidewire) are preferred for occluded lesions, often with a catheter (eg, 5-Fr hydrophilic Terumo Glide catheter) or over-the-wire balloon support. At times, coronary 0.014- or 0.018-inch guidewires are needed for particularly challenging occlusions or for smaller diameter vessels.

PTA balloon and stent selection for PEI

Balloon selection depends on guidewire compatibility (either 0.014-, 0.018-, or 0.035-inch), the reference diameter of the vessel, lesion length, and the catheter length required to reach the stenosis. Numerous angioplasty balloons are commercially available (see **Table 7**) in various diameters and lengths. The balloon diameter should reflect the vessel reference diameter; the recommended balloon diameters for various arterial segments are listed in **Table 8**. Stent selection is dependent on similar factors as for balloon angioplasty and, in addition, the lesion location, which influences the preference for self-expanding or balloon-expandable stents (see **Table 9**). Self-expanding stents are more flexible, noncrushable, and can be placed across joints [9]; however, they shorten slightly with deployment and do not have as much radial strength as balloon-expandable stents. In general, with the use of nitinol self-expanding stents, the stent diameter chosen should be ~1 mm larger than the reference balloon diameter used for the lesion segment.

Currently, there are only a few US Food and Drug Administration (FDA)-approved iliac stents in the United States: Palmaz (P308 and P3008; Cordis, Miami Lakes, FL, USA), SMART and SMART Control nitinol stents (Cordis), and Iliac Wallstent (Boston Scientific). However, there are numerous FDA-approved biliary stents currently being used for iliac or femoral artery PEI (see **Table 10**).

Technical approach to iliac and femoral artery PEI

The fundamental technical skills required for percutaneous interventions of the iliac and femoral arteries are similar to other arterial interventions. Most experienced interventionalists already possess these skills, and only need familiarity with the peripheral vascular equipment. After successfully placing the arterial sheath in the desired location (see **Vascular access for lower**

Company	Balloon
Cordis, Miami Lakes, FL, USA	Powerflex P3
	Slalom
	Opta Pro
Bard, Murray Hill, NJ, USA	Conquest
	Opti-Plast
	Centurion
Boston Scientific, Natick, MA, USA	Talon
Guidant, Indianapolis, IN, USA	Viatrac
	Agiltrac
	Blue Max

Table 7. Examples of commercially available peripheral vascular angioplasty balloons.

Lesion location	Balloon diameter (mm)
Common iliac artery	8–10
External iliac artery	6–8
Common femoral artery	5–6
Superficial femoral artery	4–6
Popliteal artery	4–5
Tibial or peroneal artery	<4

Table 8. Recommended angioplasty balloon diameters at various lesion locations.

Lesion location	Stent preference
Aorto-ostial lesions	Balloon-expandable
Common iliac bifurcation	Balloon-expandable
Common iliac across internal iliac	Self-expandable
External iliac artery	Self-expandable
Common femoral artery	Self-expandable
Superficial femoral artery	Self-expandable

Table 9. Preference of balloon-expandable or self-expandable stent based on lesion location.

extremity PEI section), the next challenge is crossing the occlusive/stenotic lesion with the appropriate guidewire (see **Guidewire selection for PEI** section). This is particularly demanding for long chronic total occlusions, with attendant risks of dissection, perforation, distal embolization, and loss of collateral circulation. Thus, proper diagnostic angiographic views should initially be taken to identify the paths of the collateral circulation, the location of distal vessel reconstitution, and the presence of a "stump", which will all help to map the correct path of the occluded vessel. A 0.035-inch hydrophilic wire should first be used for a severely stenotic or occluded lesion; otherwise, a Wholey wire is acceptable. For additional support, a 5-Fr Glide catheter

Company	Stents
Self-expandable	
Bard, Murray Hill, NJ, USA	Memotherm, Luminexx, Conformexx
Boston Scientific, Natick, MA, USA	Symphony, Wallstent, WallGraft
Cordis, Miami Lakes, FL, USA	SMART Control, Precise
Gore, Flagstaff, AZ, USA	Viabahn
Guidant, Indianapolis, IN, USA	Dynalink, Acculink
IntraTherapeutics, New Brighton, PA, USA	IntraCoil, Protégé
Medtronic, Minneapolis, MN, USA	Aurora Biliary
Balloon-expandable	
Cordis	Palmaz, Corinthian Genesis
Boston Scientific	NIR, NIROYAL, Express Biliary
Guidant	MegaLink, OmniLink, Herculink
IntraTherapeutics	DoubleStrut, IntraStent
Medtronic	Flexible Biliary, Extra Support Biliary Plus, Bridge X3 Biliary

Table 10. Stents available for iliac and femoral artery intervention.

can be used with the wire; if a straight-tipped guidewire is used, the Glide catheter tip should be angled and *vice versa*. If these strategies are not adequate for crossing the chronic occlusion, a 0.014-inch, 300-cm stiff coronary guidewire (eg, Shinobi [Cordis], Pilot [Guidant, Indianapolis, IN, USA], or Confianza [Asahi] wires) can be tried, with the support of an over-the-wire coronary angioplasty balloon. It is important to maintain an intraluminal path with the help of oblique views and "road-map" angiographic views. Although subintimal wire passage is often unavoidable, entry back into the true lumen is crucial before commencing balloon angioplasty.

The choice of balloon diameter and length depends on the lesion location and length (see **PTA balloon and stent selection for PEI** section). It is important to start with a smaller balloon diameter and lower inflation pressure to reduce the risk of perforation and dissection. The decision of whether to stent depends on the lesion location and the results of balloon angioplasty. Most interventionalists do not recommend routine stenting of femoropopliteal lesions unless the angioplasty results are suboptimal (presence of significant residual stenosis [>30%], residual pressure gradient [>5 mm Hg], or flow-limiting dissection flap), since stenting has not been shown to be superior to PTA alone in this location. However, stenting of iliac artery lesions is associated with better long-term patency and lower restenosis, and is thus generally indicated for iliac intervention (see **Results of iliac and femoral artery interventions** section, below).

PEI of the aortic bifurcation into both common iliac arteries needs to be addressed separately, since the aortic bifurcation needs to be reconstructed (elevated) using the "kissing" balloon and stenting technique. Access via both CFA retrogradely with short 7-Fr sheaths is necessary to enable crossing both common iliac arteries with the guidewires, followed by "kissing" balloon inflations simultaneously, and the deployment of balloon-expandable stents in a "kissing" fashion

(a)

(b)

(c)

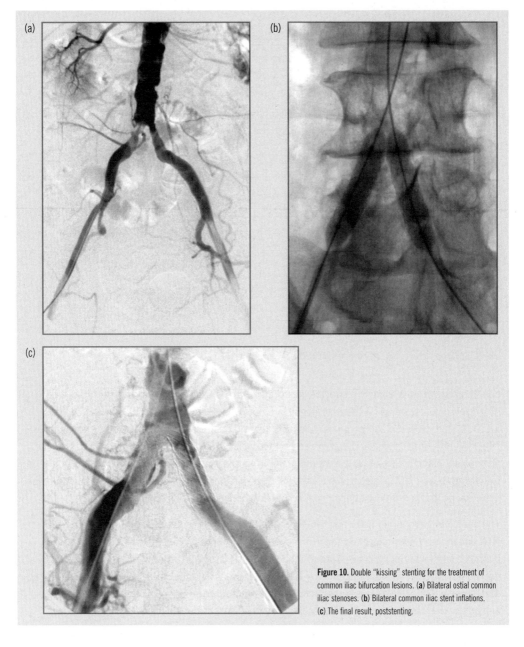

Figure 10. Double "kissing" stenting for the treatment of common iliac bifurcation lesions. (a) Bilateral ostial common iliac stenoses. (b) Bilateral common iliac stent inflations. (c) The final result, poststenting.

(see **Figure 10**). After stent deployment, it may be necessary to inflate with larger balloons to ensure adequate expansion of the aortic portion of the stents.

Novel devices for crossing chronic total occlusions are available and may be useful in particularly long and challenging lesions. The Safe-Cross guidewire and support catheter (IntraLuminal, Carlsbad, CA, USA) uses adjunctive radiofrequency microablation for intraluminal crossing of total occlusions. The Frontrunner CTO Catheter device (LuMend, Redwood City, CA, USA) utilizes the controlled blunt dissection technique to cross total occlusions. The SilverHawk System

(FoxHollow Technologies, Redwood City, CA, USA) uses a carbide blade for plaque atherectomy of total occlusions. In contrast, the CrossPoint TransAccess Catheter (TransVascular, Menlo Park, CA, USA) utilizes intravascular ultrasound to identify the true lumen and a 24-gauge needle to access it, using a 0.014-inch guidewire that has been entrapped in the subintimal passage.

Percutaneous aortic interventions

Percutaneous interventions of the aorta for both occlusive and aneurysmal disorders have also been successfully performed. Endovascular aneurysm repair by the placement of an aortic stent graft was first described by Parodi et al. in 1991 [10]. Since the approval of commercial aortic stents by the FDA in 2000, thousands of stent grafts have been placed for thoracic descending and abdominal aortic aneurysms. The aim of such stent grafts is to exclude the aneurysm, thus preventing transmission of systemic blood pressure to the aneurysm wall, which may curb expansion and rupture. However, these procedures are primarily performed by surgeons, since the current devices are bulky and require introduction via a large arterial lumen (>20 Fr) through surgical cut-down.

In contrast, percutaneous treatment of aortic stenosis lies more within the domain of endovascular interventionalists, since balloon and stent deployment can be achieved via an 8- to 10-Fr femoral arterial sheath. Either balloon-expandable (eg, Palmaz) or self-expanding stents (eg, Wallstent) can be deployed for aortic stenoses, following predilatation with large peripheral balloons (diameter 8–12 mm) [11]. However, there is no clear consensus with respect to the optimal interventional strategy – ie, primary stenting, provisional stenting, or angioplasty alone – for the treatment of aortic occlusive disease [11,12].

Complications of lower extremity PEI

In a review by Becker et al., the incidence of major complications (prolonged hospitalization, permanent adverse sequelae, or death) in 4,662 PTA procedures was 5.6%; 2.5% required surgery, 0.2% suffered limb loss, and 0.2% died [13]. Similarly, Matsi et al. found a 5% major complication rate among 410 lower extremity PTA procedures, with 2% requiring surgery [14]. Such complications include access-site injury (eg, hematoma, false aneurysm, bleeding) and those related to the angioplasty site (eg, distal embolization, dissection, acute thrombosis, perforation, rupture, occlusion).

Subacute arterial thrombosis can occur hours to days after the procedure, but the incidence has declined with the use of dual antiplatelet therapy (aspirin and a thienopyridine). Late thrombosis with the use of stenting and adjunctive brachytherapy can be prevented with prolonged dual antiplatelet therapy (>12 months). External stent compression or deformation is no longer a concern since the introduction of self-expanding stents; however, both balloon-expandable and self-expanding stents can fracture when placed across flexion joints [15,16]. Arterial perforation and rupture (typically from over-dilatation, and most commonly involving a heavily calcified iliac artery) is uncommon, but can rapidly lead to hemorrhagic death or compartment syndrome. Immediate balloon tamponade is crucial, simultaneously with reversal of anticoagulation. Prompt surgical repair is often necessary unless the tear is minor or unless it can be treated with a covered stent (eg, Wallgraft [Boston Scientfic], Viabahn [Gore, Flagstaff, AZ, USA], Hemobahn [Gore]).

Results of iliac and femoral artery interventions

PEI of the iliac artery is feasible, with a procedural success rate of >95% for PTA/stent and a 2- to 4-year patency rate of 82%–89% [17–21]. Two randomized studies have compared PTA with stenting (using the Palmaz balloon-expandable stent). Richter et al. showed superior results with stenting in 185 patients: the 4-year patency rate was 94% with stenting versus 69% with PTA [22]. In contrast, the Dutch Iliac Stent Trial, which enrolled 279 patients, showed no difference between PTA with provisional stenting (57% did not require stenting) versus routine stenting with respect to the initial hemodynamic success (improvement in ABI by >0.1), cumulative patency rates (71% vs 70%), or 2-year clinical success (78% vs 77%) [23]. However, a meta-analysis by Bosch et al. showed that iliac stenting has superior technical success and long-term patency compared with PTA for occlusive arterial disease [24]. Overall, most interventionalists would favor stenting for the majority of iliac artery stenoses.

Unlike in the iliac artery, the long-term patency of more distal endovascular stenting is less optimal. A retrospective case series showed an increasing 6-month restenosis rate with more caudal vessels: 0.5% for iliac, 11% for SFA, and 20% for popliteal lesions. The 4-year primary patency rates were 86%, 65%, and 50%, respectively [25]. The procedural success rate of femoropopliteal PTA is >90% [26,27], but the long-term patency at 3–5 years is only around 50%–70% [27–31]. Earlier small randomized trials (each <60 patients) that compared the use of stents versus PTA alone showed no added benefit with stenting in terms of 1-year patency [32–34]. A more recent trial by Cejna et al. randomized 141 patients to PTA alone versus Palmaz stents for femoropopliteal occlusions. The initial technical success was superior with stenting (99% vs 84%, $P=0.009$), but again there was no difference in primary or secondary patency rates at 1 or 2 years [35]. Thus, the current recommended approach for femoropopliteal PEI is PTA alone, with provisional stenting when PTA results are suboptimal (residual diameter stenosis >30%, residual pressure gradient >5 mm Hg, or a flow-limiting dissection) or when restenosis occurs after PTA.

The high restenosis rates associated with conventional PTA and stenting of femoropopliteal vessels prompted the development of adjunctive and novel devices to curb restenosis. Gamma brachytherapy has been successfully used for both *de novo* and restenotic lesions. Small pilot and randomized trials have demonstrated superiority over angioplasty alone (see **Table 11**) [36–40]. Data from the ongoing Phase III VIENNA-3, VIENNA-5, and PARIS trials will further elucidate the role of brachytherapy in the treatment of femoropopliteal lesions.

The use of a drug-eluting stent was studied in a small feasibility trial (SIROCCO), which randomized 36 patients with SFA disease to sirolimus-coated versus bare-metal SMART® stents. This study, although not adequately powered, showed no statistically significant difference in the 6-month in-lesion (0% sirolimus vs 23.5% bare-metal, $P=0.10$) or in-stent (0% sirolimus vs 17.6% bare-metal, $P=0.23$) restenosis rate. The use of "cryoplasty" with the PolarCath system (which uses nitrous oxide to lower the inflating balloon temperature

Study	Design	N	Lesion type	Treatment	Results
Liermann et al. [36]	Nonrandomized feasibility trial	40	Restenosis	PTA + BT	Restenosis at up to 7 years: 18%
VIENNA-1 [37]	Nonrandomized feasibility trial	10	Restenosis	PTA + BT	Restenosis at 12 months: 40%
VIENNA-2 [38]	Randomized Phase III trial	113	Restenosis or de novo	(a) PTA + BT (b) PTA alone	Restenosis at 6 months: (a) 28%, (b) 54%, P<0.05. Patency at 12 months: (a) 64%, (b) 35%, P<0.005
VIENNA-4 [39]	Nonrandomized feasibility trial	33	De novo	PTA + stent + BT (clopidogrel 75 mg/day for 1 month)	Restenosis at 6 months: 30%. Late stent thrombosis (>1 month): 21%
PARIS Pilot [40]	Nonrandomized feasibility trial	40	De novo	PTA + BT (no stenting) (5/40 did not receive BT)	Restenosis – angiographic at 6 months: 17%; clinical at 12 months: 13%

Table 11. Clinical trials using gamma iridium-192 brachytherapy (BT) for femoropopliteal arteries. PTA: percutaneous transluminal angioplasty.

to −10°C; CryoVascular Systems, Los Gatos, CA, USA) appears to be promising, mitigating balloon-related dissections in femoropopliteal vessels with a potential reduction in target-lesion revascularization. A 102-patient registry study, PVD-CHILL, is ongoing.

Conclusion

PEI of symptomatic iliac and femoral arterial disease is feasible, and is an accepted first-line interventional alternative to surgical revascularization. Major technological advances in percutaneous equipment (eg, catheters, guidewires, angioplasty balloon, balloon-expandable stents, and self-expanding stents) have improved the procedural and long-term success rates for lower extremity arterial interventions. These techniques utilize fundamental principles similar to those of percutaneous coronary interventions, with the exception of larger balloon diameters, 0.035-inch guidewires, and the frequent use of self-expanding stents. Novel devices have been developed to cross particularly challenging chronic total occlusions and are likely to improve procedural success. Ongoing randomized trials are evaluating the use of brachytherapy, drug-eluting stents, and other novel devices to improve long-term patency. Thus, PEI is evolving rapidly. Its application in lower extremity arterial intervention will continue to have a dominant role and is expected to increase progressively.

References

1. American Heart Association. *Heart Disease and Stroke Statistics – 2003 Update*. Dallas, TX: American Heart Association, 2002.
2. Fowkes FG, Housley E, Cawood EH, et al. Edinburgh Artery Study: prevalence of asymptomatic and symptomatic peripheral arterial disease in the general population. *Int J Epidemiol* 1991;20:384–92.
3. Wilt TJ. Current strategies in the diagnosis and management of lower extremity peripheral vascular disease. *J Gen Intern Med* 1992;7:87–101.
4. Dormandy J, Mahir M, Ascady G, et al. Fate of the patient with chronic leg ischaemia. A review article. *J Cardiovasc Surg (Torino)* 1989;30:50–7.
5. Dotter C, Judkins M. Transluminal treatment of arteriosclerotic obstructions: description of a new technic and a preliminary report of its application. *Circulation* 1964;30:654–70.
6. Weitz JI, Byrne J, Clagett GP, et al. Diagnosis and treatment of chronic arterial insufficiency of the lower extremities: a critical review. *Circulation* 1996;94:3026–49.
7. TransAtlantic Inter-Society Consensus (TASC). Management of peripheral arterial disease (PAD). *Eur J Vasc Endovasc Surg* 2000;19 (Suppl. A):Si–xxviii, S1–250.
8. Ogren M, Hedblad B, Isacsson SO, et al. Non-invasively detected carotid stenosis and ischaemic heart disease in men with leg arteriosclerosis. *Lancet* 1993;342:1138–41.
9. Cho L, Roffi M, Mukherjee D, et al. Superficial femoral artery occlusion: nitinol stents achieve better flow and reduce the need for medications than balloon angioplasty alone. *J Invasive Cardiol* 2003;15:198–200.
10. Parodi JC, Palmaz JC, Barone HD. Transfemoral intraluminal graft implantation for abdominal aortic aneurysms. *Ann Vasc Surg* 1991;5:491–9.
11. Stoeckelhuber BM, Meissner O, Stoeckelhuber M, et al. Primary endovascular stent placement for focal infrarenal aortic stenosis: initial and midterm results. *J Vasc Interv Radiol* 2003;14:1443–7.
12. Nyman U, Uher P, Lindh M, et al. Primary stenting in infrarenal aortic occlusive disease. *Cardiovasc Intervent Radiol* 2000;23:97–108.
13. Becker GJ, Katzen BT, Dake MD. Noncoronary angioplasty. *Radiology* 1989;170:921–40.
14. Matsi PJ, Manninen HI. Complications of lower-limb percutaneous transluminal angioplasty: a prospective analysis of 410 procedures on 295 consecutive patients. *Cardiovasc Intervent Radiol* 1998;21:361–6.
15. Babalik E, Gulbaran M, Gurmen T, et al. Fracture of popliteal artery stents. *Circ J* 2003;67:643–5.
16. Sacks BA, Miller A, Gottlieb M. Fracture of an iliac artery Palmaz stent. *J Vasc Interv Radiol* 1996;7:53–5.
17. Gruntzig A, Kumpe DA. Technique of percutaneous transluminal angioplasty with the Gruntzig balloon catheter. *AJR Am J Roentgenol* 1979;132:547–52.
18. Spence RK, Freiman DB, Gatenby R, et al. Long-term results of transluminal angioplasty of the iliac and femoral arteries. *Arch Surg* 1981;116:1377–86.
19. Schwarten DE. Percutaneous transluminal angioplasty of the iliac arteries: intravenous digital subtraction angiography for follow-up. *Radiology* 1984;150:363–7.
20. Gallino A, Mahler F, Probst P, et al. [Early and late results in 250 cases of percutaneous transluminal dilatation in the lower extremities]. *Vasa* 1982;11:319–21 (in German).
21. Palmaz JC, Laborde JC, Rivera FJ, et al. Stenting of the iliac arteries with the Palmaz stent: experience from a multicenter trial. *Cardiovasc Intervent Radiol* 1992;15:291–7.
22. Richter GM, Roeren T, Noeldge G, et al. [Initial long-term results of a randomized 5-year study: iliac stent implantation versus PTA]. *Vasa Suppl* 1992;35:192–3 (in German).
23. Tetteroo E, van der Graaf Y, Bosch JL, et al. Randomised comparison of primary stent placement versus primary angioplasty followed by selective stent placement in patients with iliac-artery occlusive disease. Dutch Iliac Stent Trial Study Group. *Lancet* 1998;351:1153–9.
24. Bosch JL, Hunink MG. Meta-analysis of the results of percutaneous transluminal angioplasty and stent placement for aortoiliac occlusive disease. *Radiology* 1997;204:87–96.
25. Henry M, Amor M, Ethevenot G, et al. Palmaz stent placement in iliac and femoropopliteal arteries: primary and secondary patency in 310 patients with 2–4-year follow-up. *Radiology* 1995;197:167–74.
26. Morgenstern BR, Getrajdman GI, Laffey KJ, et al. Total occlusions of the femoropopliteal artery: high technical success rate of conventional balloon angioplasty. *Radiology* 1989;172:937–40.
27. Capek P, McLean GK, Berkowitz HD. Femoropopliteal angioplasty. Factors influencing long-term success. *Circulation* 1991;83(2 Suppl.):I70–80.
28. Adar R, Critchfield GC, Eddy DM. A confidence profile analysis of the results of femoropopliteal percutaneous transluminal angioplasty in the treatment of lower extremity ischemia. *J Vasc Surg* 1989;10:57–67.
29. Gallino A, Mahler F, Probst P, et al. Percutaneous transluminal angioplasty of the arteries of the lower limbs: a 5 year follow-up. *Circulation* 1984;70:619–23.

30. Hewes RC, White RI Jr, Murray RR, et al. Long-term results of superficial femoral artery angioplasty. *AJR Am J Roentgenol* 1986;146:1025–9.

31. Krepel VM, van Andel GJ, van Erp WF, et al. Percutaneous transluminal angioplasty of the femoropopliteal artery: initial and long-term results. *Radiology* 1985;156:325–8.

32. Do-dai-Do, Triller J, Walpoth BH, et al. A comparison study of self-expandable stents vs balloon angioplasty alone in femoropopliteal artery occlusions. *Cardiovasc Intervent Radiol* 1992;15:306–12.

33. Vroegindeweij D, Vos LD, Tielbeek AV, et al. Balloon angioplasty combined with primary stenting versus balloon angioplasty alone in femoropopliteal obstructions: A comparative randomized study. *Cardiovasc Intervent Radiol* 1997;20:420–5.

34. Zdanowski Z, Albrechtsson U, Lundin A, et al. Percutaneous transluminal angioplasty with or without stenting for femoropopliteal occlusions? A randomized controlled study. *Int Angiol* 1999;18:251–5.

35. Cejna M, Thurnher S, Illiasch H, et al. PTA versus Palmaz stent placement in femoropopliteal artery obstructions: a multicenter prospective randomized study. *J Vasc Interv Radiol* 2001;12:23–31.

36. Liermann D, Kirchner J, Bauernsachs R, et al. Brachytherapy with iridium-192 HDR to prevent from restenosis in peripheral arteries. An update. *Herz* 1998;23:394–400.

37. Minar E, Pokrajac B, Ahmadi R, et al. Brachytherapy for prophylaxis of restenosis after long-segment femoropopliteal angioplasty: pilot study. *Radiology* 1998;208:173–9.

38. Minar E, Pokrajac B, Maca T, et al. Endovascular brachytherapy for prophylaxis of restenosis after femoropopliteal angioplasty: results of a prospective randomized study. *Circulation* 2000;102:2694–9.

39. Wolfram RM, Pokrajac B, Ahmadi R, et al. Endovascular brachytherapy for prophylaxis against restenosis after long-segment femoropopliteal placement of stents: initial results. *Radiology* 2001;220:724–9.

40. Waksman R, Laird JR, Jurkovitz CT, et al. Intravascular radiation therapy after balloon angioplasty of narrowed femoropopliteal arteries to prevent restenosis: results of the PARIS feasibility clinical trial. *J Vasc Interv Radiol* 2001;12:915–21.

6 Infrapopliteal intervention and limb salvage

Michael H Wholey

Introduction

With the rise of peripheral vascular disease in the general population, there has been an increased awareness of severe atherosclerotic disease affecting the lower extremities. The disease progression is complex and can be multifactorial, including any level of disease in the iliac, femoropopliteal, and infrapopliteal arteries, including the anterior tibial, posterior tibial, and peroneal arteries. There are many causes of atherosclerotic disease involving the lower extremities; the chief causes include genetic predisposition, smoking of tobacco, diabetes, and cholesterol [1].

The objective of this chapter is for the reader to gain a better understanding of infrapopliteal disease, anatomy, and the interventional options in treating this disease.

Anatomy

The popliteal artery originates from the superficial femoral artery (SFA) at the level of the adductor canal. It courses inferior to the femur, crossing the knee joint. Here, it undergoes a short descent and bifurcates into the anterior tibial artery laterally and the continuation of the tibialperoneal trunk (see **Figures 1** and **2**). This short trunk bifurcates into the peroneal and posterior tibial arteries. The anterior tibial artery courses along the anterior–lateral aspect of the leg, parallel to the fibula, where it crosses the ankle and forms the pedal dorsalis artery. The posterior tibial artery courses in the medial–posterior compartment, crosses the ankle and calcaneous, and forms the medial and lateral plantar branches. These branches join with the pedal dorsalis artery, forming the plantar arch. The peroneal artery flows to the ankle and stops, with collateral vessels to the anterior and posterior tibial arteries.

A few anatomical variants occur. Occasionally, the anterior tibial artery is hypoplastic with the peroneal artery forming the pedal dorsalis artery (see **Figure 3**).

Methods

Angiographic technique

Either the antegrade or retrograde femoral approach can effectively demonstrate the lower extremity run-off. We routinely gain access in the common femoral artery in the standard retrograde manner. When performing interventions in the popliteal and infrapopliteal arteries, we frequently choose an antegrade puncture; we seek to have the needle (usually a 5-Fr micropuncture set) enter the femoral artery in the bottom third of the femoral head. We anesthetize the skin based upon fluoroscopic findings and landmarks. Frequently, the guidewire will enter the profunda femoral branch. If so, we place a short 4- or 5-Fr sheath and inject a small amount of contrast to locate the bifurcation and then redirect the guidewire. Also, we have been using ultrasound for assistance in entering some femoral arteries.

When a retrograde approach is chosen, we frequently use a pigtail catheter, such as the Omniflush catheter (Cook, Bloomington, IN, USA), to study the abdominal aorta and pull it down

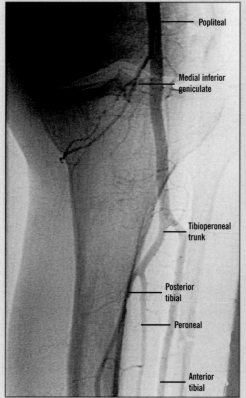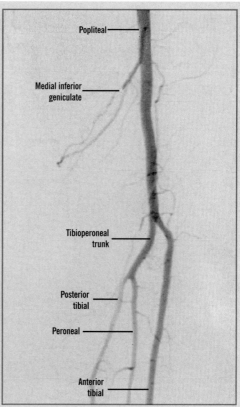

Figure 1. Left infrapopliteal artery injection.

for the pelvis oblique views, followed by selection of the external iliac artery. In these retrograde approaches, the best pictures are achieved with the catheter tip selected in the external iliac artery, if clinically possible. In order to perform safe and effective angiography of the extremities, digital subtraction and at least 14-inch image intensifiers must be used.

Once in place, we use the following injection rates with an angiographic injector:

- 8 cc/s for a total volume of 10–12 cc for the upper leg (common femoral artery, SFA, profunda femoral artery)

- 8 cc/s for a total volume of 12–20 cc for the lower femur

- 8 cc/s for a total volume of 15–25 cc for the knee, with a slight obliquity to see the trifurcation vessels

- 8–11 cc/s for a total volume of 20–35 cc for the lateral foot

We dilute the contrast mixture: generally, two thirds contrast media and one third saline. In patients with elevated creatinine levels, we perform the steps outlined below.

Good hydration the night before

With repeat labs the following morning if needed.

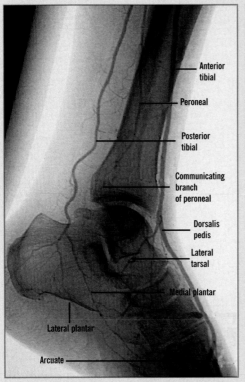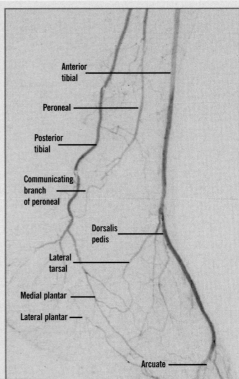

Figure 2. Infrapopliteal artery injection.

Medications

- Mucomyst (*N*-acetyl cysteine, 600 mg PO bid the day before, the morning of, and day of the procedure; AstraZeneca, Wilmington, DE, USA)

- Fenoldopam (Corlopam; Abbott, IL, USA)

Fenoldopam is a dopamine agonist that helps to improve renal flow. It is a catecholamine structurally related to dopamine and dobutamine, and does not cross the blood–brain barrier. It has vasodilatory effects in the peripheral circulation, including the renal artery bed. It is very short lasting (5 minutes) and is given intravenously at least 20 minutes prior to the study and for 4 hours afterwards. Blood pressure monitoring is performed to taper the drug. We administer 0.01–1.60 µg/kg/min. Blood pressures are checked every 15 minutes. However, a recent trial failed to find benefit with this agent.

Alternative contrast agents

Carbon dioxide is a fairly effective agent in the iliac arteries and upper legs (see **Figure 4**). It is less effective in extremities below the knee. Gadolinium has been used as a magnetic resonance imaging agent, but we have been using it as an angiographic agent in abdominal and lower extremity angiograms. It can be detected on digital subtractional angiography, especially with newer systems. It can be injected undiluted or in a mixture: we have achieved good results with a mixture of one third gadolinium, one third contrast media, and one third saline (see **Figure 5**). The maximum amount of gadolinium injected is approximately 60 cc.

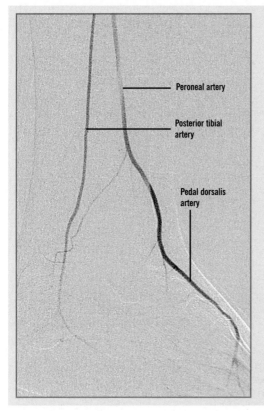

Peroneal artery

Posterior tibial
artery

Pedal dorsalis
artery

Figure 3. An anatomical variant of the peroneal artery that communicates
with the pedal dorsalis artery.

Diagnosis

Arterial occlusive disease of the infrapopliteal artery is easily diagnosed with the presence of arterial stenoses and occlusions. The degree, length, and location of stenoses and occlusions must all be documented in order to develop a treatment plan. Occasionally, other findings will be detected, such as aneurysms, trauma, arteriovenous fistulae, or other causes of the peripheral vascular symptomatology.

A physical examination, including ankle brachial indices, noninvasive studies, and clinical history, should be performed beforehand. Hence, clinical history, physical examinations, and imaging studies (including angiographic findings) are all relevant in developing a proper treatment strategy.

Interventional techniques
for high-grade stenosis

Patient selection is dependent upon several factors, the most important of which is location. We frequently intervene on femoropopliteal lesions in order to increase flow to treat nonhealing ulcers, rest pain, and severe claudicants. Our criteria for intervening on infrapopliteal lesions

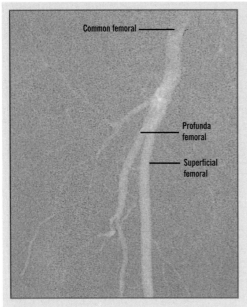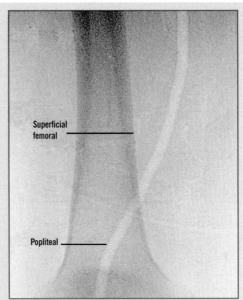

Common femoral

Profunda
femoral

Superficial
femoral

Superficial
femoral

Popliteal

Figure 4. Carbon dioxide injection of a lower extremity angiogram.

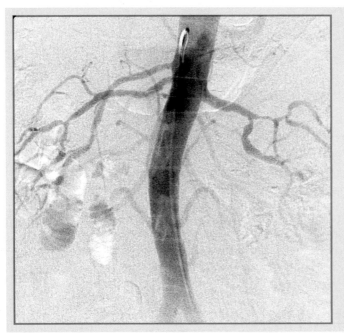

Figure 5. Abdominal angiogram performed with
a mixture of one third gadolinium, one third
contrast media, and one third saline at 15 cc/s
for a total of 30 cc.

are more stringent, and intervention is generally reserved for limb salvage (categories 4–6
SVS/SCVIR) [2]. Unfortunately, the patient population has severe comorbidities. The average
patient age is 69 years, with serious risk factors. They have a 5-year survival of 50% due to
stroke or myocardial infarction, and diabetes is present in 63%–91% of patients undergoing
tibial interventions [3,4].

Standard angioplasty of popliteal and infrapopliteal arteries

A focal lesion in the popliteal artery, tibial peroneal trunk, or the run-off vessels of the peroneal, anterior, or posterior tibial arteries is a relatively common finding in patients with peripheral vascular disease. How you approach each of these lesions depends on its severity, location, and the size of the vessel (see **Figure 6**). We use the following general angioplasty techniques:

- common femoral artery access, either antegrade (very important for a truly infrapopliteal lesion) or retrograde via a 6- to 7-Fr sheath up and over the aortic bifurcation. Contraindications to the antegrade approach are primarily based on obesity

- heparinize the patient and use nitroglycerin 150–200 µg intra-arterially, as needed

- elect the SFA with a 100-cm, 5-Fr diagnostic catheter with a 0.035-inch steerable wire

- under roadmap (images that allow for advancement of catheters and guidewires into vessels outlined by digital subtraction), visualize the lesion and then cross with a 0.014-inch guidewire

- angioplasty with a balloon sized to the vessel: for popliteal arteries, we use 3- to 4-mm percutaneous transluminal coronary angioplasty (PTCA) balloons; for tibial and peroneal arteries, we use 2- to 3-mm PTCA balloons, either monorail or coaxial

- leave the inflation balloon expanded for approximately 30 seconds and then deflate slowly

- assess with an angiogram for further intervention

Posttreatment, patients should be placed on clopidogrel (Plavix; Bristol-Myers Squibb, NY, USA) and aspirin for at least 1 month. Cholesterol-lowering agents may also be considered.

The long-term success of popliteal and infrapopliteal lesion angioplasty is determined by several factors. In the STAR (SCVIR Transluminal Angioplasty and Revascularization) registry for femoropopliteal angioplasty, the following criteria were found to affect long-term patency [5]:

- lesion length: lesions >3 cm had a relative risk of patency loss of 2.0 compared with lesions ≤3 cm ($P=0.022$)

- the status of tibial run-off: a single tibial vessel with 50%–99% stenosis or occlusion of all three run-off vessels had a relative risk of patency loss of 8.5

- limbs with multiple percutaneous transluminal angioplasty (PTA): compared with limbs with a single angioplasty site, limbs with multiple PTA had a relative risk of primary patency loss of 2.6 ($P=0.004$)

The presence of an intimal flap was not predictive of outcome ($P=0.53$).

The primary patency of femoropopliteal lesions has been found to vary from 46% to 86% at 1-year follow-up, and from 46% to 69% at 3-year follow-up (see **Table 1**) [5–10].

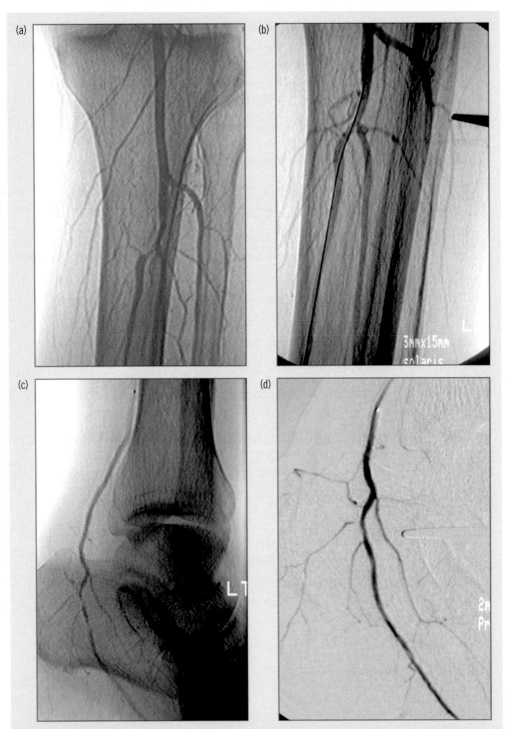

Figure 6. Angioplasty of a high-grade anterior tibial lesion and posterior tibial artery. (**a**) Angiogram in a patient with a nonhealing ulcer with high-grade lesions of the left posterior tibial artery at origin. Once the lesion has been crossed with a 0.014-inch wire, dilatation is performed with a 3-mm × 15-mm percutaneous transluminal coronary angioplasty (PTCA) balloon to 8 atm for 30 seconds. (**b**) Final angiogram of a treated anterior tibial artery showing improved flow to the right foot. (**c**) The same patient with a high-grade lesion of the posterior tibial artery. (**d**) Successful angioplasty with a 2-mm PTCA balloon catheter.

Author(s)	N	Primary patency (%)			
		1 year	2 years	3 years	5 years
STAR registry, 2001 [5]	205	86	80	69	–
Johnston et al., 1987 [6]	254	–	–	–	36
Capek et al., 1991 [7]	217	81	–	61	58
Jamsen et al., 2002 [8]	173	46	–	–	25
Karch et al., 2000 [9]	85	74	62	57	52
Becker, 1991 [10]	4,304	–	67 (review)	–	–

Table 1. Primary patency of angioplasty results for femoropopliteal lesions.

Important trends in treating infrapopliteal lesions

Over the last few years, there have been several important trends in the treatment of infrapopliteal lesions. Many of these have resulted from the transfer of technology and equipment used to treat coronary arteries. Though similar in vessel size, the infrapopliteal arteries are plagued by slow flow, poor distal run-off, and other differences, making long-term patency poor at best. The following trends may offer significant future improvements.

Drugs

Newer drugs, including clopidogrel and aspirin (new in this application), have been very helpful in maintaining patency immediately, but few studies have assessed their long-term benefits. Strecker et al. found primary patency rates of 76% at 1 year and 70% at 2 years in a clopidogrel plus aspirin group [11]. These were better than in the aspirin-only group, which had primary patency rates of 75% at 1 year and 50% at 2 years [11].

Stents

To stent or not to stent infrapopliteal arteries has been a long-standing debate. At our institution, there has been little difference in long-term results whether we stent or perform standard angioplasty [12]. We refrain from stenting the popliteal artery at the knee joint because of the severe mechanical stress that self-expandable stents experience at that site. As importantly, the popliteal artery is easily accessible for our vascular surgeons to perform necessary bypasses.

The proximal popliteal artery near the adductor canal can be stented with a self-expandable stent, but is also susceptible to stress (see **Figure 7**). To avoid the devastating results of distal embolization, we prefer to stent if the patient is at high risk for embolization (based on the characteristics of the lesion, such as heavy calcification) or is on hemodialysis (see **Figure 8**). The new stent profiles (5–6 Fr) allow for easy deployment in the SFA and proximal popliteal artery. We generally postdilate these stents with a balloon matched to the vessel diameter.

A sirolimus-coated femoral stent trial in Europe found several fractured nitinol stents in the SFA location. Though the findings did not lead to altered medical management, they are still somewhat concerning [13] – some investigators have discovered complications from popliteal stent fractures [14]. In the European trial, the in-stent mean lumen diameter was significantly larger in the sirolimus-eluting stent group than in the uncoated stent group (4.95 mm vs 4.31 mm, $P=0.047$). Developments in stent technology, especially with drug coatings,

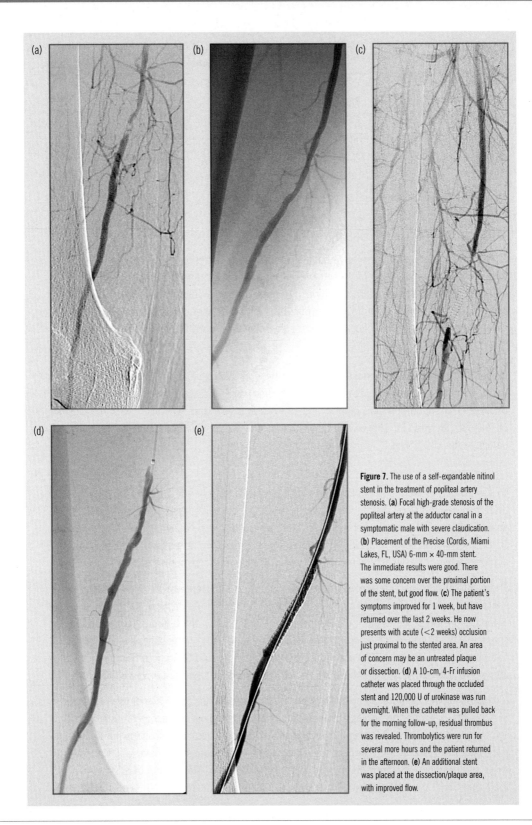

Figure 7. The use of a self-expandable nitinol stent in the treatment of popliteal artery stenosis. (**a**) Focal high-grade stenosis of the popliteal artery at the adductor canal in a symptomatic male with severe claudication. (**b**) Placement of the Precise (Cordis, Miami Lakes, FL, USA) 6-mm × 40-mm stent. The immediate results were good. There was some concern over the proximal portion of the stent, but good flow. (**c**) The patient's symptoms improved for 1 week, but have returned over the last 2 weeks. He now presents with acute (<2 weeks) occlusion just proximal to the stented area. An area of concern may be an untreated plaque or dissection. (**d**) A 10-cm, 4-Fr infusion catheter was placed through the occluded stent and 120,000 U of urokinase was run overnight. When the catheter was pulled back for the morning follow-up, residual thrombus was revealed. Thrombolytics were run for several more hours and the patient returned in the afternoon. (**e**) An additional stent was placed at the dissection/plaque area, with improved flow.

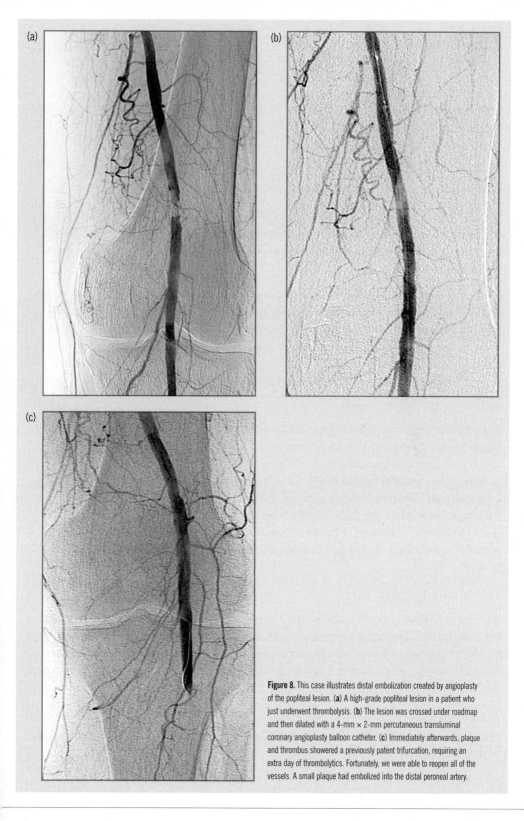

(a)

(b)

(c)

Figure 8. This case illustrates distal embolization created by angioplasty of the popliteal lesion. (**a**) A high-grade popliteal lesion in a patient who just underwent thrombolysis. (**b**) The lesion was crossed under roadmap and then dilated with a 4-mm × 2-mm percutaneous transluminal coronary angioplasty balloon catheter. (**c**) Immediately afterwards, plaque and thrombus showered a previously patent trifurcation, requiring an extra day of thrombolytics. Fortunately, we were able to reopen all of the vessels. A small plaque had embolized into the distal peroneal artery.

Author(s)	N	Primary patency (%)		
		1 year	2 years	3 years
Chatelard and Guibourt, 1996 [15]	35	80	75	–
Bergeron et al., 1995 [16]	39	–	75	–
Gordon et al., 2001 [17]	57	55	–	30
Conroy et al., 2000 [18][a]	48	79	72	70
Strecker et al., 1997 [19]	80	–	51	48
Lugmayr et al., 2002 [20]	44	–	–	76

Table 2. Primary patency of stent-assisted angioplasty results for femoropopliteal lesions.
[a]This study treated chronic occlusions.

should make stenting of these small vessels safer and improve long-term results. Randomized trials of drug-eluting stents in coronary arteries have already shown quite significant reductions in restenosis.

Because of their size, we prefer to use angioplasty for tibial and peroneal arteries, but we will stent if there is a poor response from angioplasty or if a significant dissection develops. We prefer to use self-expanding stents, usually 1–2 mm more than the diameter of the vessel. Some centers have reported good results with balloon-mounted stents. The rate of primary patency of stent-assisted angioplasty for femoropopliteal lesions has varied from 55% to 80% at 1-year follow-up, and from 30% to 76% at 3-year follow-up (see **Table 2**) [15–20].

Embolic protection devices

The advent of distal protection devices, including balloon occlusion and embolic filters (see **Figure 9**), will dramatically alter the intervention of many high-grade lesions in both the periphery and in thrombolytic interventional cases. Distal embolic protection devices have been found to be extremely useful in treating saphenous vein bypass grafts and carotid artery lesions, and should be used in treating high-risk lesions in the infrapopliteal arteries. Distal embolization of the infrapopliteal lesions has been reported in approximately 1%–5% of cases, but is probably much more frequent. Because of the direct flow from the popliteal artery to the trifurcation, occlusion of the important tibial and peroneal arteries can occur suddenly and can be difficult to treat.

Cutting balloon angioplasty

Acceptance is growing for the use of cutting balloons in treating infrapopliteal lesions. Although the currently available cutting balloons in the US only go up to 4 mm, which limits some cases, the use of a cutting balloon to treat femoropopliteal lesions is also growing. Some centers have had good early experience with this new technology provided by IVT (Interventional Therapeutics; Boston Scientific, Natick, MA, USA) (see **Figure 10**).

Cryogenic balloon angioplasty

Little is known about the effects of cryogenic balloon angioplasty. Studies of this new technology have recently begun.

(a)

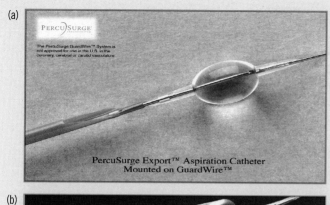

PercuSurge Export™ Aspiration Catheter
Mounted on GuardWire™

(b)

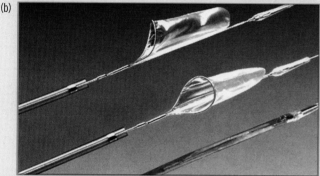

(c)

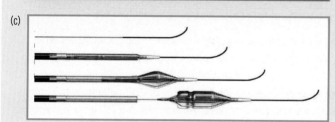

Figure 9. Several of the distal protection devices that may become useful in performing interventions in the infrapopliteal region. (a) PercuSurge Export Aspiration catheter mounted on a GuardWire (Medtronic, Minneapolis, MN, USA); (b) FilterWire (EPI; Boston Scientific, Natick, MA, USA); (c) MedNova (Abbott, IL, USA).

Interventional techniques for chronic total occlusions

Treatment of occlusions of the infrapopliteal arteries depends upon the lesion's location, its length, and the clinical status of the patient. When confronted with a total occlusion, the major question is over the status of the extremity: is it an acute or chronic process? The clinical presentation and physical examination of the disease process are crucial. Likewise, the presence of collaterals with distal run-off to the foot and the absence of an arterial clot lead to the diagnosis of chronic occlusive disease.

There are several techniques for treating chronic occlusive disease of the SFA, popliteal, and infrapopliteal arteries. We have had good technical success in recanalizing short SFA and popliteal lesions with the use of a 0.035-inch hydrophilic glidewire (Terumo Medical, Somerset,

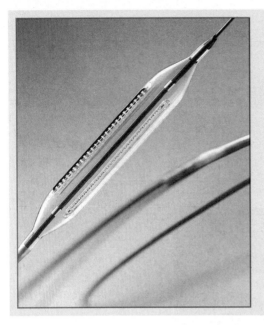

Figure 10. Cutting balloon by IVT (Boston Scientific, Natick, MA, USA).

NJ, USA) and a 4- to 5-Fr diagnostic catheter. We use roadmap techniques to carefully cross short focal lesions and then place a small, self-expanding stent. We prefer to come from above with an antegrade puncture, though some centers use the popliteal approach, in which the popliteal artery is accessed using ultrasound assistance and a micropuncture set.

Another approach is to place an infusion catheter or guidewire at or in the occluded vessel and begin thrombolytic therapy. We infuse urokinase at approximately 120,000 U/h in addition to heparinization, with the goal of reopening the vessel and reducing lesion length. We then proceed with angioplasty and possible stent placement. In a series of 250 patients with chronic arterial occlusions of the iliac and femoropopliteal arteries, we achieved a 77% technical success rate in reopening these vessels with thrombolytic therapy. The development of new mechanical thrombectomy catheters, such as from Bacchus Vascular (Santa Clara, CA, USA), may speed the current, usually overnight, process.

Newer devices transferred from coronary recanalization offer promise for the treatment of longer lesions and possibly in improving long-term results. There have been positive reports from the use of lasers in recanalizing long lesions [21,22]. Likewise, there have been good reports with use of the LuMend Frontrunner catheter (Redwood City, CA, USA) and the IntraLuminal catheter system (Carlsbad, CA, USA). Whichever recanalization technique is used – whether a wire, laser, or other device – maintenance of patency is imperative, with good and frequent surveillance and reintervention.

Interventional techniques in acute occlusions of infrapopliteal arteries

Acute arterial occlusive disease of the infrapopliteal arteries carries a high risk of morbidity and mortality. It is important to try to prevent this stage from occurring through better screening of patients with severe peripheral vascular disease. With improved noninvasive imaging by ultrasound, magnetic resonance angiography, and computed tomography angiograms, this should happen in the near future. Likewise, in patients with bypass grafts, improved follow-up by noninvasive testing is already reducing the numbers of patients with acute ischemic limbs at our institution.

Once a patient with an ischemic limb arrives in the emergency room or in your office, time is of the essence. We work closely with our vascular surgeon to decide what we can safely accomplish in a certain period of time. Our approach for a cold extremity is summarized below.

* Access the contralateral artery with a micropuncture set or single wall needle, place a 5- to 6-Fr sheath, and then perform abdominal and pelvic angiograms to assess inflow.

* Select the contralateral external iliac artery and do a complete angiogram of the leg, including flow (if any) to the foot.

* Identify the level of occlusion and the presence of any collateral flow distally.

* If the patient has occluded his or her bypass graft, gain access to the graft and begin thrombolytic therapy. We have used mechanical thrombectomy devices to speed the process, but with mixed success. We have had similar rates of success with bypass grafts as with native arteries, though many centers report a greater success rate with native vessels. In our experience, the most important indicator of success with thrombolysis of graft and native vessels is the status of the distal run-off. Other factors include the status of the patient, inflow disease, end-stage renal disease, lesion length, and location of the lesion [23,24].

* For native arteries, we carefully select the occluded vessel and begin thrombolytic therapy with possible mechanical thrombectomy. For occlusions in the popliteal lesion, we prefer to cross the occlusion and place a 4- to 5-Fr infusion catheter with sideholes throughout the clot. For lesions at the trifurcation, there are several approaches (see **Figure 11**). Some interventionalists will cross the occlusion and place an infusion guidewire into the posterior, anterior tibial, or peroneal artery. There is a risk of spasm reducing inflow, which could result in worsened flow to the foot. This is especially true when a catheter is placed in the small vessels near the foot. There is also a risk of dissection in small vessels and of occluding the other infrapopliteal vessels. We often use the more conservative approach of leaving an infusion catheter or guidewire in the popliteal artery. Occasionally, we make a channel through the occlusion with a steerable guidewire, leaving the infusion catheter parked in the popliteal artery. Treatment of occlusions in the infrapopliteal has been debated for years. Much is dependent upon your level of experience and equipment, as well as the condition of the patient.

* The dosage of urokinase will be a 250,000 U bolus or 4 hours of 240,000 U/h with reassessment and possible catheter repositioning. We mix 250,000 U of urokinase with

(a)

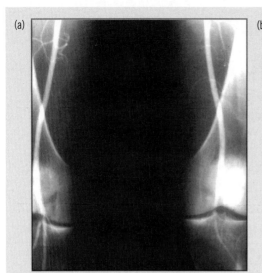

(b)

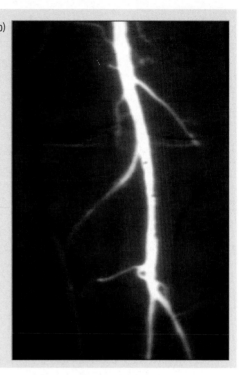

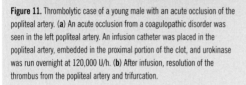

Figure 11. Thrombolytic case of a young male with an acute occlusion of the popliteal artery. (a) An acute occlusion from a coagulopathic disorder was seen in the left popliteal artery. An infusion catheter was placed in the popliteal artery, embedded in the proximal portion of the clot, and urokinase was run overnight at 120,000 U/h. (b) After infusion, resolution of the thrombus from the popliteal artery and trifurcation.

250 cc normal saline and run the pump at 300 cc/h for a total dose of 120,000 U/h for the remaining night, with reassessment in the morning. We also heparinize the patient at 800–1000 U/h through a peripheral vein. We administer meperidine (Demerol), diphenhydramine (Benadryl), cimetidine IV, and acetaminophen (Tylenol) PO to counter possible allergic reactions to urokinase.

• The endpoint for thrombolysis is resolution of the occlusion with restored arterial flow. Occasionally, distal embolization occurs, requiring continued thrombolysis. We try to maintain 24 hours as the maximum time period for thrombolysis, but will occasionally continue thrombolysis for 2 days, if needed. Complications with thrombolysis do occur; the most concerning is cerebral hemorrhage, which occurs in approximately 1% of patients. Other major complications include bleeding at the groin or from recent surgery. Failure of thrombolytics can vary from 0% to 14%. Poor distal run-off has been our major factor for failure (see **Figure 12**). Other factors, such as poor limb viability, location and severity of lesions, and identification of underlying stenosis, are all major determinants of the effectiveness of thrombolytic therapy. It is imperative to maintain a good regimen of follow-up for all patients who have undergone thrombolytic therapy. In our experience, approximately 70% will require further intervention, such as angioplasty or stenting, immediately or with elective surgery. After discharge, we will follow these patients with noninvasive labs, such as Doppler and computed tomography angiograms, every 6–12 months.

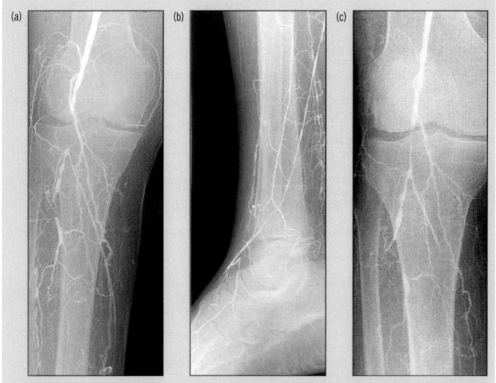

Figure 12. Illustration of thrombolytic failure, probably due to poor distal run-off. (**a**) This was a case of a failing bypass graft in a 75-year-old patient who presented with severe ischemia in his right foot, which had lost motor function and most sensory function. The initial angiogram shows occlusions of the native popliteal artery and a small caliber popliteal-to-anterior tibial bypass graft. (**b**) An initial angiogram of the lateral right foot showed poor distal run-off provided by the pedal dorsalis artery. We placed an infusion catheter in the popliteal artery and began thrombolytics. (**c**) After overnight infusion, we were able to reopen the distal popliteal artery, but unable to maintain patency of the bypass graft. The patient's foot worsened and required amputation. This case illustrates the importance of distal run-off in trying to perform thrombolysis, and also highlights the need for patients to begin therapy before motor and sensory deficits occur.

Conclusion

Though intervention of infrapopliteal peripheral vascular disease has been established for the past 20 years, recent advances in stent technology with various coatings, the application of cutting balloon technology, and medical management all promise to increase the patency of these vessels. High technical success has been very useful in treating infrapopliteal lesions and helping to treat nonhealing ulcers. However, the poor long-term patency of these interventions has limited the appeal of infrapopliteal angioplasty. This will hopefully change within the next decade. Regardless, careful and timely clinical follow-up is crucial in maintaining secondary patency for infrapopliteal lesions.

References

1. Dankner R, Goldbourt U, Boyko V, et al. Predictors of cardiac and noncardiac mortality among 14,697 patients with coronary heart disease. *Am J Cardiol* 2003;91:121–7.
2. Rutherford RB. Standards for evaluating results of interventional therapy for peripheral vascular disease. *Circulation* 1991;83(2 Suppl.):I6–11.
3. Kram HB, Gupta SK, Veith FJ, et al. Late results of two hundred seventeen femoropopliteal bypasses to isolated popliteal artery segments. *J Vasc Surg* 1991;14:386–90.
4. Lyon RT, Veith FJ, Marsan BU, et al. Eleven-year experience with tibiotibial bypass: an unusual but effective solution to distal tibial artery occlusive disease and limited autologous vein. *J Vasc Surg* 1994;20:61–8; discussion 68–9.
5. Clark TW, Groffsky JL, Soulen MC. Predictors of long-term patency after femoropopliteal angioplasty: results from the STAR registry. *J Vasc Interv Radiol* 2001;12:923–33.
6. Johnston KW, Rae M, Hogg-Johnston SA, et al. 5-year results of a prospective study of percutaneous transluminal angioplasty. *Ann Surg* 1987;206:403–13.
7. Capek P, McLean GK, Berkowitz HD. Femoropopliteal angioplasty. Factors influencing long-term success. *Circulation* 1991;83(2 Suppl.):I70–80.
8. Jamsen TS, Manninen HI, Jaakkola PA, et al. Long-term outcome of patients with claudication after balloon angioplasty of the femoropopliteal arteries. *Radiology* 2002;225:345–52.
9. Karch LA, Mattos MA, Henretta JP, et al. Clinical failure after percutaneous transluminal angioplasty of the superficial femoral and popliteal arteries. *J Vasc Surg* 2000;31:880–7.
10. Becker GJ. Intravascular stents. General principles and status of lower-extremity arterial applications. *Circulation* 1991;83(2 Suppl.):I122–36.
11. Strecker EP, Boos IB, Gottmann D, et al. Clopidogrel plus long-term aspirin after femoro-popliteal stenting. The CLAFS project: 1- and 2-year results. *Eur Radiol* 2003 (Epub. ahead of print).
12. Grimm J, Muller-Hulsbeck S, Jahnke T, et al. Randomized study to compare PTA alone versus PTA with Palmaz stent placement for femoropopliteal lesions. *J Vasc Interv Radiol* 2001;12:935–42.
13. Duda SH, Pusich B, Richter G, et al. Sirolimus-eluting stents for the treatment of obstructive superficial femoral artery disease: six-month results. *Circulation* 2002;106:1505–9.
14. Babalik E, Gulbaran M, Gurmen T, et al. Fracture of popliteal artery stents. *Circ J* 2003;67:643–5.
15. Chatelard P, Guibourt C. Long-term results with a Palmaz stent in the femoropopliteal arteries. *J Cardiovasc Surg (Torino)* 1996;37(3 Suppl. 1):67–72.
16. Bergeron P, Pinot JJ, Poyen V, et al. Long-term results with the Palmaz stent in the superficial femoral artery. *J Endovasc Surg* 1995;2:161–7.
17. Gordon IL, Conroy RM, Arefi M, et al. Three-year outcome of endovascular treatment of superficial femoral artery occlusion. *Arch Surg* 2001;136:221–8.
18. Conroy RM, Gordon IL, Tobis JM, et al. Angioplasty and stent placement in chronic occlusion of the superficial femoral artery: technique and results. *J Vasc Interv Radiol* 2000;11:1009–20.
19. Strecker EP, Boos IB, Gottmann D. Femoropopliteal artery stent placement: evaluation of long-term success. *Radiology* 1997;205:375–83.
20. Lugmayr HF, Holzer H, Kastner M, et al. Treatment of complex arteriosclerotic lesions with nitinol stents in the superficial femoral and popliteal arteries: a midterm follow-up. *Radiology* 2002;222:37–43.
21. Das TS. Percutaneous peripheral revascularisation with excimer laser: equipment, technique and results. *Lasers Med Sci* 2001;16:101–7.
22. Scheinert D, Laird JR Jr, Schroder M, et al. Excimer laser-assisted recanalization of long, chronic superficial femoral artery occlusions. *J Endovasc Ther* 2001;8:156–66.
23. Ouriel K, Veith FJ. Acute lower limb ischemia: determinants of outcome. *Surgery* 1998;124:336–41; discussion 341–2.
24. Ouriel K, Veith FJ, Sasahara AA. Thrombolysis or peripheral arterial surgery: phase I results. TOPAS Investigators. *J Vasc Surg* 1996;23:64–73; discussion 74–5.

7 Renal and mesenteric artery intervention

Debabrata Mukherjee and Leslie Cho

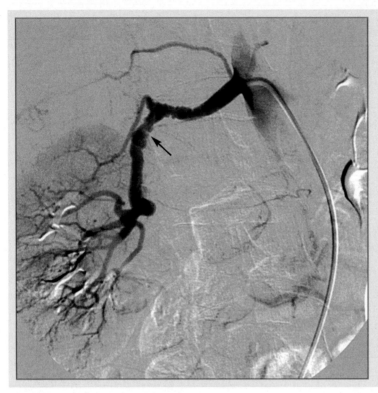

Figure 1. Selective right renal angiogram showing fibromuscular dysplasia in a 66-year-old female with new-onset hypertension. Note the characteristic beaded appearance. (Figure courtesy of Deepak L Bhatt, MD.)

Renal artery stenosis

Renal artery stenosis (RAS) is the most common cause of secondary hypertension, and its incidence appears to be rising because of increased atherosclerosis in an aging population. RAS can cause renal insufficiency and uncontrolled hypertension, and is associated with increased cardiovascular morbidity and mortality.

There have been significant recent improvements in the noninvasive detection of RAS. At the same time, revascularization techniques have evolved and most renal artery revascularization is now performed percutaneously. Despite these improvements, controversy still exists as to which patients should be screened for RAS and the optimal treatment for individuals with RAS.

Clinical features

More than 90% of RAS cases are atherosclerotic in nature and involve the ostium and the proximal portion of the main renal artery, with plaque extending into the perirenal aorta [1]. The prevalence of atherosclerotic RAS increases with age and with the presence of diabetes, peripheral arterial disease, coronary artery disease, hypertension, and dyslipidemia. Fibromuscular dysplasia accounts for 10% of RAS cases and is typically seen in young and middle-aged females. In contrast to atherosclerotic RAS, fibromuscular dysplasia affects the distal two thirds of the main renal artery and has a characteristic beaded appearance on angiography (see **Figure 1**).

Young or middle-aged female with severe hypertension and no family history (fibromuscular dysplasia)	Recurrent flash pulmonary edema
	>1.5 cm difference in renal sizes
Uncontrolled hypertension despite at least three antihypertensive agents in adequate doses (regimen includes a diuretic)	Hypertension with hypokalemia (secondary hyperaldosteronism due to elevated renin)
Worsening blood pressure control in a compliant, long-standing hypertensive patient	Bruit over the abdominal aorta (lateralizing bruit over the renal arteries is more specific, but uncommon)
Acute renal failure or creatinine elevation with angiotensin-converting enzyme inhibitors or angiotensin receptor blockers	Hypertension and concomitant peripheral arterial disease
	Severe hypertensive retinopathy
Chronic renal insufficiency with mild proteinuria and bland urinary sediment	

Table 1. Clinical signs suggestive of renal artery stenosis.

Although often thought of as a cause of systemic hypertension, RAS is not commonly associated with mild or moderate hypertension; however, it is present in a third of patients with malignant hypertension or uncontrolled hypertension despite multiple antihypertensive agents. RAS may also present as end-stage renal failure, with or without hypertension, with a bland urinary sediment and non-nephrotic proteinuria. Patients with bilateral RAS or stenosis of an artery to a solitary kidney may present as acute renal failure if they are administered angiotensin-converting enzyme inhibitors (ACEIs) or angiotensin receptor blockers. An uncommon presentation of RAS is recurrent episodes of flash pulmonary edema. **Table 1** enumerates a number of clinical signs suggestive of RAS.

Diagnosis

The decision to evaluate a patient for RAS should be based on the clinical likelihood of that patient having RAS. The clinical signs listed in **Table 1** will help to identify individuals with a high pretest likelihood of RAS. Once the decision has been made to screen an individual, there are multiple options available.

Duplex ultrasound

Ultrasonography can provide a significant amount of useful information in the form of renal size and images of the renal arteries; it can also measure blood flow velocities and pressure waveforms. It is an ideal screening test because it is noninvasive and can predict the presence or absence of RAS with a high degree of accuracy [2]. Moreover, calculation of the end-diastolic velocity and renal artery resistance index from the flow velocities may predict clinical outcomes after renal artery revascularization. However, there is a 15%–20% rate of failure to adequately visualize the renal arteries, due to either operator inexperience or technical issues – such as obesity or the presence of bowel gas.

Captopril renal scanning

Captopril renal scanning (CRS) is another noninvasive method of detecting RAS. Huot et al. evaluated the performance characteristics (sensitivity, specificity, and predictive values) of CRS in a consecutive series of 90 patients who underwent both CRS and renal arteriography within a 6-month period [3]. CRS was found to have:

- 74% sensitivity (95% confidence interval [CI]: 62–83)

- 59% specificity (95% CI: 49–69)

- 58% positive predictive value (95% CI: 47–68)

- 75% negative predictive value (95% CI: 64–84)

This study found evidence of spectrum bias, because the sensitivity and specificity (as well as the predictive values) were different for groups with and without vascular disease. The results of CRS were substantially worse in a clinical practice setting than previously reported in research settings, despite a similar prevalence of RAS. Based on the available data, CRS should not be used as an initial screening test for RAS, even in patients with high clinical likelihood of the condition [3].

Spiral computed tomography

Spiral computed tomography (CT) provides excellent anatomical images of the renal arteries, but does not provide any physiological information, such as blood flow velocities. The requirement for significant amounts of iodinated contrast agent and radiation exposure are further disadvantages of this technique.

Magnetic resonance angiography

Magnetic resonance angiography (MRA) is a promising imaging modality that provides images of the renal arteries and permits reconstruction of the images in different planes. Newer machines allow characterization of the plaque, and flow-dependent imaging complements the morphologic images of contrast-enhanced MRA by providing hemodynamic information. Gadolinium, which is non-nephrotoxic, is used as the contrast agent. However, costs and availability limit the widespread use of MRA as a screening tool.

Contrast angiography

The widely available technique of contrast angiography remains the gold standard for diagnosing RAS. Hemodynamic assessment of the lesion may be performed at the same time, and a pressure gradient >20 mm Hg may identify individuals suitable for revascularization [4]. However, there is a risk of worsening renal function related to the contrast agent or atheroemboli. In individuals with marked renal insufficiency, either carbon dioxide or gadolinium may be used for digital subtraction aortography in lieu of an iodinated contrast agent.

Management

In addition to consideration of revascularization, patients with RAS should be targeted for appropriate secondary prevention of cardiovascular events. Optimal therapy includes good blood pressure control (according to the guidelines of the sixth Joint National Committee on blood pressure), modification of cardiovascular risk factors, and appropriate use of antiplatelet therapy, lipid-lowering therapy, and beta-blockers. Patients undergoing peripheral arterial and renal artery interventions have significantly improved outcomes if treated with appropriate evidence-based secondary preventive therapy. For blood pressure control, ACEIs are especially useful in patients with unilateral RAS.

Resistant or poorly controlled hypertension and unilateral or bilateral renal artery stenosis
Renal artery stenosis and recurrent flash pulmonary edema for which there is no readily explainable cause
Dialysis-dependent renal failure and bilateral renal artery stenosis or renal artery stenosis to a solitary functioning kidney
Chronic renal insufficiency (creatinine >2 mg/dL) and ≥75% bilateral renal artery stenosis or unilateral renal artery stenosis with a solitary functioning kidney

Table 2. Current indications for renal artery revascularization.

Revascularization options include either surgical or percutaneous revascularization. The currently accepted indications for renal revascularization are listed in **Table 2**. Surgical revascularization is rarely performed except in the presence of abdominal aortic aneurysms, dissections, or aneurysm of the renal arteries. Angioplasty has become the revascularization modality of choice. Following Gruntzig's initial 1978 report of successful balloon angioplasty of RAS with a resultant improvement in blood pressure control and enhanced renal perfusion, there have been a number of studies on the efficacy of percutaneous revascularization for the treatment of RAS. Most interventionalists would agree that the technical aspects of renal revascularization have become easier with an expanding arsenal of low-profile balloons, self-mounted stents, and 6-Fr systems. No longer are we limited by the complexity of the lesion – now, the burden lies in deciding whether revascularization will provide clinical benefit over continued medical therapy.

Van Jaarsveld et al. reported the largest trial comparing balloon angioplasty with medical therapy for the treatment of RAS [5]. This was a prospective, randomized, multicenter trial that included patients ($N = 106$) with >50% stenosis of one or both renal arteries, serum creatinine ≤2.3 mg/dL, diastolic blood pressure ≥95 mm Hg on at least two antihypertensive medications, and a 0.2 mg/dL increase in serum creatinine during treatment with an ACEI. Based on an intention-to-treat analysis, renal angioplasty provided little advantage over antihypertensive drug therapy in this study.

Although this is the largest randomized study to date, it suffered from several major limitations, including a relatively small sample size and the use of angioplasty without stenting, which partially resulted in the 47.9% restenosis rate. In addition, 22 of 50 patients assigned to the medical therapy group subsequently underwent angioplasty due to refractory hypertension at 3 months' follow-up and were analyzed in an intention-to-treat manner, thus potentially diluting the difference in long-term outcome. In contrast to these results, White et al. reported significant reductions in systolic and diastolic blood pressure and in the number of medications needed in a prospective cohort of 100 patients treated with balloon-expandable stents [6].

These discordant results have raised the question of whether it is possible to predict which patients will improve after renal stenting. A simple, valid test would improve outcomes in patients undergoing renal revascularization and decrease the number of futile procedures. Radermacher et al. demonstrated that a renal artery resistance index ([1 − end-diastolic velocity / maximal systolic velocity] × 100) value of at least 80 reliably identifies patients with RAS in whom angioplasty or surgery will not improve renal function, blood pressure, or kidney survival [7].

Mukherjee et al. subsequently demonstrated that a preprocedural end-diastolic velocity >90 and resistance index <75 identifies individuals who are likely to benefit with improvement in creatinine or reduction in blood pressure after renal revascularization [8]. In both of these studies,

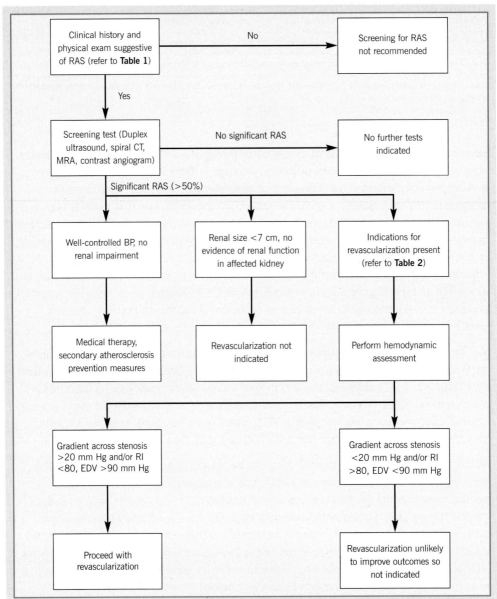

Figure 2. Algorithm for the detection and treatment of renal artery stenosis. BP: blood pressure; CT: computed tomography; EDV: end-diastolic velocity; MRA: magnetic resonance angiography; RAS: renal artery stenosis; RI: renal artery resistance index ([1 − end-diastolic velocity / maximal systolic velocity] × 100). Adapted with permission from the American College of Cardiology (Mukherjee D. Renal artery stenosis: who to screen and how to treat? *ACC Curr J Rev* 2003;12:70–5).

a resistance index >80 was a very strong predictor for lack of benefit after revascularization. **Figure 2** depicts a simplified algorithm for the screening and treatment of RAS.

Angiography

Renal angiography is usually performed as a prelude to renal artery revascularization. Other indications for renal angiography include the evaluation of prospective renal donors to define

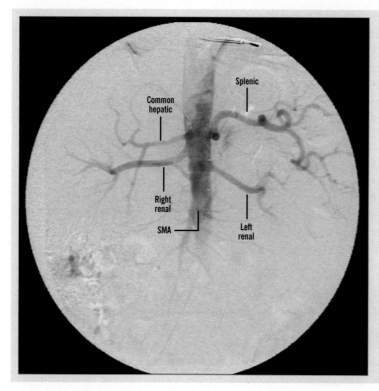

Figure 3. An anteroposterior abdominal aortogram to visualize the mesenteric and renal arteries. SMA: superior mesenteric artery.

arterial supply, and assessing vascularity in renal tumors. An abdominal aortogram is initially performed with a straight pigtail catheter (see **Figure 3**) placed at the level of the L1 vertebra. We typically use digital subtraction angiography (DSA) and inject a total of 10 cc of contrast for an abdominal aortogram (20 mL/s and 0.5 seconds injection). This allows the origin of the main renal arteries to be visualized (typically arising at the L1/L2 level), and accessory renal arteries (if present). The anteroposterior abdominal aortogram is a good "scout" shot – it is useful in gaining orientation of the renal ostium, but can miss true focal ostial stenosis as renal ostia come off a few degrees posteriorly.

Selective renal artery cannulation can usually be performed with a Judkin's Right (JR)4 catheter. However, arteries with unusual or angulated take-offs may need to be cannulated with an SOS or Cobra catheter. For renal arteries with a downward take-off, a left internal mammary artery (LIMA) catheter may be used. Selective renal angiograms are performed with 3–4 cc of contrast, hand-injected using DSA in an ipsilateral oblique projection (right anterior oblique 20°–30° for right renal artery, etc). One should stay on cine for delayed imaging to visualize the nephrogram and ascertain the renal size.

If there is significant angiographic stenosis of the renal artery, a pressure gradient should be measured prior to consideration of revascularization. A gradient >20 mm Hg suggests hemodynamically significant stenosis. A clinical benefit of using a 5-Fr SOS catheter for selective cannulation is that by withdrawing the catheter slightly, the tip advances beyond the proximal portion of the renal artery and a gradient can be measured directly.

Renal angiograms can be performed from either the brachial or the femoral approach, although the femoral approach is preferred by many operators. The brachial approach may be the preferred approach for a very steep downward take-off of the renal arteries, particularly if intervention is planned. Techniques to minimize embolization and other complications during a renal angiogram include using a 5-Fr system and reforming the SOS catheter in the suprarenal aorta to minimize scraping of the renal arteries.

Intervention

Renal revascularization can be performed using either the femoral or the brachial approach, with the femoral approach being preferred. Currently, a guiding catheter is the most commonly employed instrument as it considerably facilitates stent implantation. Available guide catheters include the hockey stick, multipurpose, renal double curve (RDC)1, and RDC catheters in 6–8 Fr sizes. With improvements in balloon and stent profiles, most operators now use a 6 Fr guide catheter. Use of a smaller catheter may decrease access site vascular complications and potentially reduce renal artery embolic complications.

Initial reports of renal angioplasty and stenting used 0.035-inch or 0.018-inch guidewires to allow advancement of bulky balloon catheters and stents, but a 0.014-inch guidewire is currently preferred. A 0.014-inch guidewire minimizes traumatization of small branch vessels. Once an appropriate guide is seated in the ostium, unfractionated heparin is administered at 60 U/kg to achieve an activated clotting time of 200–250 seconds. The stenosis is crossed with a 0.014-inch guidewire and predilated with an appropriately sized balloon catheter (5–5.5 mm diameter for most renal arteries). Following dilatation, an appropriately sized stent (typically 6–7 mm diameter) is advanced and deployed to cover the entire lesion, with 1–2 mm of the stent extending into the aorta to ensure complete coverage of the ostium. A stent with good radial strength should be chosen to prevent recoil of the ostium; we have successfully used the PALMAZ GENESIS (Cordis, Miami Lakes, FL, USA), and the HERCULINK PLUS stent (Guidant, Indianapolis, USA) for renal artery stenting (see **Figure 4**).

The ostium is typically postdilated with the stent balloon partially in the aorta at higher atmospheres to flare the ostium. One should be careful to align the balloon catheter coaxially during postdilatation to avoid creating aortic dissections. Potential complications of renal artery stenting include renal atheroembolization, aortic dissections, blue-toe syndrome from peripheral embolization, and perinephric hematomas related to branch-vessel perforation. Avoiding larger diameter wires and hydrophilic guidewires significantly reduces the risk of perinephric hematomas. Postprocedure, patients should receive lifelong aspirin and clopidogrel for 1–12 months.

Emerging technologies

The absence of a consistent benefit across studies and the occasional increase in creatinine after endovascular intervention of the renal arteries can possibly be attributed to atheroembolism due to debris generated during the intervention. Studies have demonstrated atheroembolism after either endovascular or surgical revascularization of renal arteries. It has also been demonstrated that atheroembolic renal disease after revascularization for atherosclerotic RAS is associated with decreased survival and an increased incidence of atherosclerotic morbid events [9].

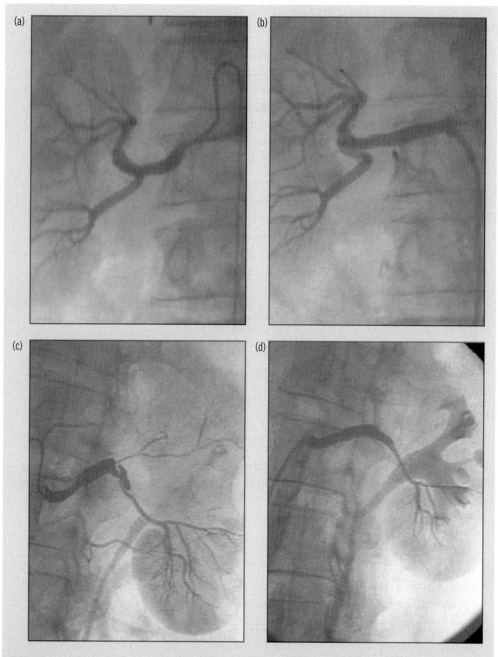

Figure 4. Two cases of severe renal artery stenosis treated with renal artery stenting. (**a,b**) Case 1 was a 72-year-old female who was transferred from an outside hospital for recurrent episodes of pulmonary edema and rising creatinine. She was severely hypertensive despite five antihypertensive drugs. Her creatinine at presentation was 4.3 mg/dL and she needed hemofiltration for hypervolemia on the day of admission. She underwent renal angiography the following day, which revealed severe ostial right renal artery stenosis (**a**) with 108-mm gradient across the stenosis and an occluded left renal artery with an atrophic left kidney. She underwent successful renal stenting with complete resolution of the gradient (**b**). Over the next few days her creatinine stabilized at 1.6 mg/dL and her episodes of pulmonary edema resolved. (**c,d**) Case 2 was a 39-year-old male with severe hypertriglyceridemia and refractory hypertension despite four antihypertensive agents. Renal angiography revealed an ulcerated plaque in the inferior division of the left renal artery (**c**) and mild atherosclerosis of the right renal artery without hemodynamically significant stenosis. This was successfully treated with renal stenting (**d**). On follow-up, his blood pressure was well-controlled with two antihypertensive agents.

Thus, it makes sense to protect the renal microvasculature from atherosclerotic debris during revascularization, which in turn may prevent worsening of renal function.

A pilot study has demonstrated the efficacy of emboli protection devices (PercuSurge GuardWire, Medtronic, Minneapolis, MN, USA) during percutaneous angioplasty and stenting for RAS [10]. Visible debris was extracted from all patients in this study. These preliminary results suggest that protected renal artery angioplasty and stenting may be a safe method to decrease the risk of renal atheroembolism during the procedure and to protect against renal function deterioration [11,12]. Several ongoing trials are assessing the safety and efficacy of filter-based emboli protection devices as an adjunct to renal artery stenting.

Technological advances such as emboli protection devices and drug-eluting stents may improve the immediate and long-term outcomes of renal artery stenting. An ongoing trial (RESIST) is evaluating the combination of a glycoprotein IIb/IIIa inhibitor and emboli protection devices during renal stenting, and a safety and efficacy trial of 100 patients has been announced to compare the sirolimus-eluting, stainless-steel, balloon-expandable stent with a bare metal stent for renal revascularization (the GREAT trial).

Mesenteric artery stenosis

Chronic mesenteric ischemia is usually related to progressive atherosclerotic narrowing of the mesenteric arteries. Due to the wide range of causes, mesenteric ischemia often goes undiagnosed and untreated, leading to high morbidity and mortality.

Mesenteric arterial anatomy

An understanding of mesenteric arterial anatomy is crucial to understanding and managing these patients. The gastrointestinal tract is supplied by the celiac trunk, the superior mesenteric artery (SMA), and the inferior mesenteric artery (IMA) [13]. The celiac trunk originates from the anterior aorta just below the diaphragm at the level of the thoracic vertebrae 12 (T12) or the first lumbar vertebra. It branches into the common hepatic, splenic, and left gastric arteries.

- The left gastric artery supplies the lesser curvature of the stomach and collateralizes with the right gastric artery branch of the hepatic artery.

- Brances of the common hepatic artery include the hepatic and gastroduodenal arteries; the latter supplies the distal stomach and duodenum.

- The gastroduodenal artery supplies the greater curvature of the stomach via the right gastroepiploic artery.

The SMA is located a few centimeters below the celiac artery, usually around the first lumbar vertebra at 20°–30° caudal angulation. It supplies the pancreas, duodenum, jejunum, and the right half of the colon. The branches of the SMA are the inferior pancreaticoduodenal artery, the jejunal and ileal braches, the ileocolic artery, the right colic artery, and the middle colic artery.

The IMA originates from the mid to distal infrarenal aorta around the third lumbar vertebra, which is usually ≥5 cm below the origin of the SMA. It supplies the distal transverse, left, and

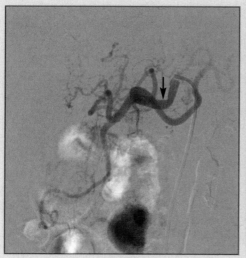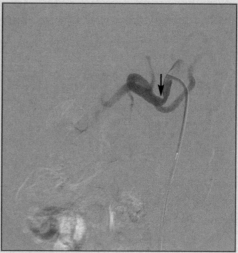

Figure 5. A celiac artery with (**a**) minimal narrowing, (**b**) accentuated to a moderate degree by deep expiration. (Figure courtesy of Deepak L Bhatt, MD.)

sigmoid portions of the colon and the rectum. Its branches are the left colic artery, the sigmoid (inferior left colic) arteries, and the superior rectal artery. The SMA and IMA collateralize via the marginal artery of Drummond and the meandering mesenteric artery.

Arcuate ligament syndrome

Arcuate ligament syndrome is caused by compression of the celiac trunk by the median arcuate ligament of the diaphragm and is typically seen in middle-aged, female patients. Individuals complain of abdominal pain with eating, postprandial emesis, and may present with marked weight loss. The pain is usually less severe than intestinal ischemic pain. Bruit may be heard in the upper abdomen during a physical exam. On angiography with the image intensifier in the lateral position, the median arcuate ligament is seen to compress the celiac axis; this is accentuated by deep expiration (see **Figure 5**). The historical treatment is surgical division of the median arcuate ligament. This is curative, although surgical bypass is sometimes necessary.

Clinical features

Mesenteric artery stenosis results in insufficient blood flow to the small intestine, causing intestinal ischemia. Chronic mesenteric ischemia is usually due to atherosclerosis, but is rarely caused by extensive fibromuscular disease or trauma. The celiac trunk, SMA, and IMA usually have ostial disease and occlusions are typically found in the proximal few centimeters of these arteries. Chronic mesenteric ischemia results when at least two of the three major splanchnic arteries have severe stenosis. The SMA is almost always involved in symptomatic cases. At rest, patients have sufficient intestinal blood flow to maintain gut viability and prevent symptom development. However, the increased demand on mesenteric circulation after a meal may overwhelm the compensatory ability of the collateral circulation, thereby causing postprandial intestinal angina.

Patients with chronic mesenteric ischemia typically present in the fifth or sixth decades of life [14,15]. They often have atherosclerotic disease elsewhere, such as peripheral vascular disease, coronary artery disease, and/or cerebrovascular disease. Females are more likely to be affected than males. Most patients complain of postprandial abdominal pain. The classic description is crampy or colicky pain located in the epigastric area that begins 15–30 minutes following eating, lasts for 2–3 hours, and gradually subsides. The postprandial pain can result in fear of food (sitophobia) [16]. Patients may compensate by eating smaller portions. Most patients with chronic mesenteric ischemia have marked weight loss. A physical examination often reveals weight loss and generalized signs of atherosclerosis. Rarely, patients have an abdominal bruit. Most often, patients initially receive a malignancy work-up.

Diagnosis

Plain abdominal x-ray, CT, and endoscopy are insensitive in diagnosing chronic mesenteric ischemia, but can rule out other diseases (such as malignancy). Duplex ultrasound requires excellent technical skills and a well-prepared patient. Vessel tortuosity, respiratory motion, and the presence of bowel gas impede good visualization.

Velocity parameters used to determine the presence of ≥70% stenosis (peak systolic velocity >275 cm/s for the celiac artery and >200 cm/s for the SMA) have been reported with sensitivities and specificities of around 90% compared with angiography. Therefore, duplex ultrasound is fairly reliable in excluding the diagnosis of chronic mesenteric ischemia.

Gadolinium-enhanced MRA has also been used in the diagnosis of mesenteric artery stenosis. Biplanar aortography, including selective engagement of the celiac trunk, SMA, and IMA, remains the diagnostic test of choice. Lateral abdominal aortograms are optimal to visualize the origin and the proximal portion of the mesenteric arteries. In addition to defining the extent of the disease, angiography determines collateral flow. Chronic mesenteric ischemia requires flow-limiting stenosis or occlusion of at least two of the three mesenteric arteries. In general, large collaterals (such as the wandering artery of Drummond from the IMA to the SMA in the case of SMA stenosis) are present and help to confirm the presence of lesions that are suspected to be flow limiting.

Management

Patients with chronic mesenteric ischemia have traditionally been treated with mesenteric vascular surgical revascularization [17,18]. Overall, the operative mortality remains high (approximately 7.5%–10%) [16]. There are several surgical revascularization strategies, including visceral endarterectomy, antegrade supraceliac aorta to visceral bypass, and retrograde infrarenal aorta to visceral bypass. Before surgical revascularization, the patient may benefit from total parenteral nutrition (TPN). Although there is controversy regarding the length and benefit of TPN, improving the nutritional status of the patient prior to surgery seems rational.

Transaortic visceral endarterectomy is a technically challenging procedure that requires extensive retroperitoneal vascular exposure. This technique also has a greater risk of paraplegia because of supraceliac aortic cross-clamping. Endarterectomy may be particularly beneficial in cases where the patient has both visceral stenosis and RAS. Endarterectomy is very difficult in patients with extensive aortic atherosclerosis and an alternative technique may be considered.

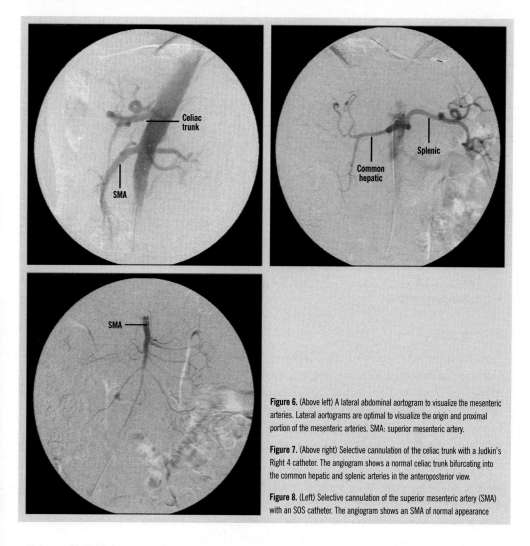

Figure 6. (Above left) A lateral abdominal aortogram to visualize the mesenteric arteries. Lateral aortograms are optimal to visualize the origin and proximal portion of the mesenteric arteries. SMA: superior mesenteric artery.

Figure 7. (Above right) Selective cannulation of the celiac trunk with a Judkin's Right 4 catheter. The angiogram shows a normal celiac trunk bifurcating into the common hepatic and splenic arteries in the anteroposterior view.

Figure 8. (Left) Selective cannulation of the superior mesenteric artery (SMA) with an SOS catheter. The angiogram shows an SMA of normal appearance

Retrograde SMA bypass is the most commonly performed visceral bypass procedure. The simplicity of the approach to the infrarenal aorta and infrapancreatic SMA makes this procedure attractive to surgeons. With retrograde bypass, care must be taken to configure a graft that will not kink. Antegrade bypass is the procedure of choice when there is marked infrarenal aortic atherosclerosis. Endarterectomy appears to have the lowest recurrence rate, followed by antegrade bypass reconstruction, and finally retrograde reconstruction.

Endovascular treatment is becoming the first-line therapy for chronic mesenteric ischemia at many experienced centers. Early studies found high restenosis rates; however, stenting has significantly improved outcomes. Visceral surgical revascularization in a malnourished patient, even in specialized centers, leads to significant morbidity and mortality in comparison with endovascular treatment. The endovascular approach is less invasive and compares favorably with surgery in terms of clinical success, complications, and long-term outcomes. Steimetz et al. demonstrated that endovascular therapy for mesenteric artery stenosis is efficient in both the short and long-term [19].

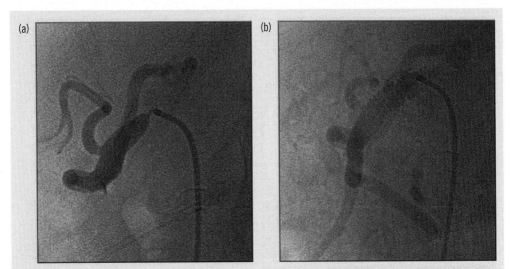

Figure 9. Successful endovascular stenting of superior mesenteric artery stenosis for chronic mesenteric ischemia. (**a**) Pre-stenting; (**b**) Post-stenting. (Figure courtesy of Deepak L Bhatt, MD.)

Angiography

Typical indications for mesenteric angiography include chronic mesenteric ischemia or intestinal angina, acute mesenteric ischemia, and uncontrolled gastrointestinal bleeding. Initially, lateral aortography should be performed to identify the origin of the mesenteric vessels (see **Figure 6**). Selective cannulations of the celiac trunk (see **Figure 7**), SMA (see **Figure 8**), and IMA can usually be performed using a JR4 or LIMA catheter in the lateral projection. In some cases, catheters with longer tips, such as the SOS or Cobra catheters, may be needed for selective injections.

For good quality mesenteric angiograms without streaming, the rate of injection should match the flow rate of the vessel being studied. Typical flow rates are 10 mL/s for the celiac trunk, 8 mL/s for the SMA, and 3 mL/s for the IMA. DSA acquisition may be less helpful for mesenteric angiography due to the presence of bowel gas. In patients being evaluated for gastrointestinal bleeding, the clinically suspected vessel should be injected first.

Intervention

Mesenteric artery revascularization can be performed using either the femoral or the brachial approach, with the femoral approach being preferred. Many of the concepts discussed in the section on renal artery intervention also apply to mesenteric artery revascularization, including the use of similar guide catheters, such as the Hockey Stick, Multipurpose, JR4, and RDC catheters in 6–8 Fr sizes. Most operators currently use a 6-inch Fr guide catheter and a 0.014-inch guidewire system.

Once an appropriate guide is seated in the ostium, unfractionated heparin is administered at 60 U/kg to achieve an activated clotting time of 200–250 seconds. The stenosis is crossed with a 0.014-inch guidewire and predilated with an appropriately sized balloon catheter (5–6 mm diameter for most mesenteric arteries). Mesenteric angioplasty has a good technical success rate but a high rate of restenosis [20], and routine stenting is recommended. Following dilatation, an appropriately sized stent (typically 6–7 mm diameter) is advanced and deployed to cover the entire lesion, with 1–2 mm of the stent extending into the aorta to ensure complete coverage of the ostium (see **Figure 9**).

A major consideration in the choice of the stent is that it has good radial strength to prevent recoil of the ostium for mesenteric artery stenting. The ostium is typically then postdilated with the stent balloon partially in the aorta at higher atmospheres to flare the ostium. Similarly to in renal stenting, care should be taken to align the balloon catheter coaxially during postdilatation to avoid creating aortic dissections. Potential complications of mesenteric artery stenting include atheroembolization, aortic dissections, and access site vascular complications. Postprocedure, patients should receive lifelong aspirin and clopidogrel for 1–12 months. In the future, emboli protection devices and drug-eluting stents may further improve the safety and durability of endovascular mesenteric artery revascularization.

References

1. McLaughlin K, Jardine AG, Moss JG. ABC of arterial and venous disease. Renal artery stenosis. *Br Med J* 2000;320:1124–7.
2. Olin JW, Piedmonte MR, Young JR, et al. The utility of duplex ultrasound scanning of the renal arteries for diagnosing significant renal artery stenosis. *Ann Intern Med* 1995;122:833–8.
3. Huot SJ, Hansson JH, Dey H, et al. Utility of captopril renal scans for detecting renal artery stenosis. *Arch Intern Med* 2002;162:1981–4.
4. Gross CM, Kramer J, Weingartner O, et al. Determination of renal arterial stenosis severity: comparison of pressure gradient and vessel diameter. *Radiology* 2001;220:751–6.
5. van Jaarsveld BC, Krijnen P, Pieterman H, et al. The effect of balloon angioplasty on hypertension in atherosclerotic renal-artery stenosis. Dutch Renal Artery Stenosis Intervention Cooperative Study Group. *N Engl J Med* 2000;342:1007–14.
6. White CJ, Ramee SR, Collins TJ, et al. Renal artery stent placement: utility in lesions difficult to treat with balloon angioplasty. *J Am Coll Cardiol* 1997;30:1445–50.
7. Radermacher J, Chavan A, Bleck J, et al. Use of Doppler ultrasonography to predict the outcome of therapy for renal-artery stenosis. *N Engl J Med* 2001;344:410–7.
8. Mukherjee D, Bhatt DL, Robbins M, et al. Renal artery end-diastolic velocity and renal artery resistance index as predictors of outcome after renal stenting. *Am J Cardiol* 2001;88:1064–6.
9. Krishnamurthi V, Novick AC, Myles JL. Atheroembolic renal disease: effect on morbidity and survival after revascularization for atherosclerotic renal artery stenosis. *J Urol* 1999;161:1093–6.
10. Henry M, Klonaris C, Henry I, et al. Protected renal stenting with the PercuSurge GuardWire device: a pilot study. *J Endovasc Ther* 2001;8:227–37.
11. Dorros G, Jaff M, Mathiak L, et al. Renal function and survival after renal artery stent revascularization may be influenced by embolic debris. *J Invasive Cardiol* 2004;16:189–95.
12. Bhatt DL. Embolization – a pathological mechanism in renal artery stenosis. *J Invasive Cardiol* 2004;16:196–7.
13. Rosenblum JD, Boyle CM, Schwartz LB. The mesenteric circulation. Anatomy and physiology. *Surg Clin North Am* 1997;77:289–306.
14. Moawad J, Gewertz BL. Chronic mesenteric ischemia. Clinical presentation and diagnosis. *Surg Clin North Am* 1997;77:357–69.
15. Greenwald DA, Brandt LJ, Reinus JF. Ischemic bowel disease in the elderly. *Gastroenterol Clin North Am* 2001;30:445–73.
16. Barkhordarian S, Gusberg R. Mesenteric ischemia: identification and treatment. *ACC Curr J Rev* 2003;12:19–21.
17. Stanley JC. Mesenteric arterial occlusive and aneurysmal disease. *Cardiol Clin* 2002;20:611–22, vii.
18. Lipski D, Ernst C. Visceral ischemic syndromes. In: Moore W, editor. *Vascular Surgery: A Comprehensive Review*, 4th edition. Philadelphia: WB Saunders, 2000:543–54.
19. Steinmetz E, Tatou E, Favier-Blavoux C, et al. Endovascular treatment as first choice in chronic intestinal ischemia. *Ann Vasc Surg* 2002;16:693–9.
20. Odurny A, Sniderman KW, Colapinto RF. Intestinal angina: percutaneous transluminal angioplasty of the celiac and superior mesenteric arteries. *Radiology* 1988;167:59–62.

8 Subclavian artery and upper extremity intervention

Ivan P Casserly and Samir R Kapadia

Introduction

Endovascular intervention in the upper extremities typically represents a small fraction of an endovascular specialist's workload. This is due to the relative sparing of the upper extremity arterial vascular tree from atherosclerosis. Where there is atherosclerotic disease of an upper extremity, it is largely confined to the subclavian artery, with rare involvement of the axillary or brachial arteries. Therefore, subclavian artery intervention constitutes the bulk of upper extremity interventions.

Anatomy

As with all endovascular procedures, it is important to understand the typical angiographic anatomy and most common anomalies before embarking on an interventional procedure (see **Table 1**). We describe the entire anatomy of the upper extremities [1,2] because, occasionally, the endovascular specialist is required to perform complete upper extremity diagnostic studies.

Subclavian artery

The right and left subclavian arteries supply the arterial flow to the right and left upper extremities, respectively. Typically, the left subclavian artery arises directly from the aortic arch as the third and final of the great vessels, while the right subclavian artery arises from the bifurcation of the innominate artery (see **Figure 1**). The innominate and left subclavian arteries typically arise from the horizontal portion of the arch, although there is considerable interindividual difference in the location of, and distance between, the origins of the great vessels (see **Figure 1a–c**). With increasing age and atherosclerotic change in the aortic arch, the origins arise from the ascending portion of the arch (see **Figure 1d**). The most common anomaly of the subclavian artery origin is where the right subclavian artery originates as the terminal vessel from the descending thoracic aorta (seen in 0.5% of people) (see **Figure 2a**). A bovine origin of the left common carotid artery off the innominate artery occurs in approximately 7%–20% of people, and is relevant in angiography of the right subclavian artery (see **Figure 2b**).

The subclavian artery extends from its origin to the lateral border of the first rib. By tradition, the artery is divided into three segments based on their relationship to the scalenus anterior muscle. The most important branches arise from the first segment and include the vertebral artery, internal thoracic artery, and thyrocervical trunk (see **Figure 3**). The vertebral and internal thoracic arteries are largely constant between individuals in their origin and course, arising as the first and second branches, respectively. Typically, the right and left vertebral arteries are asymmetric in size, with a dominant vessel contributing most of the flow to the basilar artery. In contrast, the thyrocervical trunk varies tremendously between individuals in terms of the pattern and size of its various branches. The most common anomaly of the subclavian artery branches is where the left vertebral artery originates directly from the aortic arch (0.5%–6%) (see **Figure 2c**).

Axillary artery

The axillary artery is a direct continuation of the subclavian artery. It extends from the lateral border of the first rib to the inferior border of the teres major muscle (see **Figures 3** and **4**).

Artery	Subdivisions	Boundaries	Branches	Sub-branches	Supply
Subclavian	I	Origin to medial border of scalenus ant mm	Vertebral Internal thoracic Thyrocervical	 Ascending cervical Inferior thyroid Suprascapular[a] Transverse cervical	Brain Thoracic wall Neck mm Thyroid gland Scapular mm Neck mm
	II	Posterior to scalenus ant mm	Costocervical	Deep cervical Superior intercostal	Neck mm First two intercostal spaces
	III	Lateral border of scalenus ant mm to lateral border first rib	Suprascapular		Scapular mm
Axillary	I	Lateral border of first rib to medial margin of pectoralis minor mm	Superior thoracic		First two intercostal spaces
	II	Posterior to pectoralis minor mm	Thoracoacromial	Acromial Deltoid Pectoral Clavicular	
	III	Lateral border of pectoralis minor mm to inferior border of teres major mm	Lateral thoracic Subscapular Ant cx humeral Post cx humeral	 Cx scapular Thoracodorsal	Pectoral mm, mam gland Scapular mm Latissimus dorsi mm Upper arm mm Upper arm mm
Brachial		Inferior border of teres major mm to neck of radius	Profunda brachial Nutrient Superior ulnar collateral Inferior ulnar collateral Multiple muscular br	Ant descending br Post descending br	Elbow collateral Elbow collateral Humerus Elbow collateral Elbow collateral Arm mm
Radial		Neck of radius to styloid process of radius	Radial recurrent Multiple muscular br Palmar carpal Dorsal carpal Superficial palmar		Elbow collateral Forearm mm Wrist Wrist Hand
Ulnar		Neck of radius to pisiform carpal bone	Ant ulnar recurrent Post ulnar recurrent Common interosseous Palmar carpal Dorsal carpal Deep carpal Muscular br	 Ant interosseous Post interosseous	Elbow collateral Elbow collateral Forearm mm Forearm mm, elbow collateral Wrist Wrist Hand Forearm mm

Table 1. Summary of the arterial anatomy of the upper extremity system. [a]The subscapular branch may also arise from subdivision III of the subclavian artery. ant: anterior; br: branch; cx: circumflex; mam: mammary; mm: muscle; post: posterior.

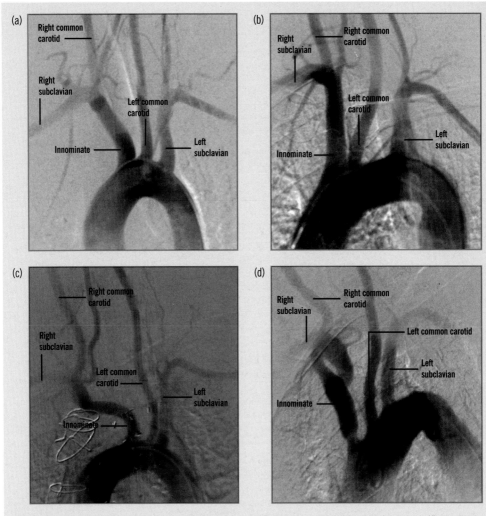

Figure 1. Normal variation in the inter-artery distance and location of the great arteries off the aortic arch. (**a,b,c**) Variations of a type I arch; (**d**) a type III arch.

The bony landmark for this inferior margin is the anatomical neck of the humerus. As with the subclavian artery, the axillary artery is divided into three anatomic segments based on their relationship to the pectoralis minor muscle. The branches of the axillary artery demonstrate significant interindividual variation and are outlined in **Table 1**.

Brachial artery

The brachial artery is the direct continuation of the axillary artery. It extends from the inferior border of the teres major muscle (anatomical neck of the humerus) to the neck of the radius (see **Figures 4** and **5**). The profunda brachii branch of the brachial artery is considerably smaller than its counterpart in the thigh. It descends posteriorly in the arm and contributes to the elbow collateral circulation. The other major branches of the brachial artery include muscular branches to the arm muscles, the nutrient artery to the humerus, and collateral vessels to the elbow.

(a)
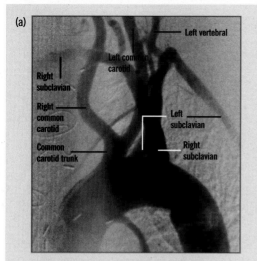

Left vertebral

Left common carotid

Right subclavian

Right common carotid

Common carotid trunk

Left subclavian

Right subclavian

(b)
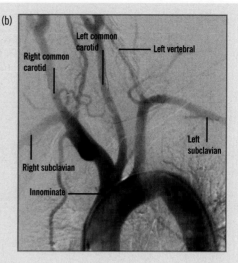

Left common carotid

Left vertebral

Right common carotid

Left subclavian

Right subclavian

Innominate

(c)
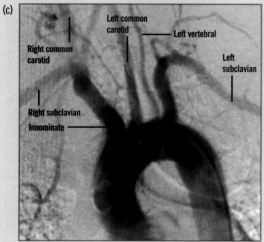

Left common carotid

Left vertebral

Right common carotid

Left subclavian

Right subclavian

Innominate

Figure 2. Common anomalies of the great vessels encountered during upper extremity angiography. (**a**) Origin of the right subclavian artery distal to the left subclavian artery. (**b**) Origin of the left common carotid artery from the innominate artery (bovine). (**c**) Direct origin of the vertebral artery from the aortic arch.

Ulnar artery

The ulnar artery is the major vessel to the forearm and is usually larger than the radial artery (see **Figure 5**). It is the equivalent of the tibioperoneal artery in the leg. It arises from the brachial artery bifurcation and extends from the neck of the radius to the pisiform carpal bone. Its main branch is the interosseous, which supplies the interosseous membrane and forearm muscles. In addition, the ulnar: supplies collateral branches to the elbow, muscular branches to the forearm, and carpal branches to the palmar and dorsal aspect of the wrist; contributes to the deep palmar arch; and continues into the hand as the major source of blood flow to the superficial palmar arch.

Radial artery

The radial artery is the smaller of the terminal branches of the brachial artery. It extends from the neck of the radius to the styloid process of the radius (see **Figure 5**). It is the equivalent of the anterior tibial artery in the leg. Like the ulnar artery, the radial artery contributes collaterals to the

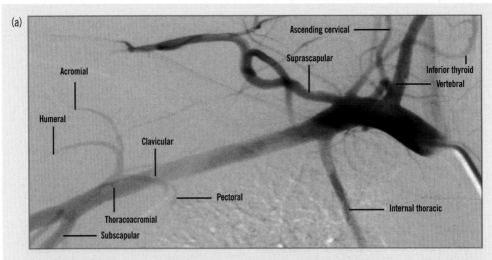

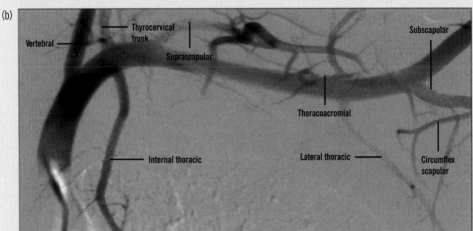

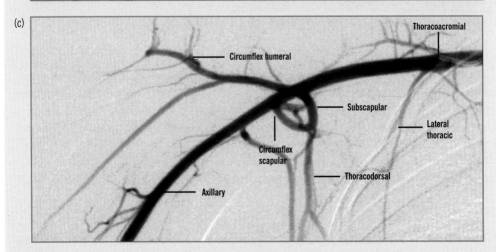

Figure 3. Angiography of the subclavian and axillary arteries and their major branches. (**a**) Right upper extremity, left anterior oblique view. (**b**) Left upper extremity, right anterior oblique view. (**c**) Right upper extremity, posteroanterior view.

(a)

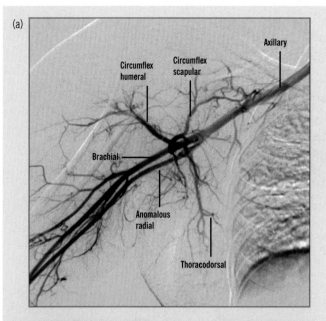

(b)

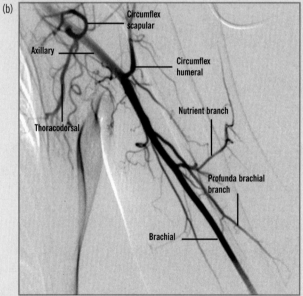

Figure 4. Angiography of the axillary and brachial arteries and their major branches. (a) Right upper extremity, posteroanterior (PA) view. Note the anomalous origin of the radial artery directly from the medial aspect of the axillary artery. (b) Left upper extremity, PA view.

elbow, muscular branches to the forearm, and carpal branches to the palmar and dorsal aspects of the wrist. In the hand, it contributes to the superficial palmar arch and continues into the hand as the major source of blood flow to the deep palmar arch.

Arterial supply to the hand

The arterial supply of the hand is provided by the superficial and deep palmar arches (see **Figure 6**). The deep arch is primarily formed from the terminal portion of the radial artery

(a)

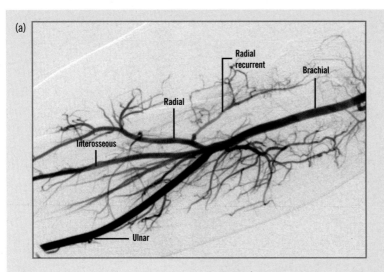

(b)

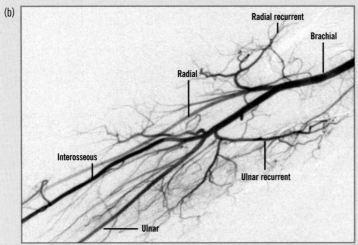

(c)

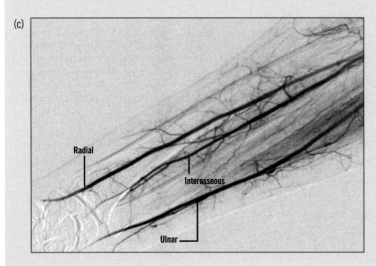

Figure 5. Angiography of the distal right arm and forearm (posteroanterior view) showing the distal portion of the brachial artery and the radial and ulnar arteries.

(a)

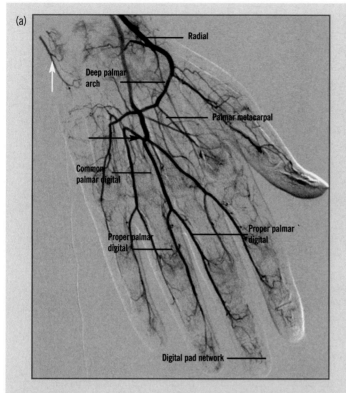

Radial

Deep palmar arch

Palmar metacarpal

Common palmar digital

Proper palmar digital

Proper palmar digital

Digital pad network

(b)

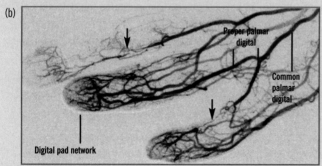

Proper palmar digital

Common palmar digital

Digital pad network

Figure 6. Angiography of the hand and digits. (a) Left hand, posteroanterior (PA) view. (b) Right little, index, and middle fingers, PA view. These angiograms are from two separate patients with small-vessel vasculitis manifested by ulnar artery occlusion (white arrow) and segmental occlusions of the proper digital arteries (short black arrows). The long black arrow indicates a superficial palmar arch.

and is complete in 95% of individuals. The superficial arch is primarily formed from the terminal portion of the ulnar artery and is complete in 80% of patients. Angiographically, the deep arch lies proximal to the superficial arch and is generally less prominent. Common palmar digital arteries arise from the superficial arch and fuse with palmar metacarpal branches from the deep arch. In the interdigital space, each of the common palmar digital arteries then divides into two proper palmar digital arteries, which run along the sides of the second to fifth digits and supply the arterial network of the finger pads. The thumb usually receives a direct branch from the terminal portion of the radial artery (princeps pollicis branch).

(a)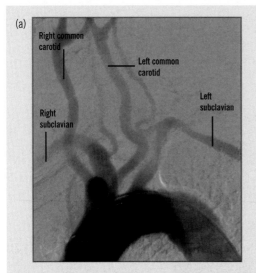

(b)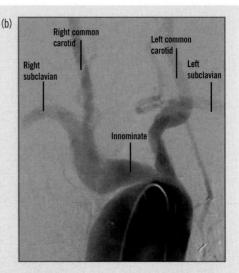

Figure 7. Arch aortogram in (**a**) the left anterior oblique (LAO) and (**b**) the right anterior oblique (RAO) projection in the same patient. Note the prominent overlap of the right subclavian, right common carotid, innominate, and left common carotid arteries in the LAO view. In the RAO view, the separate origin of the innominate artery from the aortic arch is clearly seen.

Angiography

It is prudent to perform an arch aortogram (40° left anterior oblique [LAO]) using a pigtail catheter prior to selective angiography of the upper extremities. This facilitates the detection of anomalies (eg, anomalous origin of the right subclavian artery distal to the left subclavian artery, direct origin of the vertebral artery from the arch) and of anatomical features that will increase the complexity of angiography and influence the choice of catheters and wires used to perform angiography and intervention (eg, a type III arch, tortuosity of the innominate or proximal subclavian artery). An arch aortogram in the right anterior oblique (RAO) view may be useful in rare circumstances where the vessel origins overlap in the LAO view (see **Figure 7**).

In most patients, the innominate and left subclavian arteries can be selectively engaged with a Judkins Right (JR)4 diagnostic catheter, which is advanced to the ascending aorta distal to the origin, torqued counter-clockwise such that its tip turns superiorly, and then withdrawn into the vessel ostium. An angled glide catheter can be used in a similar manner. For elderly patients with type III arches, a Vitek or Simmons catheter (both Cook, Bloomington, IN, USA) may be required. Our practice is to deliver the Vitek catheter to the descending thoracic aorta, direct the tip posteriorly, and then advance the catheter over the arch. Typically, the catheter will sequentially engage the origin of the great vessels. Withdrawal of the Vitek is achieved by first pushing forward on the catheter, which has the effect of advancing the catheter into the ascending aorta. A long wire is then passed through the catheter to straighten the curve. Finally, the catheter is removed, keeping the wire distal to the catheter tip. This technique minimizes trauma to the arch.

The Simmons catheter is more challenging to use as reshaping the catheter in the aortic arch can be difficult. Generally, the catheter is reshaped in the ascending aorta and then withdrawn into the origin of the great vessels. Trauma to the great vessel ostia may be minimized by advancing

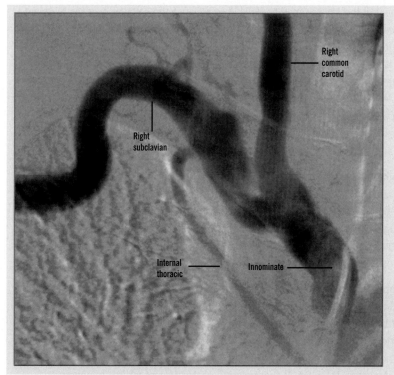

Right
common
carotid

Right
subclavian

Internal
thoracic

Innominate

Figure 8. Selective angiography of the innominate artery in the right anterior oblique projection, clearly showing the origin of the right subclavian and common carotid arteries.

a Wholey wire (Mallinckrodt, Hazelwood, MO, USA) (or other soft-tipped wire) just distal to the catheter tip prior to catheter withdrawal. The removal technique for the Simmons catheter is similar to that for the Vitek.

Selective angiography of the innominate and right subclavian arteries should be performed in orthogonal oblique projections with the patient's arm in the neutral position (ie, adducted at the patient's side). The RAO projection is particularly useful in delineating the origin of the right subclavian artery from the right common carotid artery (see **Figure 8**). The LAO projection allows accurate determination of the origin of the right vertebral and right internal mammary arteries (IMAs), which is important in assessing the suitability of a lesion for stenting and for accurate stent placement. For the left subclavian artery, the RAO projection generally allows the most accurate determination of the left vertebral and left IMA origins. When thoracic outlet syndrome (TOS) is suspected, angiography is performed in the posteroanterior (PA) projection with the arm in the neutral position, and then repeated with the shoulder in full abduction, external rotation, and retroversion (as if pitching a baseball).

Selective angiography of the axillary or brachial arteries requires initial engagement of the innominate and left subclavian artery origins with the diagnostic catheter. Thereafter, the least traumatic method is to advance a long (300-cm), soft-tipped 0.035-inch wire such as a Wholey or Magic torque wire (Medi-tech, Natick, MA, USA) into the brachial artery using the digital subtraction arteriography (DSA) roadmapping function, and advance the diagnostic catheter over this wire. When the diagnostic catheter is a JR4 or angled glide catheter, this is usually a straightforward maneuver. Where the arch anatomy necessitates the use of a Vitek or Simmons catheter for engagement of the ostia, it may be difficult to advance the catheter over the wire and these catheters can be exchanged for an angled glide or multipurpose (with sideholes) catheter. Unfortunately, the soft-tipped wires are not very steerable and it is often not possible to deliver them to the brachial artery. In contrast, the angled glidewire is a very steerable hydrophilic wire, but requires more careful manipulation so as not to cause dissection. Catheter advancement and exchanges using this wire also require more care than is required for nonhydrophilic wires in order to avoid losing wire position. Floppy glidewires may be used where support is not an issue and may minimize the risk of vessel trauma. A stiff angled glidewire will generally be required where there is type II or III arch anatomy, or where there is severe tortuosity of the proximal vessels.

Axillary artery angiography is performed with the arm in the neutral position or slightly abducted. For brachial and hand angiography, the patient's forearm is placed supine on an arm board. The fingers of the hand are splayed and taped in position. Images are generally taken in the PA projection, although angulated views may occasionally be required. Ipsilateral oblique projections of the forearm vessels can be particularly helpful in separating the course of the ulnar, interosseous, and radial arteries.

It is advisable to adopt a step-wise approach to angiography of the upper extremities, starting proximally and working distally. This method will allow the immediate detection of anomalies such as the origin of the radial artery from the axillary artery (1%–3%), or a high origin of either the radial or ulnar arteries from the brachial artery (15%–20%). Failure to use this method may lead to the erroneous diagnosis of a vessel occlusion where none exists. Visipaque (Amersham Health, Princeton, NJ, USA) is the preferred contrast agent for use in upper extremity angiography and is well tolerated by patients. Our practice is to use hand injections of 5–10 cc of contrast with DSA angiography for upper extremity angiography.

Upper extremity intervention

Subclavian artery PTA/stenting

Subclavian artery stenosis is most commonly caused by atherosclerotic disease. Stenosis typically occurs in the first part of the subclavian artery (see **Figure 9**). Within this subset, the majority of stenoses occur proximal to the origin of the vertebral artery (see **Figure 9a**). In reported series, the incidence of left subclavian artery stenosis far exceeds that of right subclavian artery stenosis, but the disparity is less apparent when innominate artery stenosis is included. When occlusion occurs, this almost always extends from the ostium of the subclavian artery to the origin of the vertebral artery (see **Figure 9e**).

Intervention is generally reserved for the treatment of symptomatic patients (see **Table 2**). Symptoms may be attributable to upper extremity, cerebral, or coronary ischemia. Upper extremity ischemic symptoms are uncommon and typically occur only during upper extremity exercise. Stenosis or occlusion distal to the vertebral artery, and in the thyrocervical or costocervical trunks, is more likely to result in ischemic symptomatology as these vessels are a rich source of collateral flow distal to proximal lesions.

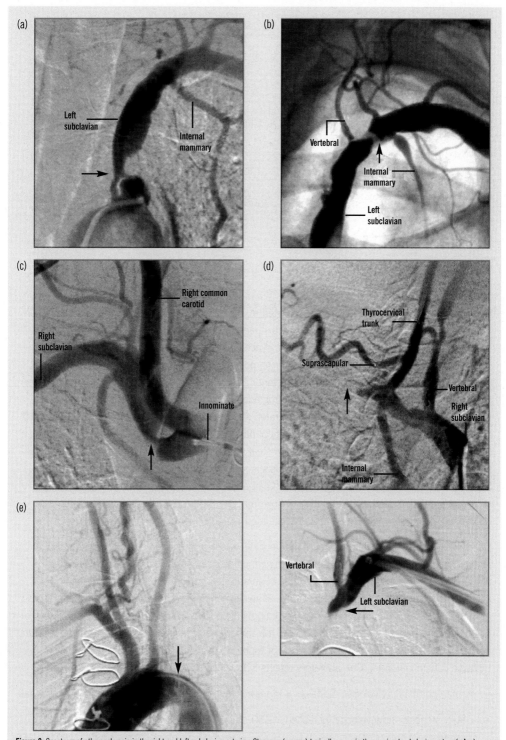

Figure 9. Spectrum of atherosclerosis in the right and left subclavian arteries. Stenoses (arrows) typically occur in the proximal subclavian artery (**a,b,c**). Occlusions may rarely occur distal to the vertebral artery (**d**), but most commonly extend from the subclavian artery ostium to the origin of the vertebral artery (**e**, arrows indicate proximal and distal extent of occlusion).

Indication
Upper limb ischemia
Vertebrobasilar symptoms
Subclavian steal syndrome
• coronary
• cerebral–posterior circulation
Protection of dialysis arteriovenous fistula
Protection of axillofemoral bypass
Protection of axilloaxillary bypass
Protection of LIMA–coronary bypass
Distal embolization

Table 2. Indications for subclavian percutaneous transluminal angioplasty/stenting of subclavian artery stenosis or occlusion. LIMA: left internal mammary artery.

Subclavian steal syndrome was initially reported in 1961 to describe posterior cerebral circulation ischemic symptomatology in patients with proximal subclavian (or innominate) artery disease. Such symptoms include diplopia, nystagmus, syncope, nausea, vertigo, or ataxia related to brainstem ischemia, and cortical blindness or homonymous hemianopsia related to posterior cerebral artery ischemia. Ischemia of the posterior circulation is caused by collateralization of the subclavian artery distal to the stenosis by retrograde flow along the vertebral artery ipsilateral to the subclavian artery stenosis, and is exaggerated during upper extremity exercise (see **Figures 10 and 11**). It is now recognized that the majority of patients with angiographic evidence of subclavian steal are clinically asymptomatic ("subclavian steal phenomenon"). Patients are more likely to be symptomatic if the proximal subclavian stenosis is ipsilateral to the dominant vertebral artery. Subclavian steal from the coronary circulation can also occur in patients with IMA grafts to the coronary circulation, where the shunting of flow from the IMA graft to the subclavian artery may result in coronary ischemia that is exaggerated during upper extremity activity.

Objective evidence of significant subclavian artery stenosis may be discerned from blood pressure recordings from both upper extremities (assuming the absence of significant contralateral disease) and Doppler ultrasound examination. The use of an arm cuff and 5-MHz continuous-wave Doppler allows brachial pressures to be determined. A difference of >15 mm Hg indicates significant disease proximal to the ipsilateral brachial artery. The innominate and subclavian arteries are easily assessed by duplex scanning and pulsed-wave Doppler. It is important to be aware that the normal flow pattern in the upper extremity may be either biphasic or triphasic; this is unlike in the leg, where only a triphasic pattern is normal. Our laboratory reports four basic findings from ultrasound data:

• normal: normal flow velocity, biphasic or triphasic waveform, clear window beneath systolic peak

• $<50\%$ stenosis: flow velocity increased <250 cm/s

• 50%–99% stenosis: flow velocity increased >250 cm/s, poststenotic color bruit

• occlusion: no flow detected

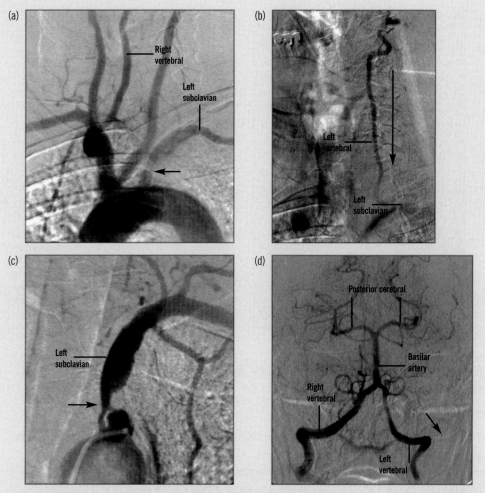

Figure 10. Subclavian artery steal phenomenon. (**a**) The early phase of a left anterior oblique (LAO) arch aortogram with absence of left vertebral artery filling and suspicion of a left subclavian artery lesion (arrow). (**b**) The late phase of an LAO arch aortogram with retrograde filling of the left vertebral artery and late filling of the left subclavian artery. The arrow indicates the direction of flow in the vertebral artery. (**c**) Selective angiography of the left subclavian artery confirms significant proximal stenosis (arrow). (**d**) Selective angiography of the right vertebral artery, showing the mechanism of steal: direct flow from the right to the left vertebral artery at the level of the vertebrobasilar junction. The black arrow indicates the direction of flow in the vertebral artery.

Procedure

Prior to the procedure, all patients should receive 24–48 hours of aspirin therapy (325 mg/day). A preprocedural loading dose of 300–600 mg clopidogrel should also be considered. In general, the femoral approach is preferred and should be successful in close to 100% of cases where the subclavian artery is not occluded. The retrograde brachial approach can be used in some cases of subclavian occlusion (eg, flush occlusion of the left subclavian artery) or where no femoral access is available (eg, aortic occlusion).

Prior to intervention, a high-quality arch aortogram and selective angiography of the affected vessel are required. In particular, the location of the lesion with respect to the ostium of the subclavian artery and the origin of its critical branches (vertebral and IMA) needs to be clearly (a)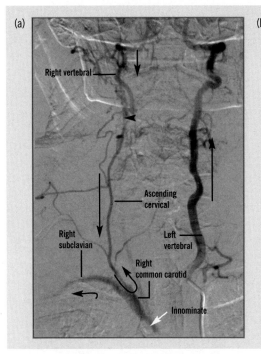

Right vertebral

Ascending
cervical

Right
subclavian

Left
vertebral

Right
common carotid

Innominate

(b)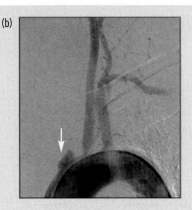

Figure 11. Subclavian steal phenomenon in a patient with innominate artery occlusion (white arrows). Selective angiography of the left vertebral artery shows antegrade flow in the left vertebral artery and retrograde flow into the right vertebral artery from the level of the vertebrobasilar junction. The right vertebral artery is occluded in the upper cervical portion of the vessel. Collateral from the right vertebral to the ascending cervical branch results in filling of the right subclavian artery and common carotid arteries. The black arrows indicate the direction of flow.

demarcated. Following the decision to intervene, heparin is administered as a bolus (70 U/kg) to achieve an ACT of 250–300 seconds.

Subclavian artery stenosis

The strategy used to treat subclavian stenoses is heavily influenced by the anatomy of the lesion, but also varies considerably between operators [3,4]. For nonocclusive stenoses, we prefer to use a guide catheter-based system from the femoral access site, and to stent the lesion where possible (see **Figure 12**). The use of a guide catheter allows greater support and flexibility in strategy during the procedure. An 8-Fr sheath is placed in the femoral artery to allow easy positioning of the stent delivery systems generally required to treat subclavian stenoses. A long (ie, 125-cm) 5-Fr diagnostic catheter (JR4, Vitek) is telescoped through an 8-Fr guide catheter (H-1, multipurpose, JR4). The diagnostic catheter is used to engage the ostium of the vessel. Through the diagnostic catheter, a heavy-support 0.014-inch (Iron Man [Guidant, Indianapolis, IN, USA], Spartacor [Guidant]), 0.018-inch (Flex T [Mallinckrodt]), or soft-tipped 0.035-inch (Wholey, Magic torque) wire is advanced to cross the stenosis. If possible, the diagnostic catheter is advanced across the lesion and the guide is advanced over the diagnostic catheter and positioned proximal to the lesion. The diagnostic catheter is then withdrawn.

Balloon angioplasty is generally required prior to stenting. Where stenting is intended regardless of the angioplasty result, it is wise to be conservative in balloon sizing in order to reduce the risk of distal dissection. For most subclavian arteries, a 5–6 mm × 20–40 mm balloon will allow adequate predilation prior to stenting. For proximal subclavian lesions, the use of balloon-expandable stents is advised because of the need for accurate placement and the high rate of restenosis and stent compression associated with self-expanding stents at this location.

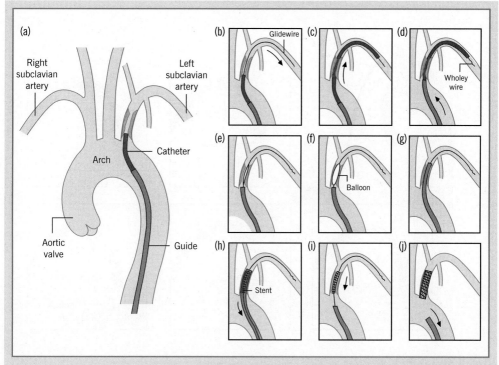

Figure 12. Interventional technique for percutaneous transluminal angioplasty/stenting for stenoses of the subclavian arteries. See text for details.

Balloon-expandable stents in the subclavian artery should be conservatively sized to the vessel size as vessel perforation in this location results in intrathoracic hemorrhage and significant morbidity. Stent sizes will generally vary between 6–8 mm in diameter and 20–40 mm in length. If the lesion involves the subclavian ostium, it is important to ensure that the ostium is adequately covered by the stent. For the left and right subclavian arteries, this is best achieved by angiography in the LAO and RAO views, respectively. It is also advisable not to cover the origins of the vertebral and IMA arteries with the stent. The relation of the stent to these vessels is best determined by using the RAO and LAO views for the left and right subclavian arteries, respectively.

Following angioplasty, some operators will advance the guide across the lesion. The stent is delivered into the guide and positioned across the lesion. The guide is then withdrawn, leaving the stent in position for deployment. This method is likely to reduce the risk of stent embolization, which can occur when the undeployed stent is withdrawn back into the guide. The onset of pain during stent deployment is a sign that further expansion may be associated with an increased risk of dissection or perforation. Final angiography should be performed to confirm the angiographic result and the absence of complications.

Subclavian artery occlusion

Subclavian artery occlusions represent a more challenging technical subset. Most operators prefer to use the retrograde brachial approach, although it is possible to attempt the procedure from the

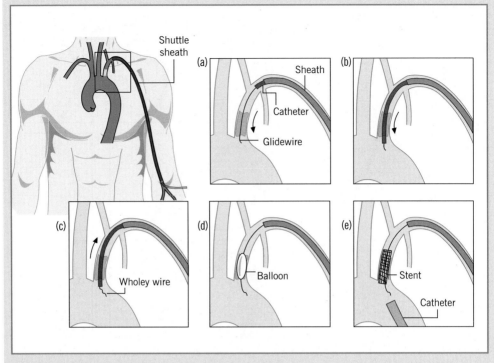

Figure 13. Interventional technique for percutaneous transluminal angioplasty/stenting for occlusions of the subclavian arteries. See text for details.

femoral approach, provided there is a stump that can be engaged with a guide catheter. Typically, we access the brachial artery and position a 6-Fr shuttle sheath (55-cm length) distal to the occlusion (see **Figure 13**). Great care is warranted in delivering this sheath past the subclavian–axillary artery junction as we have found a propensity for dissection at this site. Delivery of the sheath over a stiff Amplatz wire may reduce this risk. Successful crossing of subclavian occlusions generally requires a 0.035-inch glidewire (straight/angled) supported by a glide catheter (angled/sraight) or diagnostic catheter (eg, multipurpose). The use of very steerable stiff 0.014-inch wires (eg, Cross-IT 400XT [Guidant], ASAHI Confianza [Abbott Vascular]) may also be of some benefit in crossing these occlusions. It is imperative to confirm the intraluminal position of the wire immediately distal to the occlusion. If a subclavian artery stump exists, positioning a diagnostic catheter in the stump will give the operator a target to aim for, which should help to maintain an intraluminal position for the wire.

Having crossed the lesion, the technique is similar to that outlined above for nonocclusive stenosis. Positioning of the stent at the ostium of the subclavian artery may be difficult with brachial artery access alone, and some operators will perform angiography in the arch or innominate artery from an additional access site (usually femoral) to aid accurate stent positioning.

Outcomes

The outcome of subclavian artery percutaneous revascularization has been exclusively reported from retrospective case series [5–11]. No randomized studies have compared the outcome of percutaneous versus surgical revascularization, or the outcome for patients treated with angioplasty versus stenting.

Table 3 summarizes the largest of the case series reported. The evolution in technique from angioplasty alone, to angioplasty with provisional stenting, and finally to angioplasty and stenting in all cases reflects the improved outcomes achieved with stenting. The technical success rate in contemporary series approaches 100%. The success rate for total occlusions remains significantly less, but has dramatically improved over the last decade and can approach 90% for experienced operators.

The risk of cerebral embolization or embolization to the ipsilateral limb or IMA artery has been consistently low (<1%) or absent in all of these series. The rarity of embolism to the vertebral artery is probably explained by the delay in the re-establishment of antegrade flow following relief of the proximal obstruction (20 seconds to 20 minutes) [12]. In fact, when cerebral events occur, they are more often related to manipulation of the aortic arch than stenting of the subclavian artery itself. Limb embolization typically occurs in the digits.

Access-site complications are the most common serious adverse events reported (0%–7%), and are closely related to the use of the brachial artery for access. Complications include hematoma formation, thrombosis, and pseudoaneurysm formation. Approximately half of these complications will require operative repair. Stent migration is a real but uncommon complication. Although not specifically reported in all of these series, stent migration probably encompasses the rare event of stent dislodgement off the balloon delivery system and the migration of the stent during deployment, particularly of self-expanding stents. The latter event may result in the vertebral artery ostium being covered. The consequence of this will depend on whether there is resultant plaque shift into the vertebral ostium with compromise of antegrade flow. In addition, the dominance of the ipsilateral vertebral artery and the status of the contralateral vertebral artery will influence the neurological sequelae of any compromise in vertebral artery flow.

The major long-term risk of subclavian artery intervention is restenosis. Stenting appears to have significantly reduced the rate of restenosis, from ~15%–20% with angioplasty to 0%–10%. The treatment for restenosis will depend on its etiology. Failure to cover the ostium of the vessel will require angioplasty of the restenotic area and repeat stenting of the ostium. Inadequate stent expansion may be treated with repeat angioplasty and, sometimes, re-stenting. In the absence of either of these factors, repeat angioplasty with brachytherapy is a reasonable option. Alternatively, surgical revascularization using an extrathoracic approach (carotid–subclavian, axilloaxillary) is a reasonable option in a symptomatic patient who is an operative candidate (see **Figure 14**).

Author	Year	No. patients/ lesions	Lesion type	Procedural success (%)	Interventional strategy	Stent type	Mean follow-up (months)	Restenosis (%)	Complications, n (%) CVA/ TIA	Limb/IMA embolization	Access-site complication	Stent migration
Becker[a,b]	1989	418/423	N/R	92	PTA	N/A	N/R	19	~1%	~1%	N/R	N/A
Millaire	1993	50/50	Occlusion Stenosis	90	PTA	N/A	41	14	1 (2)	0	2 (4)	N/A
Mathias	1993	46/46	Occlusion	83	PTA alone PTA/stent	Wallstent	33	8	0	0	0	0
Kumar	1995	27/31	Occlusion Stenosis	100	PTA/stent	Palmaz	N/R	N/R	0	0	2 (6)	1 (3)
Martinez[c]	1997	17/17	Occlusion	94	Stent	Palmaz Wallstent Strecker	19.4	6	0	0	1 (6)	1 (6)
Sullivan	1998	66/66	Occlusion Stenosis	94	PTA/stent	Palmaz	12.9	5	0	2 (3)	6 (7)	2 (3)
Rodreguez-Lopez	1999	69/69	Occlusion Stenosis	96	PTA/stent	Palmaz Wallstent Strecker	13	10	1 (1.4)	0	4 (6)	1 (1.4)
Al-Mubarak	1999	38/38	Occlusion Stenosis	92	PTA/stent	Palmaz Wallstent	20	6	0	0	0	0

Table 3. Summary of outcomes following subclavian artery percutaneous intervention. [a]Includes patients undergoing innominate and common carotid artery intervention. [b]Data obtained from >13 individual studies. [c]These 17 patients were included in the subsequent series by Rodriguez-Lopez. CVA: cerebrovascular accident; IMA: internal mammary artery; N/A: not applicable; N/R: not reported; PTA: percutaneous transluminal angioplasty; TIA: transient ischemic attack.

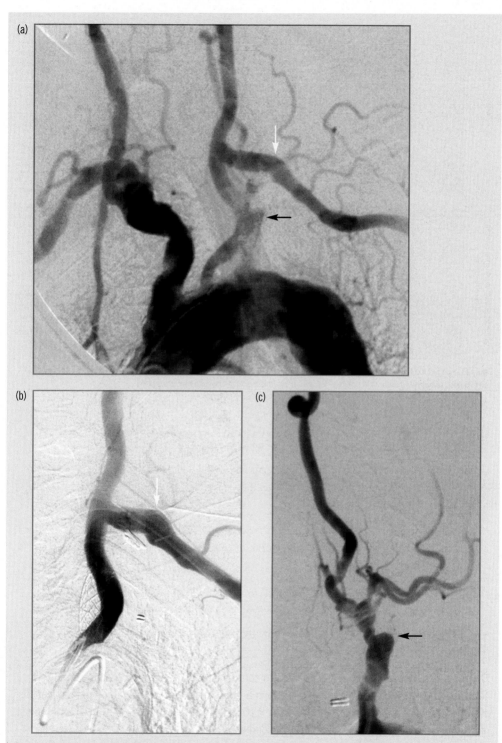

Figure 14. (**a**) Arch aortogram, (**b**) selective left common carotid artery angiogram, and (**c**) selective left subclavian artery angiogram from a patient with occlusive in-stent restenosis of the left subclavian artery who underwent surgical revascularization with an extrathoracic left common carotid to left subclavian artery bypass. Black arrows indicate subclavian artery occlusion. The white arrow indicates the left common carotid to left subclavian artery bypass.

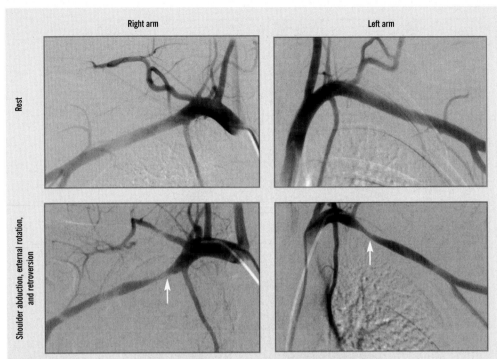

Figure 15. Angiographic illustration of bilateral subclavian artery compression in an 18-year-old male athlete (quarterback) who presented with right subclavian vein thrombosis secondary to thoracic outlet syndrome. The white arrows indicate sites of subclavian artery compression.

Vascular thoracic outlet syndrome

Thoracic outlet syndrome (TOS) refers to compression of the neurovascular structures of the arm (brachial plexus, subclavian artery, and vein) as they leave the thoracic outlet [13]. This outlet is comprised of three separate spaces [14]:

- the scalene triangle, which is bordered by the scalenus anterior (anterior) and medius (posterior) muscles, and the first rib (inferior) – only the brachial plexus and subclavian artery pass through this space

- the costoclavicular space, which is bordered by the first rib (inferior), clavicle (superior), costoclavicular ligament (medial), and scalenus medius muscle (lateral)

- the subcoracoid space, which is bordered by the pectoralis minor muscle (anterior), ribs (posterior), and coracoid process (superior)

Thus, a number of etiologies may contribute to compression of the vascular structures, and compression may occur at more than one site in a given individual. While vascular complications of this syndrome are uncommon, occurring in <10% of patients with TOS, they account for most of the serious morbidity associated with this condition.

Compression of the subclavian artery is usually described in the scalene triangle, but may also occur in the subcoracoid space (see **Figure 15**). A high incidence (>50%) of cervical

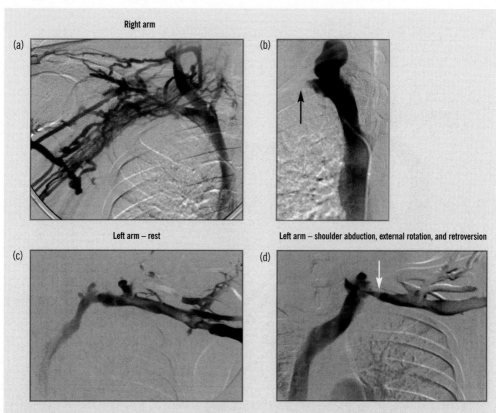

Right arm

(a)

(b)

Left arm – rest

Left arm – shoulder abduction, external rotation, and retroversion

(c)

(d)

Figure 16. Venography from a 23-year-old bowler who presented with right upper extremity swelling. **(a)** Injection of contrast in the right antecubital vein demonstrates features consistent with chronic occlusion of the left subclavian vein with prominent bridging collateral formation. **(b)** Selective venography with a catheter in the right innominate vein showing occlusion of the right subclavian vein (black arrow). **(c,d)** Left antecubital vein injection demonstrating normal filling of the left subclavian vein with the arm in a neutral position, and evidence of compression (white arrow) during shoulder abduction, external rotation, and retroversion.

ribs or anomalous ligamentous bands has been reported in patients with subclavian arterial compression [15]. Trauma to the artery leads to progressive stenosis and occlusion. Typically, there is poststenotic dilatation and aneurysm formation. Mural thrombus may form at the site of the compression or in the aneurysmal segment; the most typical clinical presentation of these patients is thromboembolism to the forearm and digits. Because of collateral formation, ischemic symptoms may be mild or absent. Angiography is useful to confirm the site of the stenosis/occlusion and the presence of aneurysm formation, and to document the presence of distal embolization. Treatment for subclavian artery complications of thoracic outlet compression usually involves surgical decompression of the artery (by release of the scalene muscles and removal of any abnormal bony structures) and surgical repair of any structural damage to the artery.

Subclavian vein complications of TOS are more common than arterial complications, and typically present as subclavian vein thrombosis with pain, edema, and cyanosis in the affected limb (see **Figure 16**). Embolization to the pulmonary circulation is uncommon, but has been reported. The acute treatment involves thrombolysis, followed by anticoagulation. There is general agreement that surgical decompression should be performed in these cases, although the timing (immediate versus delayed) is debated.

(a)

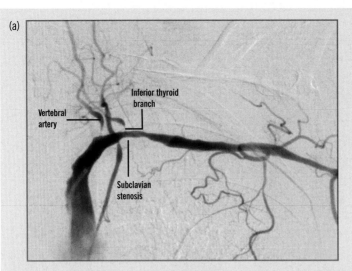

(b)

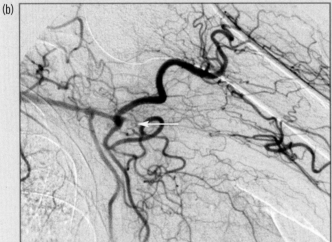

(c)

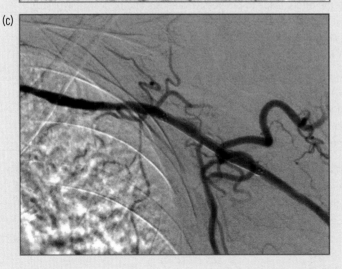

Figure 17. Subclavian and axillary artery angiography in a 63-year-old female with temporal arteritis and critical left hand ischemia. (**a**) Left subclavian and axillary artery, posteroanterior view. Note the smooth ostial lesions in the vertebral and inferior thyroid artery and the smooth, moderate subclavian artery stenosis. (**b**) Left axillary artery, left anterior oblique view. Note the axillary artery occlusion (arrow) and extensive collateralization. (**c**) Left axillary artery following angioplasty and placement of a self-expanding stent for a flow-limiting dissection. The patient had an excellent clinical response with relief of hand ischemia.

Vasculitis type	Vessel(s) involvement	Typical angiographic features
Scleroderma [1]	Small vessels and capillary bed	Multiple focal stenoses and occlusions of ulnar, palmar, and proper digital arteries
		Sparse collateral formation
		Relative sparing of radial artery
Thromboangiitis obliterans [20]	Small and medium-sized arteries and veins	Multiple areas of stenosis and occlusions of palmar, digital, ulnar, and radial arteries
		Extensive collateral formation
		Relative sparing of interosseous artery
Systemic lupus erythematosus [1]	Small arteries and arterioles	Nonspecific angiographic appearance
		Stenoses and occlusions of palmar and digital arteries
Rheumatoid arthritis [20]	Small and medium-sized vessels	Stenoses and occlusions of digital arteries
		Areas of hypervascularization adjacent to affected joints
Temporal arteritis [21]	Large and medium-sized vessels	Stenosis or occlusions with a smooth, tapered appearance
		Predilection for subclavian, axillary, and brachial arteries
		Aneurysmal lesions are uncommon
Takayasu's arteritis [22,23]	Large vessels	Stenosis, occlusions, and aneurysmal formation in affected vessels
		Predilection for arch and its branches (including right and left subclavian arteries)
		Calcification of arterial wall is a typical late feature
		Ostial lesions are common

Table 4. Typical vessel involvement and angiographic features of most common vasculitides.

Vasculitis

Endovascular specialists are infrequently asked to perform upper extremity angiography/ intervention in patients with suspected vasculitis. In patients with large-vessel vasculitis (eg, temporal arteritis, Takayasu's arteritis), angiography is reserved for those with critical ischemia and is helpful to define the extent of disease involvement and the suitability for any revascularization procedure (see **Figure 17**). Revascularization in vasculitis patients is a controversial topic. In the setting of acute vasculitis, medical therapy with immunosuppression is favored, although percutaneous revascularization is indicated if there is impending tissue loss. In the chronic or quiescent phase, revascularization is indicated for symptomatic lesions. Angioplasty or stenting in the setting of vasculitis are thought to be associated with an increased rate of restenosis. Despite the absence of randomized data, the popularity of stent-supported angioplasty in patients with large-vessel vasculitis is increasing [16–19].

Angiography may be helpful in patients with small-vessel vasculitis in whom there is doubt regarding the diagnosis. The most common clinical scenario involves patients with atherosclerotic risk factors and asymmetric acronecrosis. The absence of proximal lesions with thromboembolic potential and the presence of a symmetric bilateral process in the small vessels of the hand is strong supportive evidence of vasculitis. It should be stressed that, apart from defining the vessel size affected, angiography is rarely helpful in differentiating between the various vasculitic processes. Possible exceptions to this rule include the angiographic appearance found in scleroderma, rheumatoid arthritis, and Buerger's disease (see **Table 4**).

References

1. Kadir S. Arteriography of the upper extremities. In: Kadir S, editor. *Diagnostic Angiography*, 1st edn. Philadelphia, PA: WB Saunders Company, 1986:172–206.
2. Moore KL. The upper limb. In: Moore KL, Dalley AF, editors. *Clinically Oriented Anatomy*, 2nd edn. Baltimore, MD: Lippincott, Williams and Wilkins, 1985:626–793.
3. Motarjeme A. Percutaneous transluminal angioplasty of supra-aortic vessels. *J Endovasc Surg* 1996;3:171–81.
4. Zeitler E, Huttl K, Mathias KD. Subclavian and brachial artery diseases. In: Zeitler E, editor. *Radiology of Peripheral Vascular Diseases*, 1st edn. Berlin, Heidelberg, New York: Springer-Verlag, 2000:591–623.
5. Millaire A, Trinca M, Marache P, et al. Subclavian angioplasty: immediate and late results in 50 patients. *Cathet Cardiovasc Diagn* 1993;29:8–17.
6. Mathias KD, Luth I, Haarmann P. Percutaneous transluminal angioplasty of proximal subclavian artery occlusions. *Cardiovasc Intervent Radiol* 1993;16:214–8.
7. Martinez R, Rodriguez-Lopez J, Torruella L, et al. Stenting for occlusion of the subclavian arteries. Technical aspects and follow-up results. *Tex Heart Inst J* 1997;24:23–7.
8. Sullivan TM, Gray BH, Bacharach JM, et al. Angioplasty and primary stenting of the subclavian, innominate, and common carotid arteries in 83 patients. *J Vasc Surg* 1998;28:1059–65.
9. Al-Mubarak N, Liu MW, Dean LS, et al. Immediate and late outcomes of subclavian artery stenting. *Catheter Cardiovasc Interv* 1999;46:169–72.
10. Rodriguez-Lopez JA, Werner A, Martinez R, et al. Stenting for atherosclerotic occlusive disease of the subclavian artery. *Ann Vasc Surg* 1999;13:254–60.
11. Kumar K, Dorros G, Bates MC, et al. Primary stent deployment in occlusive subclavian artery disease. *Cathet Cardiovasc Diagn* 1995;34:281–5.
12. Ringelstein EB, Zeumer H. Delayed reversal of vertebral artery blood flow following percutaneous transluminal angioplasty for subclavian steal syndrome. *Neuroradiology* 1984;26:189–98.
13. Mackinnon SE, Novak CB. Thoracic outlet syndrome. *Curr Probl Surg* 2002;39:1070–145.
14. Novak CB. Thoracic outlet syndrome. *Clin Plast Surg* 2003;30:175–88.
15. Hood DB, Kuehne J, Yellin AE, et al. Vascular complications of thoracic outlet syndrome. *Am Surg* 1997;63:913–7.
16. Nomura M, Kida S, Yamashima T, et al. Percutaneous transluminal angioplasty and stent placement for subclavian and brachiocephalic artery stenosis in aortitis syndrome. *Cardiovasc Intervent Radiol* 1999;22:427–32.
17. Bali HK, Jain S, Jain A, et al. Stent supported angioplasty in Takayasu arteritis. *Int J Cardiol* 1998;66(Suppl. 1): S213–7; discussion S219–20.
18. Maskovic J, Jankovic S, Lusic I, et al. Subclavian artery stenosis caused by non-specific arteritis (Takayasu disease): treatment with Palmaz stent. *Eur J Radiol* 1999;31:193–6.
19. Sharma BK, Jain S, Bali HK, et al. A follow-up study of balloon angioplasty and de-novo stenting in Takayasu arteritis. *Int J Cardiol* 2000;75(Suppl. 1):S147–52.
20. Berger H, Pickel P. Radio-ulnar and hand artery diseases. In: Zeitler E, editor. *Radiology of Peripheral Vascular Diseases*, 1st edn. Berlin, Heidelberg, New York: Springer-Verlag, 2000:625–31.
21. Garcia Vazquez JM, Carreira JM, Seoane C, et al. Superior and inferior limb ischaemia in giant cell arteritis: angiography follow-up. *Clin Rheumatol* 1999;18:61–5.
22. Stanson AW. Imaging findings in extracranial (giant cell) temporal arteritis. *Clin Exp Rheumatol* 2000;18(4 Suppl. 20): S43–8.
23. Sheikhzadeh A, Tettenborn I, Noohi F, et al. Occlusive thromboaortopathy (Takayasu disease): clinical and angiographic features and a brief review of literature. *Angiology* 2002;53:29–40.

9 Carotid and vertebral artery intervention

J Emilio Exaire and Jay S Yadav

Epidemiology of carotid and vertebral disease

Stroke is the third leading cause of death in the USA: approximately 700,000 people will experience a stroke each year, and 20% of the victims will need institutional care for at least 3 months after the event. Nearly 25% of stroke patients will die within a year of the event [1]. The economic burden of this surpasses $50 billion/year in the USA alone.

Ischemic strokes, mostly caused by atherosclerotic vascular stenosis, account for almost 90% of cases. Approximately 75% of ischemic strokes involve the middle cerebral and anterior circulation; the remainder of the events involve the posterior or vertebrobasilar circulation [2].

Basic anatomy

Common carotid artery

The right common carotid artery (CCA) originates at the bifurcation of the brachiocephalic trunk, while the left CCA originates directly from the aorta. A bovine arch, in which the left CCA arises from the innominate artery, occurs in approximately 7%–20% of patients. The CCA bifurcates into the internal carotid artery (ICA) and the external carotid artery (ECA) at the level of the C4–C5 intervertebral space.

Internal carotid artery

The ICA is divided into the prepetrous, petrous, cavernous, and supraclinoid segments (see **Figure 1**). Its first major branch is the ophthalmic artery. The ICA bifurcates into the anterior and middle cerebral arteries in the subarachnoid space. The carotid sinus (containing mechanoreceptors that are responsible for the carotid sinus reflex) is located in the ICA just distal to the bifurcation of the CCA. In most adults, the carotid sinus measures approximately 7 mm in diameter.

External carotid artery

The ECA has an extensive collateral network. Therefore, unilateral stenosis is rarely symptomatic. In patients with contralateral occlusion, however, severe obstruction may cause jaw and tongue claudication. The branches of the ECA are divided into:

- anterior – including the superior thyroid, lingual, and external maxillary
- posterior – including the occipital and posterior auricular
- ascending – ascending pharyngeal
- terminal – including the internal maxillary and superficial temporal arteries

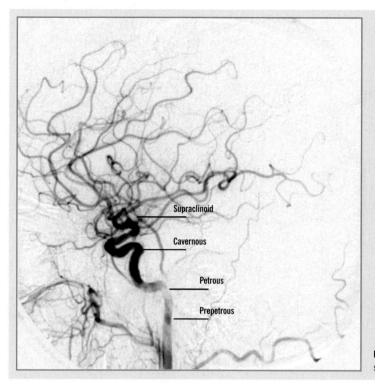

Figure 1. Internal carotid artery segments in a lateral angiogram.

Vertebral artery

The vertebral artery arises from the supraposterior aspect of the first part of the subclavian artery. The left vertebral artery arises directly from the aortic arch in approximately 0.5%–6% of patients. The vertebral artery is divided into three extracranial parts and an intracranial portion, known as V1–V4 (see **Figure 2**) [2]. V1 starts from the origin of the vertebral artery and extends to the fifth or the sixth cervical vertebra, where it enters the transverse foramina. V2 courses within the intervertebral foramina and is known as V3 when behind the atlas. V4 pierces the dura and arachnoid mater at the base of the skull and ends as it meets its opposite vertebral artery to form the midline basilar artery. The V4 segment gives rise to the posterior inferior cerebellar artery (PICA). If compromised, this branch can cause cerebellar and medullary symptoms.

Clinical evaluation

Before intervention, it is important to take a complete history and to conduct a detailed neurological examination. Although the majority of strokes are secondary to carotid or vertebral atherosclerotic disease, other stroke etiologies, such as cardioembolic events, should be thoroughly ruled out. Any pre-existing neurological deficit needs to be carefully assessed when considering intervention. Patients who have experienced a large stroke have an increased risk for postprocedural intracranial hemorrhage. It is advisable to wait 2–4 weeks after a major stroke before performing carotid intervention.

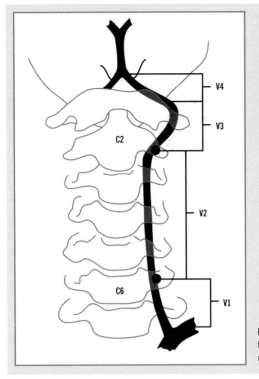

Figure 2. Anatomy of the vertebral artery. Reproduced with permission from Oxford University Press (Cloud GC, Markus HS. Diagnosis and management of vertebral artery stenosis. *QJM* 2003;96:27–54).

Diagnostic studies

Ultrasound

Duplex ultrasonography is the standard noninvasive method for the evaluation of carotid artery stenosis [3–7]. NASCET (North American Symptomatic Carotid Endarterectomy Trial) showed a low sensitivity and specificity for ultrasound (68% and 67%, respectively) [8]; however, ACAS (Asymptomatic Carotid Atherosclerosis Study) increased the specificity to 95% by adopting a standard protocol that correlated abnormal Doppler measurements with carotid arteriography [9].

Ultrasound scans are limited in several ways. Firstly, they are technician dependent and can either overestimate or underestimate the stenosis. Secondly, extensive and calcified disease may obstruct distal visualization. Likewise, tortuous vessels and contralateral disease may result in a false increase in velocity [10].

Vertebral ultrasound

Almost the whole length of the vertebral arteries can be assessed with Doppler ultrasound. However, the artery origin can only be imaged in 60% of subjects [2]. Transcranial Doppler ultrasound can be used to detect intracranial vertebral stenosis, but it often underestimates the severity of the lesion. Ultrasound has a sensitivity of ~76% in detecting vertebral artery stenosis.

Magnetic resonance angiography

Two-dimensional time-of-flight (TOF) and three-dimensional multislab TOF magnetic resonance angiography (MRA) techniques can evaluate the extracranial carotid artery up to its bifurcation. This segment is relatively motionless, superficial, and large enough for visualization. These techniques also, however, have their limitations. Turbulent flow can cause pseudostenosis in a normal bulbous bifurcation. Likewise, a tight focal stenosis can cause distal turbulence with a large flow gap, mimicking a long stenosis. Swallowing can also cause marked artifacts. Finally, any metal, such as a stent or clips, can degrade the image.

Three-dimensional contrast-enhanced MRA provides reliable imaging of the carotids from their origin to the intracranial branches [11]. MRA has a sensitivity of 75% and specificity of 88%. Concordant noninvasive testing with Doppler ultrasound and MRA improves both the sensitivity and specificity (96% and 85%, respectively) [12]. Contrast-enhanced MRA is limited by interference from contrast in the jugular vein, which may impair visualization of the carotid artery.

Vertebral magnetic resonance angiography

The posterior circulation can be assessed by gadolinium-enhanced MRA. This has high sensitivity and specificity (97% and 99%, respectively) [11].

Angiography

Angiography remains the gold standard in assessing both the severity and the characteristics of vascular stenosis. It allows simultaneous study of the origin of the neck vessels and the intracranial circulation. The collateral circulation can also be easily assessed. This is helpful, especially in predicting the safety of temporary carotid occlusion associated with stenting. Risks associated with angiography include embolization and dissection, but these seldom occur, particularly when angiography is performed with meticulous technique in the cardiac catheterization laboratory [13].

Angiographic diagnostic images

The first picture to be obtained is an aortic arch angiogram (45° left anterior oblique) with an adequate field to view the origin of the innominate artery and both carotid bifurcations. This can be performed using a 5-Fr pigtail catheter with 30 cc of nonionic contrast injected over 2 seconds. Selective engagement of both carotids is then performed, obtaining both an ipsilateral 30° oblique and lateral angiogram. Next, intracranial views of both carotids are obtained using both the posteroanterior (PA) – with slight cranial angulation – and lateral views.

The vertebral arteries are better viewed in contralateral oblique projections, which allow visualization of the ostia. The dominant vertebral artery should be assessed with a nonselective injection, obtaining intracranial views of the vertebrobasilar system in lateral and steep PA cranial projections. An inflated blood pressure cuff on the ipsilateral arm is helpful during nonselective vertebral injections. The collateral circulation to the brain hemisphere of interest needs to be defined. It also needs to be assessed before using occlusive emboli protection devices (EPDs), since an absence of collaterals may predict intraprocedural neurological symptoms.

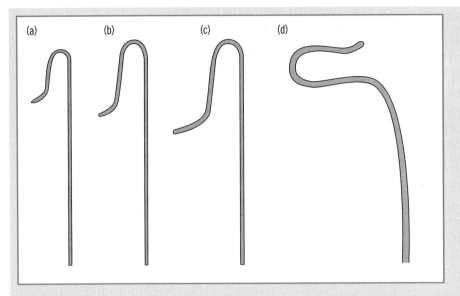

Figure 3. Diagnostic catheters for cerebral angiography: **(a)** Simmons 1; **(b)** Simmons 2; **(c)** Simmons 3; **(d)** Vitek (Cook, Bloomington, IN, USA).

Depending on the aortic arch configuration, several catheters may be used to perform cerebral angiography (see **Figure 3**). The aortic arch can be classified into three types based on the distance of the origin of the innominate artery from the top of the arch. The widest diameter of the left CCA is used as a reference unit. In a type I arch, the innominate artery originates within one diameter length from the top of the arch. In a type II arch, the innominate artery originates within two diameter lengths from the top of the arch. In a type III arch, the innominate artery originates more than two diameter lengths from the top of the arch (see **Figure 4**).

Patient selection

Procedural complications are more frequent in patients with the following conditions [14,15]:

* medical – elderly, cardiac, or pulmonary patients, acute stroke, coagulopathy, or low platelets

* anatomic – lesions that are too high (eg, intracranial) or too low (eg, common carotid origin), presence of thrombus, restenosis, tortuosity, contralateral occlusion, severe calcification, or poor access [16,17]

Severely stenotic lesions with slow flow, angiographic thrombus, or heavy calcification should be avoided by inexperienced interventionalists. Generally, treatments for bilateral carotid artery stenosis should be staged at least 30 days apart. In unusual circumstances, however, both carotids can be treated during one procedure. The major risks are profound bradycardia and hypotension due to stimulation of both carotid sinuses and cerebral hyperperfusion syndrome. Careful periprocedural medical management is necessary in these challenging patients [18].

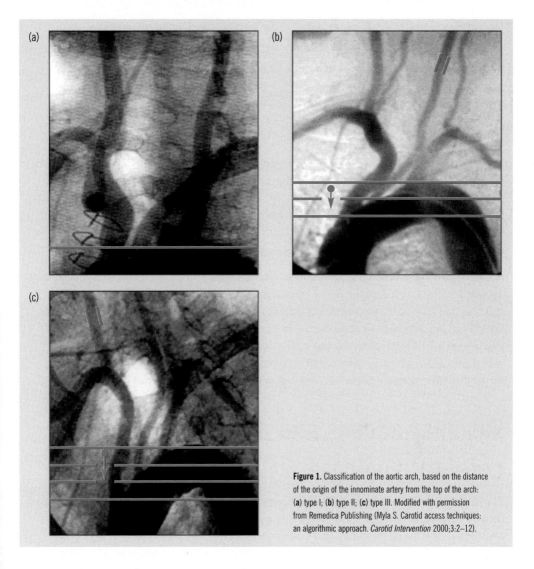

Figure 1. Classification of the aortic arch, based on the distance of the origin of the innominate artery from the top of the arch: (a) type I; (b) type II; (c) type III. Modified with permission from Remedica Publishing (Myla S. Carotid access techniques: an algorithmic approach. *Carotid Intervention* 2000;3:2–12).

Antiplatelet and anticoagulant therapy

Aspirin

Aspirin should be given up to a total of 325 mg daily 3 days before the procedure [19], and continued for at least 30 days after the intervention.

Clopidogrel

Clopidogrel should be given up to a total of 75 mg daily 5–7 days before the procedure, or a 600 mg loading dose should be given at least 2 hours before the procedure. Clopidogrel should be continued for at least 30 days after the intervention.

Heparin

A total of 50–100 U/kg should be given to maintain an activated clotting time (ACT) of 275–300 seconds. It is important to maintain the ACT within these limits when using EPDs, since they partially occlude blood flow and have the potential to cause thrombosis. Low molecular weight heparin is an alternative, but there are few data in this regard.

Bivalirudin

In a small study, 33 patients undergoing carotid stenting received bivalirudin (bolus of 0.75 mg/kg followed by an infusion of 1.75 mg/kg/h for the duration of the procedure) without concomitant glycoprotein (GP)IIb/IIIa receptor antagonists [20]. There were no procedural major adverse events in this small cohort. One patient suffered a major stroke after the procedure.

Glycoprotein IIb/IIIa receptor antagonists

Routinely used in the absence of EPD (but not recommended if EPDs are used), GPIIb/IIIa receptor antagonists appear to reduce the risk of periprocedural stroke [21]. Careful heparin dosage (50 U/kg and ACT ~250 seconds) is important to minimize the bleeding risk. GPIIb/IIIa receptor antagonists can potentially increase the risk of intracranial hemorrhage. In cases of emergent intervention, a GPIIb/IIIa receptor antagonists should be used while the patient is being loaded with aspirin and clopidogrel. Careful postprocedure blood pressure control is important (keeping the systolic blood pressure below 140 mm Hg) in minimizing the intracranial bleeding risk.

Vascular access and diagnostic cerebral angiography

The femoral approach is preferred. Since all currently available carotid stents have 6-Fr or smaller delivery systems, a long 6-Fr sheath or an 8-Fr guiding catheter should be used. In general, the approach is dictated by the nature of the aortic arch. A type I arch is relatively straightforward; type II or type III arches have more difficult access since the catheter approaching from the descending aorta will tend to prolapse into the ascending aorta as it is pushed into these deep-seated arteries [22].

Carotid selective engagement

The telescoping access system

A 125-cm long, 5-Fr JR4 or Vitek catheter (Cook, Bloomington, IN, USA) is inserted through a 90-cm long, 6-Fr Cook Shuttle sheath or an 8-Fr H1 guide (Cordis, Miami Lakes, FL, USA). The diagnostic catheter is passed through the Tuohy–Borst adaptor. An angled 0.035-inch glidewire or a Wholey wire (Mallinckrodt, Hazelwood, MO, USA) is passed through the diagnostic catheter (see **Figure 5**). The diagnostic catheter is used to engage the innominate or left CCA, and a roadmap of the carotid bifurcation is performed. The wire is then advanced through the diagnostic catheter into the distal CCA or ECA, and the diagnostic catheter is advanced into the

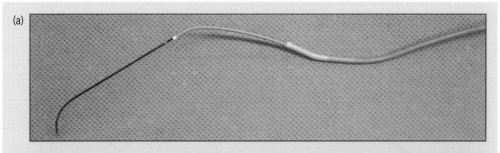

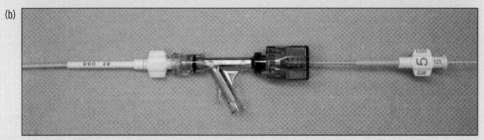

Figure 5. Telescoping access system. (**a**) Distal aspect showing the Wholey wire, 125 cm 5-Fr JR4 catheter, and H1 guide. (**b**) Proximal aspect showing the H1 guide attached to the Tuohy–Borst adaptor. The JR4 catheter passes through the Tuohy–Borst adaptor. The Wholey wire is passed through the JR4 catheter.

mid CCA over the wire. Both the diagnostic catheter and the wire are used as a rail to advance the sheath or guiding catheter into the mid CCA. The diagnostic catheter and wire are then withdrawn. Any debris should be flushed back through the Tuohy–Borst adaptor.

Approaches

For type I or II arches, a coronary approach can be used and the CCA can be directly engaged with an H1 guide catheter. This approach, however, requires a great deal of experience; the sequential approach is recommended for inexperienced interventionalists.

The sequential over-the-wire approach is the safest [23]. This technique is also useful for type III arch anatomy. A Vitek or Simmons catheter is engaged in the CCA and a roadmap is performed to separate the ECA and ICA. A 0.035-inch Glidewire (Terumo, Somerset, NJ, USA) is advanced into the ECA and the diagnostic catheter is advanced over the wire. The wire is exchanged for a stiff Amplatz wire and the diagnostic catheter is removed. A long 6-Fr sheath or an 8-Fr guide catheter with a long 5-Fr diagnostic catheter is then advanced. In cases of severe disease in the distal CCA or ECA occlusion, care should be taken to keep the wire from going through the lesion; a guide catheter approach is easier in these cases. In the presence of severe disease of the CCA ostium, the telescoping approach should not be used since the small gap between the diagnostic catheter and sheath edge may cause plaque dissection or embolization. The sheath should be advanced over the dilator to minimize trauma. With very severe ostial disease, it is necessary to treat the ostium before proceeding to the ICA. These are challenging cases and should only be treated by an experienced operator. A brachial or transradial approach can also be used (the right carotid artery should be accessed via the left brachial artery and *vice versa*). For these lesions, a 6-Fr Ansel sheath (Cook) (see **Figure 6**) is used with a Simmons 1, 1.5, or 2 catheter. The catheter is introduced into the contralateral CCA and a stiff Amplatz wire is

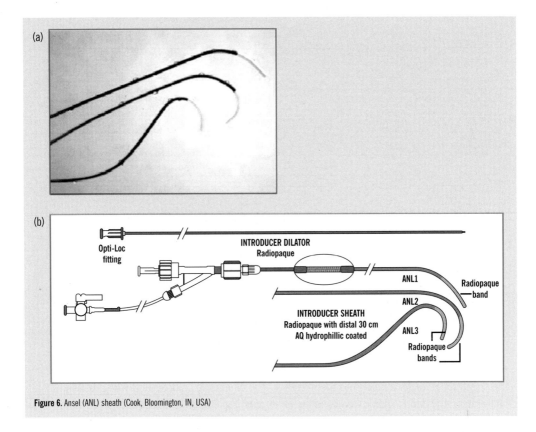

Figure 6. Ansel (ANL) sheath (Cook, Bloomington, IN, USA)

placed into the ECA. The Simmons catheter is removed and replaced with the introducer, tracking the Ansel sheath into the CCA. The curve of the Ansel sheath works well for this purpose.

For bovine arches, it is often faster to use an Amplatz left 1 guide to engage the ostium and proximal left CCA. This approach is particularly helpful when a bovine arch is combined with severe CCA disease or occlusion of the ECA such that it is not possible to move a 0.035-inch wire very far into the left CCA. It is occasionally necessary to place a stiff 0.014- or 0.018-inch wire in the CCA or ECA to maintain guide stability.

Vertebral selective engagement

A coronary approach using a 6-Fr JR4 internal mammary artery or multipurpose guide catheter is suitable to perform the intervention.

Emboli protection devices

Embolization occurs in every interventional procedure, but acquires more relevance for carotid and vertebral stenting [24,25]. Emboli are most commonly released after stent deployment and postdilatation [26,27]. Once the guide catheter or sheath is in place, an appropriate

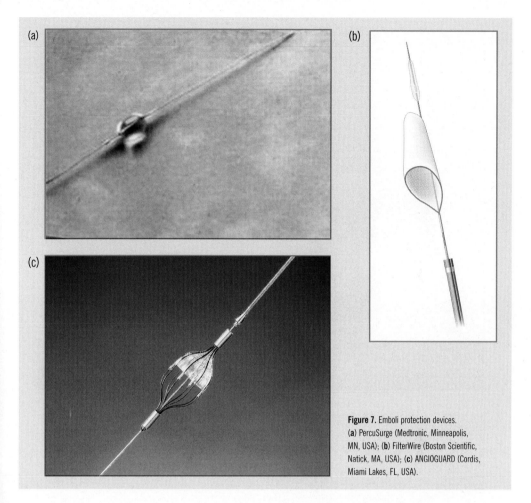

Figure 7. Emboli protection devices. (a) PercuSurge (Medtronic, Minneapolis, MN, USA); (b) FilterWire (Boston Scientific, Natick, MA, USA); (c) ANGIOGUARD (Cordis, Miami Lakes, FL, USA).

working view must be selected. This view should allow clear delineation of the lesion with minimal overlap of the ECA and ICA. At this point, the lesion is crossed with the EPD. Once the EPD reaches a straight segment of the ICA in the prepetrous portion, it is deployed. Correct apposition is then confirmed by obtaining an angiogram. The ANGIOGUARD (Cordis) will show four markers when it is fully deployed. The Filter Wire EX (Boston Scientific) needs to be checked in two different fluoroscopic projections (lateral to show the crescent, anteroposterior to show an open loop). The PercuSurge occludes flow; therefore, a stagnant column of dye will be shown when injecting dye.

EPDs can be divided into occlusive and nonocclusive devices (see **Figures 7–9**) [28–33]. Occlusive devices can be further subdivided into distal occlusion and proximal occlusion types. Nonocclusive devices include filters, which can be subdivided into those with supportive nitinol endoskeletons and those that resemble a windsock. Familiarity with a number of devices will allow the appropriate selection for a particular lesion and anatomy.

An angiogram should be performed to confirm either complete occlusion with distal occlusion devices or complete apposition of the filter wire. In lesions with thrombus, proximal occlusion

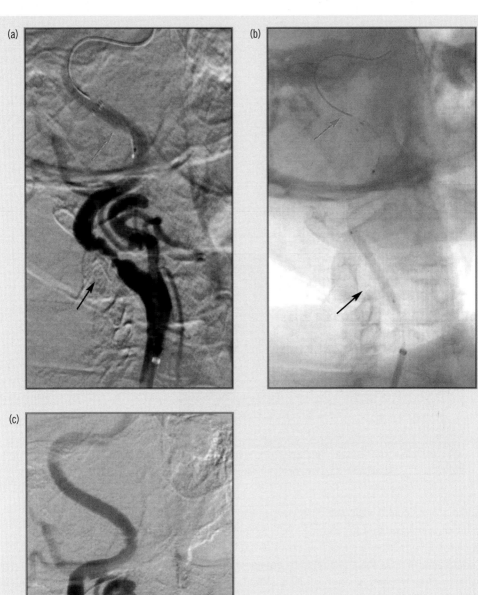

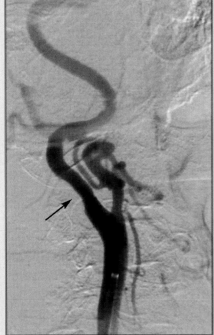

Figure 8. (**a**) A severe internal carotid artery lesion (black arrow). An ANGIOGUARD (Cordis, Miami Lakes, FL, USA) is positioned distal to the lesion (orange arrow). (**b**) Stent deployment (black arrow). Notice the ANGIOGUARD position (orange arrow). (**c**) The final result after postdilatation.

(a)

(b)

(c)

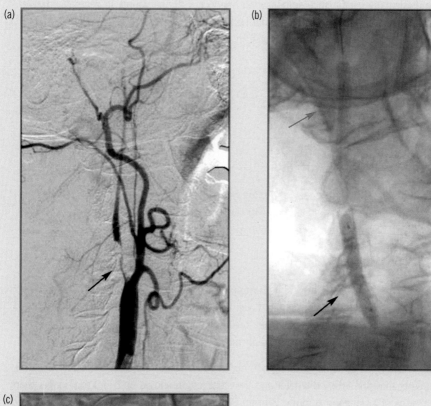
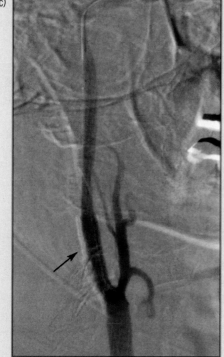

Figure 9. (a) A severe internal carotid artery lesion (arrow).
(b) A PercuSurge (Medtronic, Minneapolis, MN, USA) is inflated
distal to the lesion (orange arrow) and the stent is deployed (black
arrow). (c) The final result after aspiration and PercuSurge deflation.

devices are particularly useful since embolization may occur during wiring. In general, however, lesions with angiographic thrombus should not be treated. The patient should be placed on warfarin and the angiogram should be repeated in 4–6 weeks.

Predilatation, stent selection, and postdilatation

Predilatation

Since most carotid lesions are stenotic and often heavily calcified or have a fibrous scar from previous endarterectomy, brief predilatation (30 seconds) is almost always necessary. Usually a coronary or peripheral balloon (4-mm × 20-mm or 4-mm × 30-mm) is sufficient.

Stent selection

For most cases, the Wallstent biliary stent (Boston Scientific, Natick, MA, USA) or a nitinol stent (Precise [Cordis], Dynalink [Guidant, Indianapolis, IN, USA]) may be used. The Wallstent needs to be oversized lengthwise, since it undergoes foreshortening and has reduced radial force. A 10-mm × 20-mm size is usually adequate for most lesions.

Nitinol stents have minimal foreshortening and higher radial force; the stent diameter should be 1–2 mm greater than the artery diameter and the stent length should be 5–10 mm longer than the lesion. For most lesions, an 8-mm × 30-mm Precise nitinol stent is appropriate. Nitinol stents keep expanding after placement and, depending upon vessel compliance, will reach close to their nominal diameter over time. They should not be grossly oversized. For more discrete lesions in the mid ICA, a 7-mm × 20-mm Precise stent is usually adequate.

When selecting a stent, attention should be paid to tortuosity or kinking of the distal ICA above the lesion. Placement of a stiff sheath in the CCA accentuates the kinking by pushing up on the artery – pulling the sheath down can help to relieve it. Having the patient tilt their head back and turn their head to the contralateral side will also help to reduce the kinking. Placing a stent, however, does not reduce distal tortuosity or kinking and, indeed, usually worsens it by reducing arterial compliance. The kink can be pushed closer to the skull base, where it is even more difficult to treat. For severe carotid artery redundancy, surgical shortening of the artery is the treatment of choice.

Postdilatation

A 0.014-inch-based monorail balloon is appropriate for postdilatation, such as the Viatrac (Guidant) or the Aviator (Cordis). These balloons are available up to 6-mm diameter, which is adequate for most ICAs. Extremely aggressive postdilatation is generally not indicated since nitinol stents tend to keep expanding. Residual stenosis of 10%–20% is acceptable at the time of the procedure. Postdilatation of the stent is the most emboligenic part of the procedure; therefore, care should be taken to ensure that the EPD is in a good position and well apposed to the vessel wall.

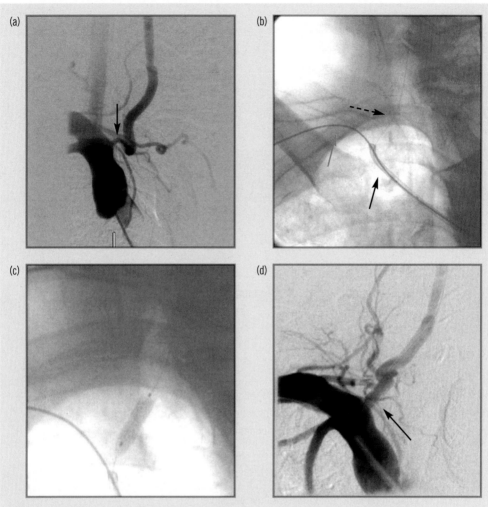

Figure 10. (a) A proximal right vertebral lesion. (b) A multipurpose A-1 guide is in position (arrow). A Wholey wire (Mallinckrodt, Hazelwood, MO, USA) is left in the subclavian artery for support (orange arrow). A coronary wire is used to cross the lesion (dashed arrow). (c) Stent deployment. (d) The final result.

Vertebral stents

Most of the time, a balloon-expandable coronary stent can be used in the vertebral circulation [34]. Predilatation and postdilatation can be safely performed with coronary balloons (see **Figure 10**). The current EPDs are relatively difficult to use in the vertebral artery and their routine use is not recommended.

Hemodynamic management

The carotid sinus reflex is generally fully activated during postdilatation of the stent. The carotid sinus contains mechanoreceptors that function as baroreceptors for blood pressure (see **Figure 11**). The receptors are located in the adventitia, and the media in the carotid sinus

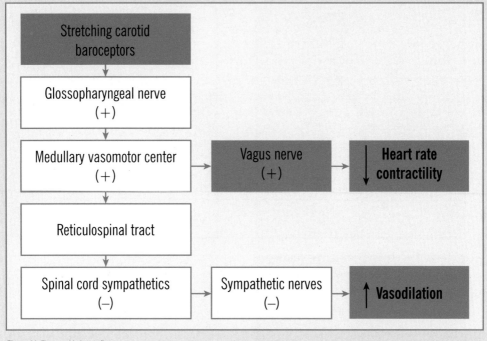

Figure 11. The carotid sinus reflex.

is thinner than in the remainder of the carotid, allowing effective transmission of intra-arterial pressure. Carotid sinus stimulation is most vigorous when the lesion is in the proximal ICA. The carotid sinus reflex has two distinct components:

- a chronotropic component, which affects the sinus and atrioventricular nodes and leads to bradycardia

- a vasodilatory component, which leads to hypotension

Bradycardia is typically short lived, but the vasodilatory response may be much more persistent. The bradycardia will typically respond to anticholinergic drugs such as atropine. Atropine should not be used routinely because it has significant side effects, particularly in elderly patients. Patients often develop urinary retention, severe dry mouth, and may become confused. Also, some patients develop significant tachycardia, which may lead to myocardial ischemia in the presence of significant coronary artery disease.

The vasodilator response is best treated with aggressive volume expansion, which should be performed prior to dilatation of the stent. In severe cases, vasoconstrictors such as pseudoephedrine, norepinephrine, or dopamine are indicated.

The routine insertion of a temporary pacemaker is not indicated. Patients with severe congestive heart failure, critical aortic stenosis, or left main disease are at particular risk for developing severe bradycardia or hypotension. A pulmonary artery catheter is indicated in these patients, with the prompt availability of a pacemaker.

EPD removal

When using the filter-type EPD, it is mandatory that an angiogram is performed to assess flow prior to collapse of the filter. When large amounts of emboli are released, the filter surface may become covered, leading to reduced or absent flow in the ICA (spasm can also reduce flow, but this is usually relieved by intra-arterial nitroglycerin). The stagnant column of blood in the ICA contains suspended particles; if the filter is collapsed at this point, these particles will be carried distally into the brain. Therefore, it is important to aspirate the ICA prior to collapse of the filter. This can be performed with a 125-cm long, 5-Fr multipurpose catheter; the aspiration catheter for the PercuSurge device can also be used.

When the EPD is withdrawn from the guide catheter, the Tuohy-Borst adaptor should be fully opened and some bleed-back allowed in case particles have been released into the guide catheter during withdrawal of the EPD. At the end of the procedure, PA and lateral intracranial views should be taken; an angiogram of the CCA should be performed when the guide catheter is being withdrawn to ascertain whether there has been any damage to the CCA.

Management of neurological complications

Brief neurological examinations should be performed after every maneuver in the carotid artery that could cause embolization – including placement of the guide catheter, traversing of the lesion with the EPD, predilatation, stent placement, postdilatation, and EPD guide catheter withdrawal. Asking the patient to speak and move the contralateral arm and leg is sufficient to assure yourself of the integrity of the major neurological pathways.

The use of EPDs has substantially reduced the risk of intraprocedural stroke. Occasionally, however, the patient will develop a neurologic deficit during the procedure. This may be related to hemodynamic ischemia resulting from flow obstruction by the EPD. In these instances, the procedure should be completed rapidly and additional heparin given if the ACT is below 300 seconds. Once the procedure is complete and the EPD removed, the patient should be reassessed. If a neurological deficit is still present, PA and lateral intracranial angiography should be performed. If there is no evidence of occlusion of the middle or anterior cerebral arteries, or one of their major branches, the patient will almost always make a full recovery within a few hours. Medical management should be started with attention to volume status and maintenance of adequate blood pressure.

If the M1 or M2 segment of the middle cerebral artery is occluded, intervention is generally required since these patients will not make a spontaneous recovery. The material involved is typically a fragment of the plaque. A mechanical approach is often effective in these rare instances. A soft hydrophilic guidewire, such as the Whisper (Guidant) or Synchro (Precision Vascular, West Valley City, UT, USA), is used to traverse the blockage; occasionally, this is sufficient to restore flow. A small 1.5- to 2.0-mm coronary balloon may also be advanced to the occlusion and gentle dilatation will often dislodge the plaque fragment. Adjuvant therapy with intra-arterial tissue plasminogen activator or a GPIIb/IIIa receptor antagonist is occasionally indicated, but care should be taken to avoid intracranial hemorrhage, particularly in the setting of a high ACT or severe hypertension. It should be remembered that patients will generally survive an ischemic stroke, but not an intracranial hemorrhage. Although unusual, it is possible for patients to embolize a few hours after placement of the stent. This can be due to plaque fragments protruding through the stent struts.

Blood pressure control

Blood pressure management is critical and the systolic blood pressure should be kept between 140 and 90 mm Hg. In hypotensive patients, volume expansion with normal saline is generally sufficient. Oral pseudoephedrine (30–120 mg every 6 hours) can be very helpful. Intravenous dopamine may sometimes be necessary. Hypertension can lead to cerebral hyperperfusion syndrome and intracranial hemorrhage. A combination of intravenous β-blockers and nitroglycerin is useful to control acute hypertension.

Since carotid stenting typically lowers the patient's blood pressure for a few days postprocedure, antihypertensive medications are often stopped in the hospital. If the patient does not restart antihypertensive medications then they may suffer an intracranial hemorrhage when their hypertension returns. It is critical that their blood pressure is checked every day after returning home and that their antihypertensive medications are restarted as it returns to baseline.

Cerebral hyperperfusion syndrome

Patients with chronic cerebral hypoperfusion have maximal dilatation of intracranial arterioles and normal cerebral autoregulation may not be restored for several days following intervention. After either surgical or percutaneous revascularization, the patient may develop cerebral hyperperfusion syndrome. The clinical picture includes a headache (ipsilateral to the carotid stent), which may progress to a focal neurologic deficit, confusion, stupor, and death. Early recognition is critical since intracranial hemorrhage occurs in 0.9% of patients. Risk factors include more than 90% stenosis, contralateral occlusions, and severe hypertension [35]. Diuretics and β-blockers are the mainstays of treatment. Vasodilators should be used cautiously since inappropriate dilation of the intracranial arteries is part of the syndrome.

Follow-up

Follow-up is scheduled at 1 month, 6 months, and yearly thereafter. Carotid ultrasound is performed at 6-month and annual visits.

Conclusion

The overall risk of major stroke, death, or myocardial infarction for carotid stenting with the use of EPD is approximately 3%, roughly half that of carotid endarterectomy. In experienced hands, this is a safe procedure with excellent acute and long-term results. In contrast to coronary intervention, in-stent restenosis occurs in <5% of carotid stents. The availability of EPD and the familiarity of the interventionalist with these devices will make carotid artery stenting the revascularization strategy of choice for occlusive carotid artery disease.

References

1. American Heart Association. *Heart Disease and Stroke Statistics – 2003 Update*. Dallas, Texas: American Heart Association, 2002.
2. Cloud GC, Markus HS. Diagnosis and management of vertebral artery stenosis. *QJM* 2003;96:27–54.
3. Erdoes LS, Marek JM, Mills JL, et al. The relative contributions of carotid duplex scanning, magnetic resonance angiography, and cerebral arteriography to clinical decisionmaking: a prospective study in patients with carotid occlusive disease. *J Vasc Surg* 1996;23:950–6.
4. Chervu A, Moore WS. Carotid endarterectomy without arteriography. *Ann Vasc Surg* 1994;8:296–302.
5. Dawson DL, Zierler RE, Strandness DE Jr, et al. The role of duplex scanning and arteriography before carotid endarterectomy: a prospective study. *J Vasc Surg* 1993;18:673–80; discussion 680–3.
6. Horn M, Michelini M, Greisler HP, et al. Carotid endarterectomy without arteriography: the preeminent role of the vascular laboratory. *Ann Vasc Surg* 1994;8:221–4.
7. Mattos MA, Hodgson KJ, Faught WE, et al. Carotid endarterectomy without angiography: is color-flow duplex scanning sufficient? *Surgery* 1994;116:776–82; discussion 782–3.
8. Eliasziw M, Rankin RN, Fox AJ, et al. Accuracy and prognostic consequences of ultrasonography in identifying severe carotid artery stenosis. North American Symptomatic Carotid Endarterectomy Trial (NASCET) Group. *Stroke* 1995;26:1747–52.
9. Howard G, Baker WH, Chambless LE, et al. An approach for the use of Doppler ultrasound as a screening tool for hemodynamically significant stenosis (despite heterogeneity of Doppler performance). A multicenter experience. Asymptomatic Carotid Atherosclerosis Study Investigators. *Stroke* 1996;27:1951–7.
10. Sidhu PS. Ultrasound of the carotid and vertebral arteries. *Br Med Bull* 2000;56:346–66.
11. Clifton AG. MR angiography. *Br Med Bull* 2000;56:367–77.
12. Johnston DC, Goldstein LB. Clinical carotid endarterectomy decision making: noninvasive vascular imaging versus angiography. *Neurology* 2001;56:1009–15.
13. Fayed AM, White CJ, Ramee SR, et al. Carotid and cerebral angiography performed by cardiologists: cerebrovascular complications. *Catheter Cardiovasc Interv* 2002;55:277–80.
14. Wholey MH, Wholey M, Matias K, et al. Global experience in cervical carotid artery stent placement. *Catheter Cardiovasc Interv* 2000;50:160–7.
15. Roubin GS, New G, Iyer SS, et al. Immediate and late clinical outcomes of carotid artery stenting in patients with symptomatic and asymptomatic carotid artery stenosis: a 5-year prospective analysis. *Circulation* 2001;103:532–7.
16. Yadav JS, Roubin GS, King P, et al. Angioplasty and stenting for restenosis after carotid endarterectomy. Initial experience. *Stroke* 1996;27:2075–9.
17. Ouriel K, Hertzer NR, Beven EG, et al. Preprocedural risk stratification: identifying an appropriate population for carotid stenting. *J Vasc Surg* 2001;33:728–32.
18. Chen MS, Bhatt DL, Mukherjee D, et al. Feasibility of simultaneous bilateral carotid artery stenting. *Catheter Cardiovasc Interv* 2004;61:437–42..
19. Bhatt DL, Kapadia SR, Bajzer CT, et al. Dual antiplatelet therapy with clopidogrel and aspirin after carotid artery stenting. *J Invasive Cardiol* 2001;13:767–71.
20. Adamyan Y, News G, Vitek J, et al. Feasibility and safety of bivalirudin during carotid stenting: results of the pilot study. *Am J Cardiol* 2002;90(Suppl. 6A):55H.
21. Kapadia SR, Bajzer CT, Ziada KM, et al. Initial experience of platelet glycoprotein IIb/IIIa inhibition with abciximab during carotid stenting: a safe and effective adjunctive therapy. *Stroke* 2001;32:2328–32.
22. Myla S. Carotid access techniques: an algorithmic approach. *Carotid Intervention* 2001;3:2–12.
23. Yoo BS, Lee SH, Kim JY, et al. A case of transradial carotid stenting in a patient with total occlusion of the distal abdominal aorta. *Catheter Cardiovasc Interv* 2002;56:243–5.
24. Topol EJ, Yadav JS. Recognition of the importance of embolization in atherosclerotic vascular disease. *Circulation* 2000;101:570–80.
25. Ohki T, Marin ML, Lyon RT, et al. Ex vivo human carotid artery bifurcation stenting: correlation of lesion characteristics with embolic potential. *J Vasc Surg* 1998;27:463–71.
26. Rapp JH, Pan XM, Sharp FR, et al. Atheroemboli to the brain: size threshold for causing acute neuronal cell death. *J Vasc Surg* 2000;32:68–76.
27. Grube E, Gerckens U, Yeung AC, et al. Prevention of distal embolization during coronary angioplasty in saphenous vein grafts and native vessels using porous filter protection. *Circulation* 2001;104:2436–41.
28. Dietz A, Berkefeld J, Theron JG, et al. Endovascular treatment of symptomatic carotid artery stenosis using stent placement: long-term follow-up of patients with a balanced surgical risk/benefit ratio. *Stroke* 2001;32:1855–9.
29. Al-Mubarak N, Roubin GS, Vitek JJ, et al. Effect of the distal-balloon protection system on microembolization during carotid stenting. *Circulation* 2001;104:1999–2002.

30. Tubler T, Schluter M, Dirsch O, et al. Balloon-protected carotid artery stenting: relationship of periprocedural neurological complications with the size of particulate debris. *Circulation* 2001;104:2791–6.

31. Reimers B, Corvaja N, Moshiri S, et al. Cerebral protection with filter devices during carotid artery stenting. *Circulation* 2001;104:12–5.

32. Angelini A, Reimers B, Della Barbera M, et al. Cerebral protection during carotid artery stenting: collection and histopathologic analysis of embolized debris. *Stroke* 2002;33:456–61.

33. Al-Mubarak N, Colombo A, Gaines PA, et al. Multicenter evaluation of carotid artery stenting with a filter protection system. *J Am Coll Cardiol* 2002;39:841–6.

34. Mukherjee D, Roffi M, Kapadia SR, et al. Percutaneous intervention for symptomatic vertebral artery stenosis using coronary stents. *J Invasive Cardiol* 2001;13:363–6.

35. Abou-Chebl A, Reginelli J, Mukherjee D, et al. Cerebral hyperperfusion and intracranial hemorrhage following internal carotid artery stenting. *J Am Coll Cardiol* 2002;39:68A.

10 Cerebrovascular intervention

Alex Abou-Chebl

Introduction

Endovascular cerebrovascular interventions are quickly becoming the preferred surgical procedure for a variety of cerebrovascular disorders. Advances in cardiac endovascular technique and equipment, along with the development of cerebrovascular-specific devices, have facilitated the transition from traditional vascular and neurosurgical procedures in a manner similar to the shift that has already occurred in the treatment of cardiovascular disorders. The cerebrovascular circulation differs in many critical ways from the cardiac and peripheral vascular circulations. These differences have greatly limited the development of cerebrovascular interventions, particularly revascularization methods such as stenting and thrombolysis.

Physicians treating patients with cerebrovascular disorders must be aware of the unique characteristics of the brain and cerebral circulation. First and foremost, the cerebral arteries and veins are histologically different from other vessels. Within 1 cm of entering the skull base, the cerebral arteries lose their adventitia and external elastic lamina. The arteries become much thinner and as a result are more easily damaged with conventional endovascular wires and balloons. Second, the large cerebral arteries run outside the brain within the subarachnoid space and are surrounded by the noncompliant skull. Dissection, perforation, or rupture of any one of the cerebral arteries is often catastrophic because intracerebral hemorrhage (subarachnoid or intraparenchymal) results in rapid and marked elevation of intracranial pressure, which cannot be easily controlled without neurosurgical decompression. Third, the brain is exquisitely sensitive to embolization; even microscopic emboli can cause devastating strokes (eg, severe hemiparesis with anterior choroidal artery occlusion). As a consequence, the neurological interventionalist should adhere to the following principles.

- Meticulous technique and attention to detail are essential.

- All air must be removed from catheters, tubes, syringes, and balloons.

- All equipment must be kept clean and free from dried blood and contrast.

- Endovascular tools should be placed in the cerebrovascular circulation for as short a period as possible.

- All saline and contrast must be heparinized.

- Stagnation of columns of blood or contrast must be avoided.

- Balloon dilation catheters and stents should never be oversized within the intracranial circulation.

- Brute force and aggressive technique are incompatible with the safe performance of cerebrovascular interventions and must be replaced by finesse and gentle technique.

- The risk of embolization and complications is proportional to the number of catheter and wire exchanges performed and the size and complexity of the endovascular equipment.

Acute ischemic stroke

Treatment overview

The concept of endovascular treatment for acute ischemic stroke (IS) is simple: the most effective means of preventing neuronal cell death and restoring function is to recanalize an occluded cerebral vessel as quickly as possible from stroke onset. To date, there has only been one randomized trial of endovascular treatment for acute stroke (PROACT [Prolyse in Acute Cerebral Thromboembolism] II, described below); as a result, there are no widely accepted techniques or pharmacological agents [1]. The approach to acute stroke treatment is further confounded by the heterogeneous nature of stroke. Unlike an acute coronary artery syndrome, which in the vast majority of patients is the result of an atherosclerotic plaque rupture and luminal compromise, acute IS is caused by (occurring roughly in equal proportions) cardiogenic embolism, atherosclerosis/thrombosis, or penetrating artery disease (ie, lipohyalinosis). In addition, in approximately 5% of patients stroke has an esoteric cause, such as dissection or a metabolic disorder. Thus, no single approach will be effective in all cases, and the guiding principle of acute IS is that treatment must be individualized for each patient, taking into account the pathophysiology of the stroke.

Intra-arterial (IA) thrombolysis, a generic term that is commonly and erroneously used to refer to all endovascular treatments for acute IS, is not a Food and Drug Administration (FDA)-approved treatment. In fact, to date there is only one FDA-approved treatment for acute IS, and that is intravenous (IV) administration of recombinant tissue plasminogen activator (rt-PA). Therefore, patients who qualify for IV rt-PA must first be offered IV treatment and given the opportunity to decline it before IA treatment is given [2]. Recanalization rates for cerebrovascular occlusions average 70% for patients treated with IA thrombolysis compared with 34% for those treated with IV thrombolysis [3]. The difference in recanalization rates is most apparent with large-vessel occlusions such as those of the internal carotid artery (ICA), which is the vessel most resistant to thrombolysis, the carotid terminus ("carotid T" or "carotid siphon") segment, the proximal (M1) segment of the middle cerebral artery (MCA), and the basilar artery (BA) (see **Figures 1** and **2**) [4,5]. There have been no randomized studies comparing recanalization rates and outcomes between IV and IA thrombolysis.

Intravenous thrombolysis

The risk of intracranial hemorrhage (ICH), which is fatal in a majority of cases, has tempered both research into and the clinical use of thrombolytic therapy for acute IS. The NINDS (National Institutes of Neurological Disorders and Stroke) trial of IV thrombolysis with rt-PA in acute stroke was the first study to show a benefit of any treatment for acute IS. This landmark study proved the efficacy and overall safety of IV rt-PA within 3 hours of stroke onset, despite a 10-fold increased risk of symptomatic brain hemorrhage (6.4% vs 0.6% with placebo) [6]. Almost 8 years after FDA approval, however, IV rt-PA utilization is very low: <5% in the USA. Although there are multiple reasons for its under-utilization, the narrow treatment window of 3 hours is the major limitation of this therapy, and is a major impetus for the continued use of IA thrombolysis.

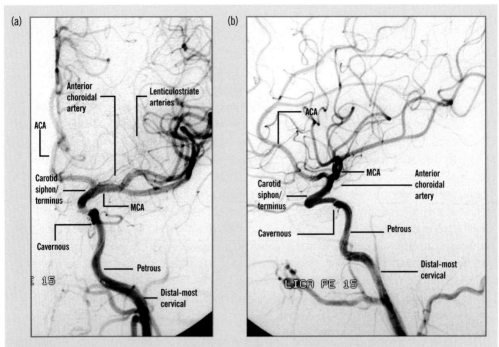

Figure 1. The normal angiographic anatomy of the anterior or internal carotid intracranial circulation, left carotid angiograms: (**a**) anteroposterior view; (**b**) lateral view. The segments of the internal carotid artery (ICA) can clearly be seen: distal-most cervical; petrous; cavernous; and carotid siphon/terminus, which is intradural. The ICA bifurcates into the middle cerebral artery (MCA), which supplies the majority of the cerebral hemispheres and is the most common location for acute ischemic large-vessel strokes, and the anterior cerebral artery (ACA). Note the anterior choroidal artery originating posteriorly from the carotid siphon before it divides into the MCA and ACA. Also note the multiple small lenticulostriate arteries, which arise from the MCA trunk.

Intra-arterial thrombolysis

In the past 15 years, several series of IS patients treated with IA thrombolysis have been reported. The results of these series suggest that IA thrombolysis is effective at recanalizing occluded cerebral vessels and that patients may derive a clinical benefit from such treatment. Firm conclusions, however, are hampered by the lack of standardization in patient selection, duration of ischemia, location and etiology of the occlusion, and the endovascular techniques and pharmacological agents used.

The only randomized trials to have evaluated the safety and efficacy of IA thrombolysis are PROACT I and PROACT II. Mechanical disruption of the clot was not permitted in either study. The first, PROACT I, was a randomized controlled safety and dose escalation trial to evaluate the safety and recanalization efficacy of recombinant pro-urokinase (r-pro-UK) in acute IS patients with MCA occlusion of <6 hours duration [7]. This study showed that a 2-hour infusion of 9 mg of r-pro-UK with a 2,000 U bolus of heparin was the safest regimen.

PROACT II, which was launched in February 1996, investigated clinical efficacy. The designers of this study realized that the weakness of previous studies was the heterogeneous nature of the patients studied and the variable treatment approach. Hence, unlike PROACT I, it excluded patients with early signs of an infarct in greater than one third of the MCA territory (the ECASS

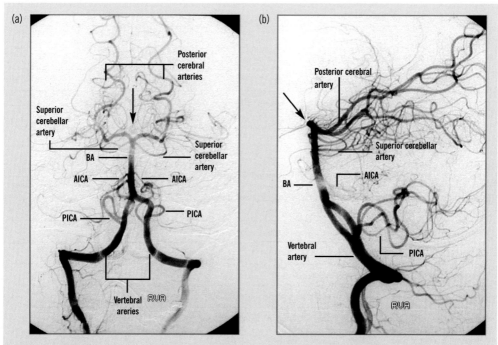

Figure 2. The normal angiographic anatomy of the posterior or vertebrobasilar circulation, selective right vertebral angiograms: (**a**) anteroposterior view; (**b**) lateral view. The vertebral arteries (VAs) are clearly seen to narrow slightly as they penetrate the dura and foramen magnum to become intracranial. The first branch of the VA is the posterior inferior cerebellar artery (PICA). The VAs join to form the single basilar artery (BA), whose first branches are the paired anterior inferior cerebellar arteries (AICAs). The AICA is typically much smaller than the PICA. The BA gives off microscopic perforating branches, which originate from its posterior portion (**b**). The final branches of the BA are the paired superior cerebellar arteries, before it divides into the paired posterior cerebral arteries. Note that the BA has multiple small arteries that arise from its apex and feed the diencephalon (arrow).

[European Cooperative Acute Stroke Study] criteria) on the initial computed tomography (CT) scan [1,8]. Furthermore, all 180 patients enrolled, both controls and those in the treatment group, received a 2,000 U IV bolus of heparin followed by 500 U/h for 4 hours (higher doses were associated with an increased risk of ICH in PROACT I). Every patient in the treatment arm also received a fixed dose of 9 mg r-pro-UK infused over 2 hours, directly into the MCA. The treatment group showed a 15% absolute benefit (58% relative benefit) in a functional outcome measure (the modified Rankin scale) at 3 months (*P*=0.04); the number needed to treat was 7. At 2 hours, the recanalization rate (TIMI [Thrombolysis in Myocardial Infarction] grade 2 or 3) was 66% for the treatment group versus 18% for the control group, but the TIMI 3 (complete recanalization) rate was only 19% with r-pro-UK versus 2% with placebo.

The risk of symptomatic brain hemorrhage was 10% in the treatment group and 2% in controls. This rate is similar to those from the major IV rt-PA trials (6% in the NINDS trial, 9% in ECASS II, and 7% in ATLANTIS [Alteplase Thrombolysis for Acute Noninterventional Therapy in Ischemic Stroke]), particularly considering the later time to treatment and greater baseline stroke severity in PROACT II [6,8–10]. Unfortunately, despite the positive results of the PROACT II trial, IA thrombolysis has to date not received FDA approval. At most major academic centers, however, IA thrombolysis with a variety of thrombolytic agents remains the *de facto* standard of care for patients with severe IS of <6 hours duration.

Acute ischemic stroke <6 hours duration
Stroke is significant, ie, disabling or life-threatening
Suspected occlusion of a large artery, ie, nonlacunar stroke syndrome
No hemorrhage on screening computed tomography scan
When IV thrombolysis carries an excessive systemic bleeding risk

Table 1. Indications for intra-arterial thrombolysis. (Nb. A patient is not a candidate for intravenous tissue plasminogen activator if stroke is >3 hours duration.)

Intracerebral hemorrhage is suspected or evident on computed tomography
History of intracerebral or subarachnoid hemorrhage, unless due to a berry aneurysm that has previously been successfully treated
History of dementia, especially of Alzheimer's type, or poor neurological function at baseline
Stroke duration is unknown or >6 hours
The patient has had a recent stroke (within 3 months)
Bleeding diathesis, elevated INR (>1.7), or thrombocytopenia (<100,000 cells/mm³)
Relative contraindications, which must be considered on an individual basis, are active treatment with: • heparin or a heparinoid • high-dose aspirin • clopidogrel • platelet glycoprotein IIb/IIIa receptor antagonists

Table 2. Contraindications to intra-arterial thrombolysis. INR: international normalization ratio.

Although 6 hours is the accepted time window for the initiation of IA treatment in most circumstances, particularly in the anterior circulation, the time window for IA thrombolysis in the vertebrobasilar (VB) circulation may be longer [11–13]. This could be due to the greater collateral blood flow in that region [14]. In all vascular territories, collateral blood flow is correlated with improved neurological outcomes after recanalization therapy [15,16].

In addition to greater recanalization efficacy and a longer time window of treatment, IA thrombolysis may also be useful in situations where IV thrombolysis carries an excessive bleeding risk, eg, recent nonintracerebral hemorrhage, surgery, arterial puncture, or in patients who are receiving systemic anticoagulation (see **Table 1**). IA thrombolysis is safer in these circumstances because smaller doses of thrombolytics can be delivered directly into the affected blood vessels [17]. The contraindications to IA thrombolysis are given in **Table 2**.

Technique

Acute stroke is a medical emergency and rapid patient evaluation and treatment are essential. Ideally, acute IS treatment should be carried out by a dedicated team of experienced physicians, nurses, and technologists. Several events must take place at once. While the patient is being prepped and draped, the thrombolytic and antithrombotic agents should be ordered from the pharmacy and the endovascular equipment should be brought into the catheterization laboratory. Immediately after access is obtained, the symptomatic artery should be quickly cannulated using a 5-Fr diagnostic catheter over a 0.035-inch hydrophilic wire. An aortic arch angiogram should be considered if the time from stroke onset is relatively short as it may simplify cannulation, but if there is only a small time window then an arch angiogram may use up precious minutes. An experienced interventionalist should be able to cannulate all of the cerebral vessels without an arch angiogram, but common arch variants, such as a shared origin of the innominate and left common carotid artery (CCA) (25% of individuals), a bovine arch with the left CCA arising from the innominate artery (7%), and a left vertebral artery (VA) arising directly from the aorta in-between the left CCA and left subclavian artery (0.5%), may make cannulation difficult and prolong the procedure.

If the ischemia is in the territory of the ICA then a CCA injection focusing on the ICA origin in two planes of view, if possible, should be performed before placing the catheter in the ICA. If the ischemia is in the VB circulation then cannulation of the left VA should be attempted first since it is easier than cannulation of the right VA. A word of caution with regards to the VAs: in many individuals, one vertebral is dominant and the other is smaller in caliber; therefore, injections in the VA must be gentle in order to avoid dissection of a very small vessel.

After the cervical angiograms, cerebral digital subtraction angiography is performed in two orthogonal planes. The standard views for optimal imaging of the MCA and intracranial ICA are a cranial AP view and a true lateral view (see **Figures 1** and **2**). The field of view should be large enough to see the entire inner table of the skull so that the venous structures are included in the angiogram. Filming should continue until the end of the venous phase. Besides an obvious vessel cut-off sign of one of the major vessels at the base of the brain, note should be made of other angiographic signs of ischemia, including:

* branch occlusions (these may be difficult to visualize)

* delayed arterial filling and emptying

* early venous shunting

Attention should also be given to whether there is a collateral blood supply and retrograde filling of the distal MCA or anterior cerebral artery (ACA) branches from pial collaterals. The presence of collaterals is a positive prognostic sign for clinical recovery and, probably, decreased risk of ICH.

After the quick screening angiogram of the symptomatic artery, the diagnostic catheter should be withdrawn and used to cannulate the contralateral carotid artery or VA, whichever is appropriate, to document collateral blood supply from the anterior communicating artery, the posterior communicating artery, or pial collaterals from the posterior cerebral artery (PCA) to the MCA or ACA or *vice versa*. Angiography should also be sufficient to exclude contraindications to thrombolysis (eg, large thrombosed aneurysms or arteriovenous malformations [AVMs]) and to help the interventionalist decide on the best method of access to the desired vessel.

Following sheath placement, a 2,000 U bolus of heparin is either given immediately or, if a longer sheath is needed, after sheath exchange has been performed. The bolus is then followed by an infusion of 500 U/h for 4 hours. This heparin regimen was developed and used in the

Description	Example
0.035-inch, 190–300 cm hydrophilic guidewire	Glidewire (Terumo)
5-Fr, 100–125 cm shaped diagnostic catheter	Berenstein, JR4, etc.
6-Fr, 100-cm soft-tipped guide catheter	Envoy (Cordis)
0.014-inch, 300-cm hydrophilic soft-tipped microguidewire	Synchro (Precision Therapeutics), Whisper (Guidant)
2.3-Fr floppy microcatheter	RapidTransit (Cordis), TurboTracker (Cordis)
6-Fr short sheath or 7–8 Fr, 70–80 cm sheath	Shuttle (Cook)
Consider	
Over-the-wire coronary angioplasty balloon	Maverick (Boston Scientific/SciMed), 1.5–2 mm diameter
Snare	Gooseneck Snare (MicroVena)

Table 3. Equipment for intra-arterial thrombolysis.

PROACT II protocol and was associated with lower rates of ICH, but at the cost of higher rates of reocclusion [1]. For the most part this is the standard regimen, but it is by no means universal and – as stressed previously – the needs of each stroke patient are unique.

Access to the occlusion site is the most critical technical issue that determines failure or success. In younger patients or those with straight vessels both proximally and distally, a 6-Fr guide catheter through a short femoral sheath placed in the distal cervical ICA or distal V2 segment of the VA provides sufficient support to allow wire and microballoon catheter access to even secondary branches of the MCA and PCA (see **Table 3**). The 6-Fr guide is used to cannulate the origin of the innominate, left CCA, or subclavian arteries and is then advanced over a 0.035-inch hydrophilic wire into the ICA or VA. Road-mapping or trace subtraction (if available) increases the margin of safety when placing the guide catheter in the distal cervical vessels. In older patients or those with severely tortuous proximal vessels or unfriendly aortic arches, I have found that a 6-Fr guide catheter is insufficient and wire placement is sometimes impossible, irrespective of guide size (see **Figure 3**). In these individuals, a modified approach using a long sheath placed in the distal CCA or subclavian arteries will often allow access.

In general, a 5-Fr diagnostic catheter is used to cannulate the origin of the great vessels and a trace subtraction image is obtained. A stiff, angled 0.035-inch hydrophilic wire is then placed in the external carotid artery (ECA) or the axillary artery. The diagnostic catheter is advanced over the wire into the ECA or axillary artery and the hydrophilic wire is exchanged for a super-stiff, nonhydrophilic wire that will effectively straighten out most tortuous segments or at least offer sufficient support to allow insertion of the sheath. With the introducer tightly secured, the sheath is inserted into the distal CCA or the subclavian artery just proximal to the VA origin. With the sheath in place and the introducer and stiff wire removed, the 6-Fr guide is inserted over the soft hydrophilic wire, using roadmapping, into the desired vessel (see **Figure 4**). It is important to use a sheath long enough to reach the desired target, but not so long that the guide catheter cannot be inserted to the desired depth.

With access secured, a 0.014-inch, hydrophilic, soft-tipped wire is loaded through a microcatheter or small angioplasty balloon catheter and advanced through the occluded segment

(a)

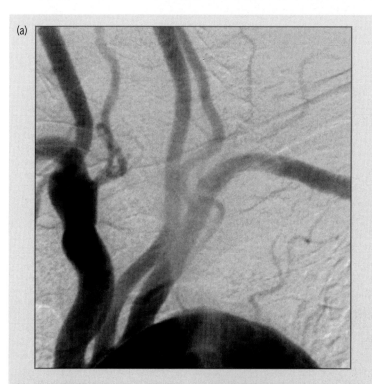

(b)

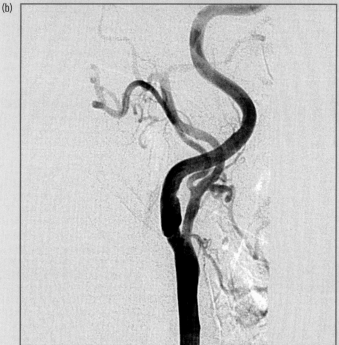

Figure 3. (a) Angiographic image showing severely tortuous great vessels (common carotids and vertebrals) and an unfriendly aortic arch. **(b)** A common carotid angiogram shows severe tortuosity of the internal carotid artery. In such cases, access to the intracranial vessels is facilitated by a long sheath placed in the distal common carotid or subclavian arteries, before advancing a guide catheter into the distal cervical vessels.

(a)

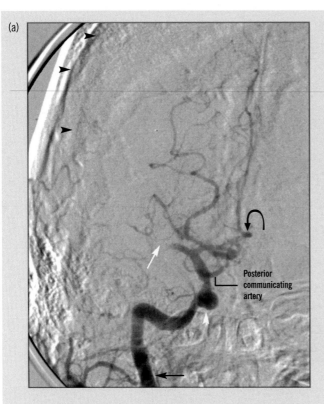

Posterior
communicating
artery

(b)

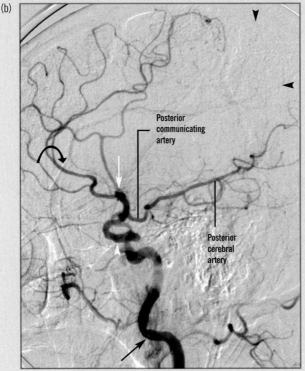

Posterior
communicating
artery

Posterior
cerebral
artery

Figure 4. A 71-year-old African-American male presented 3 hours post-onset of a dense left hemiparesis with a clinical syndrome consistent with severe right hemispheric ischemia. Urgent computed tomography of the brain was negative, so the patient was brought to the interventional suite for intra-arterial (IA) thrombolysis. An angiogram of the right common carotid artery (CCA) ([a] anteroposterior [AP] view; [b] lateral view) showed occlusion of the middle cerebral artery (MCA) trunk (white arrow in **a** and **b**) with no pial collateral flow: note the absence of MCA distal cortical branches (black arrowheads in **a** and **b**). The internal carotid artery (ICA) had severe tortuosity with an extra loop in the distal cervical segment (black arrow in **a** and **b**), as well as excessive tortuosity and diffuse atherosclerosis of the intracranial segments (white arrowheads in **a** and **b**). The anterior cerebral artery filled normally (curved arrow in **a** and **b**) and there was a large posterior communicating artery filling the posterior cerebral artery. Due to the severe tortuosity, a long 8-Fr sheath was placed in the distal CCA and a 6-Fr guide catheter was placed distally in the cervical ICA (black arrow in **c**; slight ipsilateral oblique view). The microcatheter was then guided over a 0.014-inch, hydrophilic, soft-tipped guidewire into the occluded segment of the MCA (white arrow in **c**). The patient then received 25 mg of IA tissue plasminogen activator over 20 minutes with only minimal improvement in flow. At that point, the microcatheter was exchanged for a 1.5×9 mm coronary balloon, which was used to perform percutaneous transluminal angioplasty of the occluded segment of the MCA (white arrow in **d**; slight ipsilateral oblique view). Note that the balloon has a "waist", which suggests that an underlying stenosis is the cause of the occlusion. Also note the distal placement of the microwire (black arrow in **d**) to give support for balloon advancement. Following angioplasty, there was transient TIMI 2 flow in the MCA, but by the time repeat angiography was performed the MCA had reoccluded (black arrow in **e**; slight ipsilateral oblique view). This is typical of an active atherosclerotic lesion. Angioplasty was repeated and then followed by 6 mg of abciximab infused over 5 minutes directly through the microcatheter into the stenotic segment. Fifteen minutes later, an AP angiogram (**f**) showed complete recanalization of the MCA trunk, but with an underlying residual stenosis (white arrow). Re-established flow could be seen in the distal MCA branches (black arrows in **f**). The lateral angiogram (**g**) showed filling of most of the MCA branches (white arrows), but there was persistent thrombus in one of the frontal branches (black arrow). The procedure was terminated, but the patient received aspirin and clopidogrel orally immediately at the end of the procedure. By the second postoperative day he was nearly normal, except for slight hemineglect. Magnetic resonance imaging of the brain (**h**) showed only a small insular cortex stroke (arrow); by 30 days, the patient was neurologically normal.

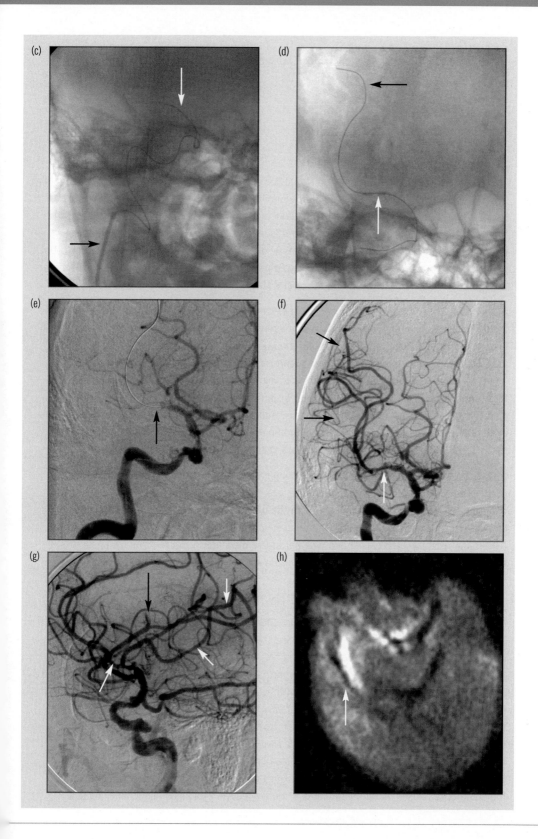

Anticoagulants	Thrombolytics	Platelet GPIIb/IIIa receptor antagonists
Heparin: 2,000 U bolus, 500 U/h × 4 h	rt-PA: 5–50 mg	Abciximab: 0.25 mg/kg bolus, 0.125 μg/kg/min × 12–24 h
	Reteplase: 1–8 U	
	Urokinase: 250,000 U	Eptifibatide: 180 μg/kg bolus, 2 μg/kg/min × 12–24 h

Table 4. The most commonly used pharmacological agents and doses during intra-arterial thrombolysis. GP: glycoprotein; rt-PA: recombinant tissue plasminogen activator.

(see **Figure 4**). Placement of the wire distal to the occluded segment must be performed carefully since the distal vessels cannot be visualized. Familiarity with the natural course of the major cerebral vessels and biplane angiography greatly facilitate this. It is important to recall that the MCA and BA perforators arise from the ventral (superior) aspect of the MCA and the dorsal (posterior) aspect of the BA trunks. Therefore, when wiring these vessels the wire tip should be pointed down or anteriorly, respectively, to avoid perforation of the small branches. With sufficient wire purchase distal to the occlusion, the microcatheter is advanced into the thrombus.

At this point in the thrombolysis procedure, there are great differences in almost every aspect of the technique among interventionalists. Some interventionalists advance the microcatheter distally enough to pass through the MCA trunk into the M2 branches (first-order MCA branches, which travel superiocaudally through the Sylvian fissure) or through the BA into the proximal PCA. The purpose behind such distal placement is to allow angiography through the microcatheter to determine the distal-most extent of the occlusion and to allow infusion of thrombolytic agent distally to lyse the "back end" of the thrombus. Alternatively, the microcatheter can be placed within the occluded segment to infuse the thrombolytic agents, because advancing the microcatheter through the thrombus and injecting contrast may produce distal embolization.

In addition to the location of the infusion catheter, there are also differences in: the choice of thrombolytic agent to infuse, the dose, the rate of infusion, and the duration of the infusion; the extent of mechanical clot disruption with the wire or microcatheter; the adjunctive use of angioplasty and possibly stenting; the adjunctive use of heparin and platelet glycoprotein (GP)IIb/IIIa receptor antagonists; and whether to use mechanical clot removal tools, such as snares and rheolytic catheters. Each of these choices will now be discussed.

Thrombolytic agents: which one, how much, how fast, for how long?

A variety of thrombolytic agents have been used for IA thrombolysis, including streptokinase, urokinase, rt-PA, reteplase, and r-pro-UK. The doses have varied depending on the agent and study [8,18–21]. **Table 4** lists the most commonly used agents and doses. Streptokinase has been associated with an excessive risk of hemorrhage and is no longer considered appropriate for stroke treatment [22]. In the PROACT II trial, a fixed dose of r-pro-UK was continuously infused over 2 hours [1]. This technique may explain why the clinical benefit in PROACT II was not as robust as had been hoped. The mean duration from presentation to the initiation of recanalization therapy was approximately 5.3 hours. Coupled with the 2-hour infusion of r-pro-UK, this meant that many patients were not actually recanalized until well past the 6-hour window. In my experience, a more rapid infusion of thrombolytics given in boluses every 5–10 minutes with the entire dose infused within 30 minutes is more effective. Prolonged, slow infusions take an inordinately long time to achieve recanalization. I also favor an adjusted dosing scheme based on several patient characteristics (see below), rather than a fixed or weight-based dose of thrombolytics as was given in PROACT II and the NINDS IV rt-PA trials, respectively. Several factors, all of which have been associated with an increased risk of ICH or poor prognosis, must be taken into account when determining the dose of thrombolytic [23]:

- patient age

- presenting blood pressure

- presenting serum glucose

- duration of ischemia

- infarct volume as measured by CT or diffusion-weighted magnetic resonance imaging (MRI) changes

- clot burden

- other extenuating circumstances (eg, elevated international normalization ratio, relative thrombocytopenia)

- intended use of other agents or aggressive mechanical manipulation

Factors that favor higher doses of thrombolytics are: younger age (generally <80 years), presenting blood pressure <185/110 mm Hg, normal blood glucose, short duration of ischemia (<4 hours), no signs of infarct on CT or MRI, moderate clot burden, and the lack of any other confounders, such as the intention to give high doses of GPIIb/IIIa receptor antagonists or to perform stenting. The converse of the above factors favors lower doses of thrombolytics, if any. In all patients, the lowest effective dose should be used, as higher doses of thrombolytics are associated with an increased risk of ICH.

Mechanical clot disruption

In addition to the infusion of thrombolytics, many interventionalists advocate mechanical clot disruption as a method of facilitating thrombolysis by increasing permeability through the thrombus. This was prohibited in the PROACT II trial, which again possibly explains the prolonged recanalization times and the generally low TIMI 3 rate (19%) at 2 hours [1]. Such mechanical manipulation can be performed with repeated passes of the microwire or microcatheter. All such maneuvers must be performed with finesse since they greatly increase the risk of vessel perforation. In my experience, this technique is helpful in cases of small clot burden or a fresh clot. Occluded ICAs or BAs are unlikely to recanalize with wire manipulation alone.

Balloon angioplasty and stenting

Balloon angioplasty

There are several reports of significant recanalization success with balloon angioplasty as an adjunct or even as the sole treatment for acute stroke [24–27]. The largest series is from Japan, where intracranial atherosclerosis and thrombotic occlusion are much more prevalent than in the general US or western European populations [25]. Nevertheless, gentle balloon inflation with an undersized coronary balloon, such as a Maverick (Boston Scientific/SciMed, Maple Grove, MN, USA), can be very effective, particularly in individuals in whom thrombotic occlusion, rather than cardioembolism, is the most likely mechanism of stroke. Such individuals include those of African-American or Asian descent and patients with diabetes mellitus. Inflations should be gentle, always keeping in mind the fragility of the intracranial vessels, and prolonged for 1–2 minutes. In patients who require percutaneous transluminal angioplasty (PTA) and who do not have adequate baseline platelet inhibition, adjuvant antiplatelet agents such as GPIIb/IIIa receptor antagonists are also given because angioplasty, even with an undersized balloon, causes endothelial injury and may actually promote platelet thrombus formation.

Stenting

There is very little published experience with stenting in the setting of acute stroke. I have treated several patients with PTA and stenting, some without any thrombolytics, with great success (unpublished data). All of the patients had what appeared to be acute thrombotic occlusion due to an underlying severe stenosis. In such patients, thrombolysis alone may be insufficient, for two reasons. Firstly, acute plaque rupture is often associated with a platelet plug/thrombus, which is less likely to respond to fibrin-specific thrombolytics. Secondly, if thrombolysis does occur, there is a continued risk of acute rethrombosis and reocclusion. This was a common event in PROACT II and has been noted in other studies, including in patients treated with IV rt-PA [1,28].

The benefits of successful stenting include the potential to minimize the use of thrombolytics and therefore decrease the risk of ICH, and to give the patient a definitive treatment that, in addition to curing the acute stroke, may prevent future events. Another benefit is that stenting has the potential to rapidly improve flow; even if the result is suboptimal, the improved flow may be sufficient to prevent further tissue ischemia.

The drawbacks are obvious and are mainly related to the increased risk of perforation or dissection with stenting. This approach is most analogous to that used in patients with acute coronary syndromes (ACS). The mechanism of stroke in patients with intracranial atherosclerosis is essentially identical to the leading cause of ACS – ie, acute plaque rupture with thrombosis. It should not be a surprise, therefore, that thrombolysis alone, which is no longer the treatment of choice for ACS, is also unlikely to be the most effective treatment for stroke patients [29]. In stroke patients who receive stents (as in ACS patients who receive stents), antiplatelet treatment is essential to prevent early stent thrombosis; patients should receive GPIIb/IIIa receptor antagonists immediately before stenting and aspirin and clopidogrel oral loads immediately after stenting. It must be emphasized that such an approach is very aggressive and has the least literature support of all of the methods that have been discussed thus far. However, as was previously stated, acute stroke is a heterogeneous disease and treatment must be adjusted to the needs of every patient – for example, stenting may not be the safest approach in an 80-year-old patient who has very calcified or tortuous vessels and in whom there is a very high risk of complications. The details of the approach to stenting and the technique are discussed in the **Intracranial angioplasty and stenting** section.

Adjunctive pharmacotherapy

Heparin

The use of heparin for interventional procedures is well founded. In the setting of acute stroke, however, the use of heparin (or the heparinoids) is associated with an increased risk of ICH [7,30]. So, should heparin be used in patients being treated with an endovascular approach for acute stroke? In PROACT I, higher doses of heparin were associated with improved recanalization rates and fewer reocclusions, but at the cost of excessive rates of ICH [7]. Since the release of the PROACT results, most interventionalists use the so-called "PROACT" heparin dose of a 2,000 U bolus at procedure onset, followed by 500 U/h for a total of 4 hours. The heparin is then discontinued and not resumed for 24 hours.

While heparin should be used cautiously, the PROACT results are not widely applicable, for several reasons.

- Firstly, the patient population in the PROACT trials consisted of patients with MCA trunk occlusion only and not patients with ICA or VB occlusions, in whom the risk of ICH may be different.

- Secondly, the PROACT trials used r-pro-UK, which requires the presence of heparin for optimal thrombolytic effect; currently available agents do not require heparin.

- Thirdly, since mechanical disruption was not permitted and r-pro-UK was infused over 2 hours, the time to recanalization in the PROACT trials may have been overly long, which would have increased the duration of ischemia and increased the risk of hemorrhagic transformation.

In my experience, some cases call for sufficient heparin to achieve an activated clotting time (ACT) of 2–2.5 times baseline. Most interventionalists begin with the PROACT bolus of 2,000 U. If angioplasty or stenting are contemplated, additional heparin is given to achieve an ACT of 250–275 (ideally). In situations where the procedure is prolonged for more than an hour, additional heparin is given in 1–2,000 U boluses. The PROACT regimen should be followed in simple cases of isolated thrombolysis where recanalization is achieved relatively quickly. Following the procedure, the heparin drip is adjusted or the heparin reversed with protamine sulfate if: the patient received GPIIb/IIIa receptor antagonists or large doses of thrombolytics; there is no underlying atherosclerotic stenosis; the patient has difficult-to-control hypertension; or a large infarct is suspected.

GPIIb/IIIa receptor antagonists

Platelet GPIIb/IIIa receptor antagonists have been successfully and safely used in the treatment of acute myocardial infarction, and there is a growing body of evidence on the use of platelet GPIIb/IIIa receptor antagonists in the treatment of acute IS. Clearly, the risk of bleeding is significant with GPIIb/IIIa receptor antagonists. However, the rate of ICH was found to be low in both a preliminary study of IV abciximab for acute IS and a small series of combined eptifibatide and IA urokinase for IS [18,31]. The addition of a GPIIb/IIIa receptor antagonist to a thrombolysis regimen may have a facilitatory effect on cerebral artery recanalization, without significantly increasing the risk of ICH. The platelet GPIIb/IIIa receptor antagonists not only inhibit new platelet thrombi from forming, but can also induce disaggregation of platelets from each other and from fibrin, resulting in a mild thrombolytic effect [32]. By exposing fibrin strands to plasmin, the thrombolytic effect of rt-PA or other agents is enhanced.

The specific agent, dose, and route to be used are highly variable (see **Table 4**). Abciximab (ReoPro; Eli Lilly, Indianapolis, Indiana, USA) has been systematically studied in the setting of acute IS [31]. As with thrombolytic agents, the lowest possible dose should be used to decrease the risk of ICH: typically, early administration of an abciximab bolus in "1/4" bolus increments, ie, 1/4 of the typical cardiac bolus regimen alternating with boluses of thrombolytic agent. However, if stenting is planned, I will administer a full weight-based bolus. Although in most of the literature on GPIIb/IIIa receptor antagonists the agents have been infused IV, I have given the boluses directly into the thrombus through a microcatheter. Theoretically, this has the benefit of saturating the thrombus and any platelets within, resulting in quicker thrombolysis.

The use of GPIIb/IIIa receptor antagonists, while promising, must be guided by knowledge of the half-lives of each agent and the lack of antidotes for their antiplatelet effect, should ICH develop. Therefore, I do not advocate their use except by physicians who have a great deal of experience with acute stroke treatment and thrombolysis.

Mechanical clot removal

Even though IV and IA thrombolysis have been proven to be effective methods of treating acute IS, both approaches have their limitations. The major limitations are the speed of recanalization and the assumption that all thrombi/emboli are amenable to thrombolysis. Also, in some circumstances, thrombolysis may be contraindicated (eg, active systemic bleeding) or associated with a higher risk of ICH (eg, recent head injury or neurosurgery). Mechanical clot removal is an alternative method of recanalization. Current approaches include microrheolytic catheters, snaring devices, and lasers.

Anecdotal reports, including my own experience, suggest that commercially available devices for foreign body removal may be effective in certain cases [33,34]. I have used a lasso-type snare designed for intravascular foreign body retrieval with good effect (unpublished data). If successful, this approach can be quite rewarding because recanalization can be achieved within seconds to a few minutes, rather than the minutes to hours that are required with pharmacological agents. There are disadvantages, however. By their very nature, mechanical devices increase the risk of vessel injury and dissection. In addition, access to the thrombosed segment is lost once the microcatheter and snare are withdrawn. If the snaring is unsuccessful on the first pass then the occluded segment must be rewired, which is not always easy or possible. I therefore save snaring for a last resort if all other measures have failed. Although clinical trials are ongoing with a variety of other embolectomy devices, none has been proven to be safe or effective and none is commercially available at this time.

The optimal technique

Given the heterogeneous nature of IS, no single agent or device will be ideal in all instances. My approach is to utilize whichever technique seems most appropriate. In fact, I often use a combination of the above agents and devices. The goal is rapid recanalization without increasing the risk of ICH. After accessing the occluded vessel, my most common approach is to initiate treatment with a pharmacological agent, often alternating doses of a thrombolytic and a GPIIb/IIIa receptor antagonist, since these agents require several minutes for their pharmacological effects to begin. If the patient is more likely to have a fibrin-rich or "red" clot (eg, the patient has underlying atrial fibrillation) then I give relatively higher doses of thrombolytic. If, on the other hand, the patient is more likely to have a platelet-rich or "white" clot (eg, thrombosis of an underlying ulcerated plaque) then higher doses of a GPIIb/IIIa receptor antagonist are given. While the agents are being infused I will consider whether a mechanical approach is needed. If so, the necessary equipment is prepped and loaded. Repeat angiography is performed and additional pharmacotherapy is given if needed – then, most often, angioplasty is performed. If that is unsuccessful, more pharmacological agents are administered and consideration is given to stenting or snaring. In this way, treatment is optimized for each patient.

Intra- and postprocedure patient management

Patient safety is the most important concern of the team. While the physician is concentrating on the intervention itself, members of the team must be constantly assessing the patient clinically. Basic life-support measures, ie, the ABCs (airway–breathing–circulation), must be attended to. Sleepy or obtunded patients who have copious secretions or who are obviously not controlling their airway should be intubated and mechanically ventilated. This is rarely necessary and I prefer not to have patients sedated and paralyzed so that the neurological exam can be used to monitor for complications and response to treatment. The cerebral vessels are quite sensitive to manipulation; headache is an important sign of vascular irritation and may be a marker for vessel injury. This is discussed further in the section on **Intracranial angioplasty and stenting**. Oxygen in the acute phase of a stroke may be of benefit and should be given to all patients [35]. Excessive oxygenation should be avoided after vessel recanalization or for more than a few hours because of the theoretical concern that it will increase reperfusion injury due to free radicals. To date, however, there are no reliable prospective data on oxygen therapy.

A more critical issue is blood pressure control. Understanding the concept of autoregulation is crucial in understanding the best approach to blood pressure control. The cerebral vessels "auto" regulate their mural tone, and therefore their diameter, so as to maintain cerebral blood flow (CBF) in a constant range over a wide range of mean arterial pressures (MAPs). Neurons have a constant, and not highly variable, demand for oxygen and nutrients that is independent of their activity. During a stroke, the arteries and arterioles of the affected brain region maximally vasodilate to maintain CBF in the face of a low perfusion pressure. Since the vessels can only vasodilate so much, the pressure–flow curve, which is essentially flat in normal circumstances, becomes linear. CBF then becomes directly proportional to MAP; as a result, extreme blood pressure elevations can greatly and rapidly increase CBF, increasing the risk of ICH. Conversely, low blood pressures can cause a marked decrease in CBF and exacerbate ischemia [36]. Blood pressure should therefore be maintained at a moderately elevated level during most of the intervention, except in patients who have a contraindication to hypertension (eg, those at very high risk for ICH, those experiencing active coronary ischemia). A safe range is to maintain systolic blood pressure values between 150 and 185 mm Hg [35]. Very short-acting beta-blockers and hydralazine are preferred agents in the acute setting since they either increase or maintain CBF without causing sedation or headache, which can confound the clinical evaluation.

All patients should be monitored in a neurological intensive care unit for at least the first 24 hours after the intervention. If a dedicated unit is unavailable then care should be given by nurses and physicians experienced in the care of neurological patients. Neurological status should be continuously assessed, or at least every 15 minutes, along with the standard critical care monitoring. Patients, staff, and even family members should all be vigilant for the occurrence of a headache, which is a common sign of ICH. Any sudden onset or crescendo headache, whether or not associated with a decline in mental status, nausea, vomiting, or worsening of focal deficits, should raise the suspicion of ICH and prompt consideration of urgent CT scanning.

Although data on the efficacy and safety of neurosurgical evacuation of an intracerebral hematoma or ventriculostomy placement for hydrocephalus following IA thrombolysis are lacking, anecdotal reports and experience suggest that such interventions may be life-saving in selected patients, although they are unlikely to improve functional outcomes [37–39]. In fact, the American Heart and Stroke Association guidelines for acute IS management recommend that all centers that perform thrombolysis have 24-hour access to a neurosurgeon and operating room [2]. Adherence to these recommendations and the management of patients in dedicated stroke and neurological critical care units has been associated with improved patient outcomes.

Intracranial atherosclerosis

Intracranial atherosclerosis is the cause of 8%–10% of all IS, but it remains a difficult clinical entity to diagnose and treat [40]. The relative lack of knowledge about the natural history of stenoses involving the cerebral vessels, the small size of the vessels, their location within the calvarium, their proximity to delicate brain tissue and cranial nerves, and the presence of small perforators further complicate and limit the therapeutic options. The intracranial vessels most commonly implicated in the pathogenesis of cerebral ischemia include the distal ICA, VA, MCA, BA, and, less commonly, the ACA and PCA. Within these vessels, the most common locations for intracranial atherosclerosis are the petrous ICA, the cavernous ICA, the clinoid or terminal ICA, the MCA trunk, the distal VA, the VB junction, and the mid BA [41]. Predisposing factors for intracranial atherosclerosis include diabetes mellitus, hypercholesterolemia, and race, with those of African-American, Hispanic, Asian, or Middle Eastern decent having the greatest risk [40].

Natural history

The risk of stroke or transient ischemic attack (TIA) in patients who have intracranial atherosclerosis has been elucidated predominantly from small and retrospective series of patients [42–48]. Amongst these series there is great variability in patient selection, evaluation, medical treatment, and the duration of follow-up. Depending on the series, the reported annual rates of stroke or TIA recurrence in patients who present with an index event vary from 3% to as high as 22% [42–49]. The average risk of recurrence falls somewhere between 6% and 10% annually. Some patients may be at higher risk of recurrence, including those with multifocal stenoses and those who have symptoms despite antithrombotic treatment [49]. Additionally, stenoses of the MCA and BA, both of which are distal to large collateral channels, may be associated with higher risks of stroke [50,51]. The MCA and BA are also unique in that small perforating arteries originate from the trunks of both vessels. The ostia of these perforators may be occluded by atherosclerosis, which may further increase the risk of ischemia.

Endarterectomy of the intracerebral vessels has been reported, but it is a very complicated and high-risk procedure and few neurosurgeons have experience with this approach. Hence, surgical bypass is the only good surgical option. However, treatment of patients with intracranial stenoses is generally limited to medical options as a result of a trial of surgical bypass in patients with MCA stenoses in which surgical patients experienced worse outcomes than those receiving medical therapy alone [45]. The mainstay of treatment is medical therapy with warfarin, although the data supporting its superiority over antiplatelet medications are weak [44].

Currently, most stroke neurologists employ combination treatments consisting of aspirin in doses varying from 50 to 1300 mg, clopidogrel, Aggrenox (a combination of aspirin and sustained-release dipyridamole) (Boehringer Ingelheim, Ridgefield, CT, USA), and warfarin. The decision to undertake endovascular treatment is often based on the recurrence of symptoms despite combination treatment, but whether endovascular repair should be performed at all remains controversial amongst neurologists [52,53]. This is because of the poorly defined natural history (although most would agree that the risk of ischemia is quite high) and the lack of a head-to-head comparison between medical and endovascular treatments. At this time, therefore, there is virtually no clinical or scientific justification for primary endovascular treatment of intracranial stenoses without an initial trial of medical treatment. More research is needed in this area, but until validated data are available every patient should be fully assessed with a multidisciplinary approach that includes a neurologist and an interventionalist, and data from anatomical and functional studies of CBF.

Clinical presentation

The clinical manifestations of intracranial atherosclerosis are varied. Ischemia is the most common presentation, and the specific symptoms depend on the particular vessel involved and brain region affected. Additionally, the mechanism of ischemia plays a role in determining the clinical manifestations. Sudden occlusion of one of the major vessels often, but not always, causes a cortical or brainstem syndrome that is frequently severe and dramatic, eg, sudden quadriplegia and coma with mid-basilar occlusion or aphasia, hemianopsia, and right-sided hemiplegia with left ICA or MCA occlusion. There may be no TIAs prior to such an event.

The stenoses may also cause hemodynamic symptoms such as transient, mild, or moderate clinical syndromes that have the same clinical features and are recurrent in nature. These spells may be related to a drop in systemic MAP, and may be positional (ie, occur with an upright posture or upon standing). In such patients, studies of CBF (eg, magnetic resonance perfusion, transcranial Doppler ultrasound [TCD]) or cerebrovascular reserve (eg, Diamox single positron emission CT [SPECT] or TCD with breath-holding) are often abnormal. Symptoms may also develop from embolization to distal small branches that may cause very focal or mild deficits, which can also be transient or recurrent. In cases of MCA or BA stenoses, clinical syndromes consistent with the classic "lacunar syndromes" may occur if there is atherosclerotic involvement of the origins of perforators [54,55]. Often, clinical symptoms occur from a combination of one of the above mechanisms. These varying clinical manifestations and their associated pathophysiological mechanisms are part of the reason that cerebral atherosclerosis is such a complicated disease to recognize and treat.

Angioplasty and stenting: techniques and results

The first report of intracranial angioplasty was reported by Sundt et al. who performed angioplasty on two patients with BA stenosis through a surgical cut down to the VA [56]. Other successes followed, and there have been many published case reports and series of PTA of the major intracranial vessels [57–75]. Most of these reports have shown favorable outcomes, but all have differed significantly in patient selection, location of stenoses, endovascular techniques, and adjuvant medical therapy. Currently, definitive conclusions about the efficacy, safety, and superiority of particular techniques or equipment cannot be made. Nonetheless, several broad concepts and techniques culled from these early series are fundamental and will be emphasized; in general, however, the techniques described in the following text are biased by my own experience.

Patient selection

Patient selection is the first important step for a successful intervention. Feasibility of the intervention in terms of vascular access is a prerequisite, and patients with tortuous cervical vessels, proximal stenoses, unfriendly aortic arches, or poor femoral access should be considered very high risk for complications with a high risk of failure. In addition, patients with recent large strokes or those who are severely disabled may not gain any benefit from an intervention if there is not enough viable and clinically relevant brain tissue at risk in the territory distal to the stenosis. Patients with recent ICH, aneurysm or AVM that are are associated with the stenosis or that are present in the distal territory, and patients with large recent strokes, may be at increased risk of ICH and their treatment should be reconsidered. The latter group of patients, particularly those with severe stenoses with poor collateral blood flow or impaired cerebrovascular reserve, may be at risk for cerebral hyperperfusion syndrome and ICH. Several series have reported hyperperfusion in such patients, in whom vigilance and aggressive blood pressure control must be maintained [76,77]. Preoperative CT scans should be considered in all patients, especially those with recent symptoms, to exclude the presence of ICH. Noncompliant individuals, those who continue to smoke and live an unhealthy lifestyle, may be at higher risk of restenosis or even acute stent thrombosis. Such individuals should be treated with caution.

Angiography

As stressed previously, thorough four-vessel angiography is essential not only for access issues, but also to define the stenotic segment(s) in multiple orthogonal views (see **Figure 5**). In general, full diagnostic angiography should be performed well in advance of the intervention to allow adequate planning of the approach and to prepare the necessary equipment. Accurate measurement of vessel size is the most critical part of the diagnostic angiogram because oversizing a balloon or stent may cause vessel rupture (as previously discussed, the cerebral vessels are quite thin and fragile).

The degree of stenosis should be defined using the WASID (Warfarin–Aspirin Symptomatic Intracranial Disease) method, which has been validated and is in common use in both medical and surgical studies [78]. The presence of side branches that originate from the region of the stenosis should also be defined prior to the intervention to allow the choice of an appropriate balloon size and stent length so as to avoid "jailing" the ostia of such branches. The critical side branches are the anterior choroidal artery arising just distal to the posterior communicating artery from the terminal ICA, the posterior inferior cerebellar artery arising from the mid segment of the intracranial VA, and the anterior inferior cerebellar artery arising from the juncture of the proximal and middle third of the BA.

Perioperative management

Platelet inhibition has been shown to be critical in preventing acute thrombus formation and platelet deposition on the damaged endothelial surface following PTA [79–81]. Foreign bodies, such as a stents, also promote platelet deposition and thrombus formation. Pretreatment with a combination of aspirin and ticlopidine or clopidogrel is an effective and essential method of preventing acute vessel thrombosis after intervention [71,75,82–84]. Clopidogrel has a lower risk of hematological side effects than ticlopidine and is the agent of choice. Treatment with this combination of agents should ideally be begun at least 4 days before intervention to allow time for adequate levels of platelet inhibition, but loading doses of clopidogrel (ranging from 300 to 600 mg) can be given within 4 hours of the intervention with good effect.

The role of platelet GPIIb/IIIa receptor antagonists in the setting of intracranial endovascular stenting procedures is unclear. These agents have been shown to be of benefit in the endovascular treatment of patients with coronary artery disease, but there are no similar data for patients undergoing endovascular intervention – in at least one series, the risk of ICH was considerable [65,73,85,86]. The use of GPIIb/IIIa receptor antagonists should not be routine; rather, they should be reserved for highly selected patients, in particular those who were not adequately pretreated with oral antiplatelet agents. A benefit of planning the intervention in advance is that pretreatment with oral antiplatelet agents can be initiated with enough time to allow the platelet inhibition to be measured with new assays of platelet receptor function. In this way, patients who have suboptimal responses to aspirin and or clopidogrel (both of which can occur in as many as 30% of patients) can be identified and corrective measures, such as increasing the doses, can be taken prior to the intervention.

Intraoperative anticoagulation is achieved with heparin via a weight-adjusted bolus followed by intermittent boluses to maintain an activated partial thromboplastin time of 1.5–2 times the normal range, or ACT between 250 and 300 seconds. Although some groups continue the heparin infusion for 12–24 hours following the procedure, there are no reliable data to justify such an approach, which may carry an excessive risk of ICH and access-site hemorrhage. The use of a fixed dose of heparin without measuring heparin activity is not appropriate.

In addition to anticoagulants, some published reports have described pretreatment of patients with antivasospasm regimens, including sublingual nifedipine [87], IA isosorbide dinitrate [61], or nitroglycerin [88]. Although in one series vasospasm was associated with poor outcomes, not all patients develop vasospasm and treatment can be reserved for those who do [89]. The potential drawback of pretreatment is that systemic arterial pressures may be decreased, which may compromise CBF.

A major issue of perioperative management, which has not received much attention in the literature, is sedation and anesthesia. Some groups commonly perform intracranial procedures under general anesthesia and tout the benefits of a secure airway, reliable control of physiological parameters, and no interference from patient movements [70,73,75]. At my institution, all cerebrovascular procedures are performed under local anesthesia – conscious sedation, achieved using low doses of IV anesthesia, is only implemented if absolutely needed. Neurological examination is not compromised by local anesthesia, and patients are able to give feedback about headache and focal deficits. With the patient awake, focal deficits due to embolization,

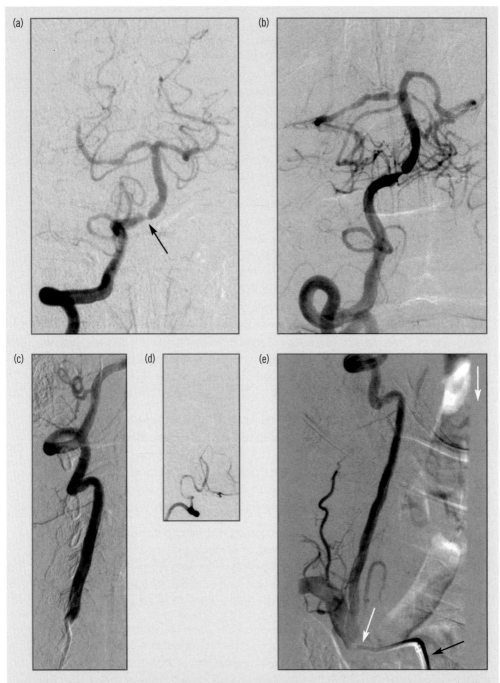

Figure 5. Angiographic images from a 62-year-old male with recurrent vertebrobasilar (VB) transient ischemic attacks (TIAs), despite treatment with warfarin and aspirin. A right vertebral artery (VA) angiogram, anteroposterior (AP) cranial view (**a**), showed a severe stenosis in the VA just proximal to the VB junction (arrow). A caudal AP view (**b**) through the open mouth (Water's view) showed the stenosis at its most severe. The cervical VA was very tortuous (**c**; lateral view), as was the aortic arch and great vessels. The left VA ended in the posterior inferior cerebellar artery (**d**; lateral view) and did not supply any collateral flow to the brainstem, which explained the recalcitrant symptoms. With the patient awake, a 7-Fr sheath (due to the tortuosity) was placed in the right subclavian artery (black arrow in **e**; right anterior oblique [RAO] view) and the 6-Fr guide catheter was advanced over the wire into the VA (white arrow in **e**) up to the C2 curve (black arrow in **f**; RAO view) for support. The soft hydrophilic wire was placed through the stenosis within the right posterior cerebral artery (PCA) for support

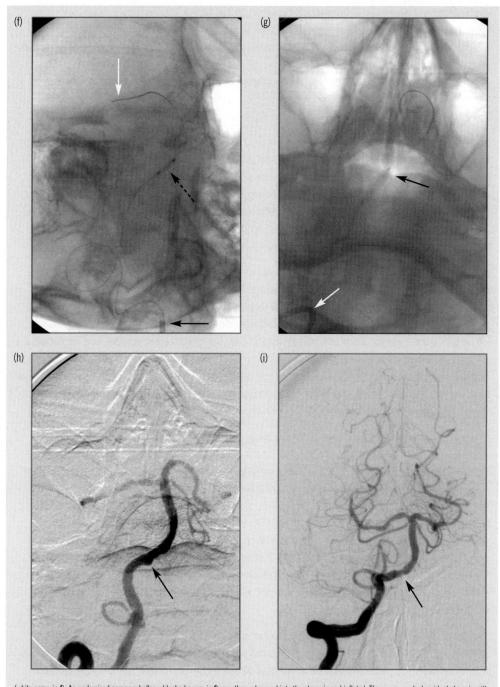

(white arrow in **f**). An undersized coronary balloon (dashed arrow in **f**) was then advanced into the stenosis and inflated. There was marked residual stenosis with recoil following percutaneous transluminal angioplasty, so a coronary stent was navigated into the stenosis (black arrow in **g**). To deliver the stent, the guide catheter was advanced even further into the VA (white arrow in **g**, Waters' view, AP caudal). This must be done with caution to avoid VA dissection. During stent deployment, the patient began to complain of a moderate headache in the back of his head. Stent deployment was immediately stopped and angiography performed. There was no extravasation of contrast or dissection. Further inflations were not performed and although angiographically there was mild residual stenosis (arrows in **h** [Waters' view, AP caudal] and **i** [Towne's view, AP cranial]), the overall result was excellent and the patient was neurologically intact. Without the patient's feedback, further stent dilatation could have resulted in vessel perforation. Following the procedure, the patient was cured of recurrent TIAs.

vasospasm, and acute vessel thrombosis can be detected earlier and corrective measures taken more quickly. Furthermore, the presence of headache or retro-orbital pain can indicate malpositioning of the microwire or an overly aggressive angioplasty [71]. Such complaints mandate a thorough reassessment of wire position and a reduction of balloon inflation pressures or cessation of inflation altogether, followed by immediate angiography to look for dissection or perforation.

Technique

Stable access to the cerebral segment is perhaps the most important technical factor in ensuring a successful procedure. As discussed in the section on acute stroke treatment, the tortuosity of the cerebral vasculature can make access to the stenotic vessel very difficult. This is even more of an issue in the case of intracranial PTA/stenting because balloon dilation catheters and stents (in particular) are much stiffer and less deliverable than the microcatheters used for thrombolysis. Therefore, without adequate and stable access to the stenotic segment, an otherwise straightforward case may be impossible to complete [90].

A femoral approach is ideal, but a brachial or radial approach is feasible, although technically challenging, especially for MCA and ICA procedures [71]. The approach is the same as for acute thrombolysis, except that in almost all cases a 6- to 8-Fr sheath should be placed in the distal CCA or subclavian artery, through which a 6-Fr guide catheter is inserted into the distal cervical ICA or VA. A 6-Fr guide catheter alone will be sufficient in only the straightest of vessels, and loss of access after wiring a tight stenosis can greatly complicate matters. It is therefore better to do all such cases, particularly those without straight vessels (ie, tortuous vessels), with a long sheath for support. Most long sheaths are too short to give support and too bulky to be safely placed in the distal cervical segments of the ICA and VA, and should not be used without a guide catheter.

There are several options for crossing the stenosis. The first option is to cross with a small (0.014-inch), hydrophilic, soft wire with an atraumatic tip, such as a Transcend (Boston Scientific/SciMed), Synchro (Precision Vascular, West Valley City, UT, USA), or Whisper (Guidant, Indianapolis, IN, USA) [71]. Balloon dilation catheters and stents can then be delivered over the hydrophilic wire. If more support is needed, the second option is to advance a hydrophilic microcatheter, such as a Rapid Transit (Cordis, Miami Lakes, FL, USA), over the hydrophilic wire across the lesion, after which the wire is exchanged for a nonhydrophilic wire that will give more support, such as a Balance Trek (Guidant) or Dasher-14 (Boston Scientific/SciMed). The microcatheter is then exchanged for a balloon dilation catheter. Crossing lesions is much easier with hydrophilic wires at the expense of less support and perhaps a greater propensity to perforate the small branches [71].

The third technique is to initially cross the lesion with a wire that gives better support, such as a Balance Trek (Guidant). The balloon catheter is advanced without exchanging wires or passing a microcatheter [61,70,91–93]. The advantage of this technique is that the lesion is crossed only once and it requires fewer catheter and wire exchanges. The disadvantage is that the stiffer support wires may increase the risk of dislodging plaque material and causing embolization. Also, patients often complain of severe headaches with this approach because of the tension that the wires place on the cerebral vessels. The best technique is whichever is most likely to succeed with the gentlest equipment, the fewest crossings of the lesion, and with as few wire and catheter exchanges as possible. With experience, the interventionalist should be able to anticipate the needs of each patient. The tip of the guidewire should be placed, with great care, distal to the stenosis to increase support. Placement in small branches or perforators originating from the main-stem MCA or the top of the BA should be avoided at all times.

After wire placement, the interventionalist must decide whether angioplasty alone is sufficient or whether stenting will be needed. Intracranial stent deployment is controversial and the stenting experience to date is limited [62,64,69–71,73,84,91,94–102]. There are three general approaches to stenting:

• direct stenting, which is the placement of the stent without initial angioplasty

• primary stenting, which is the *a priori* decision to stent after angioplasty, even if the angioplasty results are excellent

• provisional stenting, which is the *a priori* decision to stent only if the angioplasty results are suboptimal

While some advocate stent deployment as a "provisional" technique if there is a dissection, slow flow, or elastic recoil [70,71,93], others argue that stents should be deployed whenever possible [62,84,95]. The justification for stenting is that PTA carries a risk of acute failure, including elastic recoil, dissection, vasospasm, and thrombotic occlusion (platelet and/or fibrin). The potential hazards of direct stenting include an inability to deliver the stent due to lesion severity, an inability to fully deploy the stent in a rigid lesion, distal embolization, vessel injury if force is required for stent delivery, and stent embolization. On the other hand, the lesion is only crossed once with direct stenting, which decreases the risk of embolization and dissection and shortens the duration of the procedure.

Although no direct comparison has been performed between PTA and stenting in the intracranial circulation, stents have been shown to improve both short- and long-term patency in the coronary arteries, which are of similar size to the MCA, distal ICA, VA, and BA [103,104]. Stent deployment decreases the incidence of acute restenosis or rupture secondary to elastic recoil or dissection, respectively, and may also decrease the risk of acute occlusion [2,84,95,96]. Stents may also decrease the long-term risk of restenosis due to intimal hyperplasia and vascular remodeling [70]. The potential pitfalls of stenting include: added technical complexity, greater difficulty in delivery compared with balloon dilation catheters, higher risk of vessel perforation due to the higher pressures needed for full stent deployment and wall apposition, and the potential for occlusion, by the stent struts, of the ostia of small and microscopic perforators off the MCA and BA.

My approach is to perform primary stenting whenever possible. There are several reasons for this. Firstly, predilation with an undersized balloon allows for accurate sizing of the stent using the fully deployed balloon as a reference. Secondly, the patient's pain response to the dilation can be gauged and used as a guide for how aggressive to be with stent advancement and sizing. Thirdly, difficulty with balloon advancement greatly increases the probability that stent placement will fail, and can be used as an opportunity to exchange wires or to reposition the guide catheter for more support before stent placement is attempted. Lastly, if stent placement should prove to be impossible, an adequate PTA result may still be considered a technical success, with probable benefit for the patient.

When the decision to proceed with PTA has been made, the appropriate balloon should be selected. The current generation of coronary balloon catheters is well-suited for intracranial PTA. These balloons have a low profile, are semicompliant, and can be delivered through the tortuous cerebral vessels. Over-the-wire systems are the preferred balloon catheters for intracerebral interventions. Although rapid-exchange balloon systems are easier to use, they are less deliverable into tortuous vessels than over-the-wire balloons of similar crossing profile and tip flexibility. Another drawback of rapid-exchange systems is that wire exchanges cannot be performed through them, and angiography cannot be performed through their central lumen. Balloons used with success include the Open-Sail (Guidant), Predator XL or Ninja (Cordis), Ranger (Boston Scientific/SciMed), Stealth (Boston Scientific/Target Therapeutics, Fremont, CA, USA), Maverick (Boston Scientific), and Stratus (Medtronic, Minneapolis, MN, USA). Over-the-wire balloons have better trackability and are preferred to monorail balloons when vessel tortuosity is present. I prefer the Open-Sail, Ranger, or Maverick balloons for ease of deliverability. The selected balloons should be as short as possible to enhance delivery and to avoid stretching and straightening of the vessel, which could cause perforating artery injury [7]. As previously emphasized, the cerebral arteries are thin and do not have adventitial support. Vessel rupture or dissection with intraparenchymal or subarachnoid hemorrhage (SAH) is often fatal and generally there is no surgical rescue.

As a rule, balloon angioplasty catheters should always be undersized by 10%–20% [70,87,88]. Accurate measurement of vessel size is crucial. In addition, balloon inflation rates and pressures must be precisely controlled since they affect the risk of dissection and rupture. Slow inflations at low to moderate pressures (4–8 atm) for 45–60 seconds or very slow low-pressure inflation over 2–5 minutes may decrease the risk of vessel rupture [60,61,84,90,93,96]. Some investigators have advocated multiple, rapid, and brief inflations of 10 seconds duration with 7–8 atm of pressure [87,92]. Rapid inflation, particularly in calcified, noncompliant vessels, may increase the risk of rupture. During coronary angioplasty, slower inflations have been shown to be safer [105]. However, there is a risk of technical failure if gentle balloon inflation is not followed by stenting.

Angiography should be performed immediately after PTA to check for recoil, dissection, vasospasm, or distal embolization. Repeat angioplasty should be performed if there is no significant increase in lumen diameter or if there is significant recoil and if stent deployment is not planned or feasible secondary to proximal tortuosity; otherwise, a stent should be placed to maintain patency. However, the immediate PTA angiography appearance does not necessarily reflect the long-term result. For example, eventual healing of the intima and subintimal layers will sometimes lead to scar retraction and an increase in luminal diameter, giving an adequate late outcome [66,70]. Similarly, a perfect angiographic result is not always necessary for symptom resolution.

Stenting

Recent developments in coronary stent technology have resulted in low-profile, flexible stents that can be tracked intracranially. None of the commercially available stents is specifically designed for intracranial use. Commonly used coronary stents include: Bx Velocity (Cordis), GFX2 (AVE-Medtronic, Santa Rosa, CA, USA), Multilink Duet, Tetra, and Penta (Guidant). Stents that are appropriate for the intracranial circulation range in diameter from 2.5 to 4 mm, with lengths of 8–18 mm. The same rules that govern angioplasty apply to stenting. Appropriate sizing and gentle deployment are crucial. Stent placement is also critical. As previously discussed, the ostia of perforating vessels and branches should be avoided if at all possible when placing a stent. The small penetrating branches off the main-stem MCA and BA cannot be avoided, but some experimental evidence suggests that this may not be as much of an issue as previously thought [106]. The larger branches, however, such as the ophthalmic, posterior communicating, anterior choroidal, anterior cerebral, and the several cerebellar arteries arising from the VA and BA can be occluded, particularly if they originate near to, or from within, the stenotic segment. If possible, the stent should be positioned so as to avoid their origins, but the interventionalist and the patient should anticipate vessel sacrifice, which may be unavoidable and which may result in stroke.

Following stent deployment, angiography is repeated with multiple views to check for dissection, rupture, embolization, and plaque shift resulting in branch-vessel occlusion. If embolization or branch occlusion is found, the interventionalist must quickly assess the patient for a neurological deficit. If one is found then more anticoagulation may be needed or a GPIIb/IIIa receptor antagonist should be given, since platelet activation is the most likely cause of thrombosis following foreign body placement. Vessel dissection or rupture should be treated as discussed below in the **Complications** section. If there are no complications and the patient is clinically well at the end of the procedure then the heparin should not be reversed; similarly, it will not need to be continued if adequate platelet inhibition was achieved preprocedurally. Close clinical observation is necessary following the procedure because of the risk of acute thrombosis, SAH, or intracerebral hemorrhage.

Blood pressure management is critical in individuals who were recently symptomatic from a severe flow-limiting stenosis, although, as with most aspects of cerebrovascular intervention, there is no consensus on postoperative blood pressure management. Individuals who had critical stenoses with poor cerebrovascular reserve, as identified by a functional study (eg, acetazolamide SPECT or TCD), or those who had poor angiographic collaterals are at risk for hyperperfusion syndrome and ICH. In such patients, particularly those treated with GPIIb/IIIa receptor antagonists, blood pressure should be kept in the low normal range. Hypertension should be avoided in most patients, regardless of the severity of the original stenosis. In patients with multiple stenoses or in those with occlusion of a branch vessel or perforator, blood pressure management can become very complex – the risk of ICH must be balanced against the risk of ischemia induced by lower arterial pressures.

If patients are asymptomatic and their blood pressure is not difficult to control then they may be discharged 24–48 hours following the procedure. Aspirin and clopidogrel should be continued for at least 30 days, after which aspirin alone is continued indefinitely. Follow-up and vessel patency should be assessed at 30 days and then at 6–12 month intervals. Angiographic follow-up may be performed, but does carry some risk, and unless the patient is symptomatic then noninvasive methods of vascular assessment should be used, particularly TCD. Magnetic resonance angiography (MRA) and CT angiography may be inadequate for follow-up imaging: MRA is prone to susceptibility artifacts from the metal in the stents and can only indicate if there is flow restriction distal to the stent; CT angiography tends to overestimate stenoses in vessels with stents <3 mm in diameter. TCD is a noninvasive, rapid, economical, and relatively sensitive method of following most ICA siphon, MCA, VA, and BA stenoses, and can be obtained the day following the procedure. A limitation of TCD is the petrous ICA, which is also difficult to image with CT angiography because of the dense surrounding bone. If noninvasive studies suggest the presence of restenosis then angiography is justified.

Complications

Intracranial hemorrhage

The most significant potential complications of intracranial angioplasty and stenting are ICH and ischemia. ICH is the most common cause of death in published reports [65,73,107,108]. Common clinical findings of significant ICH are sudden severe headache, with or without nausea and vomiting, followed by a rapid decline in consciousness associated with extreme hypertension and bradycardia. Bleeding is usually into the subarachnoid space and occurs as a result of either rupture or dissection of the treated vessel or the tearing of branches or perforators. If ICH is suspected or if obvious extravasation of contrast is seen, anticoagulants and antiplatelets should be immediately reversed with protamine, fresh-frozen plasma, and platelet transfusions as needed. If possible, interventional measures should be performed to control the bleeding. Options include gentle prolonged angioplasty to tamponade the perforation, or stenting if a flow-limiting dissection is present. If no obvious bleeding is seen on angiography, an urgent CT of the brain should be obtained when the patient is stabilized, typically following endotracheal intubation if the ICH is significant. Urgent neurosurgical intervention may be life-saving. A lateral ventricular drain should be considered as a means to rapidly decrease intracranial pressure.

Ischemia

Ischemia can develop at any time during or following the procedure. Ischemia during the intervention may be related to vasospasm, which is common in the cerebral arteries, or due to thrombosis and embolism, which can occur if adequate levels of anticoagulation and platelet inhibition are not maintained during the procedure, especially following stent deployment. Other mechanisms of ischemia include plaque shifting and occlusion of small and often microscopic perforators of the BA and MCA.

Ischemia after completion of the intervention is commonly due to acute thrombosis of the treated vessel, either due to unrecognized dissection or inadequate platelet inhibition. If it develops, ischemia should be treated immediately with blood pressure elevation, hydration, and hemodilution to improve perfusion, and continuation of antithrombotic agents. Urgent angiography should be strongly considered to reassess the treated vessel for acute thrombosis or vasospasm. Acute thrombosis can be treated with repeat angioplasty, but will often respond to GPIIb/IIIa receptor antagonists (if ICH has been excluded with certainty on CT). IA thrombolytics can be used, but they greatly increase the risk of ICH. Vasospasm can be treated with IA nitroglycerin. In either circumstance – ICH or ischemia – the treatments are not ideal.

Outcomes

The technical and clinical outcomes of intracranial angioplasty and stenting are generally favorable; however, there have been no controlled clinical trials and results from existing studies must be interpreted cautiously. Angioplasty alone has an approximately 78% technical success rate, with stroke and death rates of 13% and 1.6%, respectively [58,70,88,89,92,93,109–111]. Dissection and arterial rupture occur in 0%–30% of patients. Data on restenosis are not available from all of the series and the duration of follow-up has varied greatly between the different series. From the data that are available, however, the restenosis rate is 30% within 1 year.

Although it is not possible to generalize from the small number of patients, some have suggested that technical success appears to be greater and complications lower with stenting [84,96]. A review of all of the published series, however, reveals that outcomes are not significantly different with angioplasty alone or stenting [62,64,69–71,73,84,91,94–102,107,108]. Technical success is slightly better with stenting, but stroke and mortality rates may be higher. The rate of dissection or rupture does appear to be lower with stenting. Restenosis data are even scarcer for patients treated with stenting and no worthwhile conclusion can be made at this time.

Many factors may affect the technical and clinical success of intracranial interventions. Operator experience, technical advances, patient selection, lesion characteristics, perioperative antithrombotic and antiplatelet medical treatment, and method and duration of follow-up will all affect outcomes.

Intracranial arteriovenous malformations

AVMs of the brain are the third most common cause of ICH. In young adults, AVMs are one of the most common causes of parenchymal hemorrhage. Until 30 years ago, surgical therapy for AVMs was frequently complicated and often unsuccessful. As with therapy for intracranial aneurysms, the development of modern microvascular neurosurgical techniques has allowed the successful management of most patients. However, large lesions with a deep vascular supply have remained a formidable surgical challenge. With the aid of endovascular therapy, patients with previously untreatable AVMs may now have a treatment option other than observation. Unlike endovascular therapy of aneurysms, however, endovascular therapy of AVMs is usually adjunctive to definitive surgical excision, rather than a separate therapeutic option.

Epidemiology

The frequency of AVMs is 0.5% in autopsy series, with an annual incidence of one seventh to one tenth that of aneurysms and a range of 0.15%–3% [112]. There is a slight male preponderance [113]. Most AVMs become symptomatic by the age of 40 years, with the peak risk of hemorrhage in the 15- to 20-year-old age group [112,113].

AVMs can occur throughout the brain and have three morphologic components:

• the feeding artery or arteries

• the draining veins

• the dysplastic nidus (an abnormal connection between arteries and veins; ie, there is no intervening capillary bed)

AVMs are classified using the Spetzler–Martin classification scheme (see **Table 5**), which is based on three radiological characteristics: size, location (eloquence of the surrounding brain), and the pattern of venous drainage, either deep or superficial [114]. A total of 15%–20% of AVMs have associated intracranial aneurysms.

Characteristic	Points assigned
Size of AVM	
Small (<3 cm)	1
Medium (3–6 cm)	2
Large (>6 cm)	3
Location	
Noneloquent site	0
Eloquent site	1
Sensorimotor, language, visual cortex, hypothalamus, thalamus, brain stem, cerebellar nuclei, or regions directly adjacent to these structures	
Direction of venous drainage	
Superficial	0
Deep (any)	1

Table 5. The Spetzler–Martin scale for evaluating risk of neurological deterioration following surgery for arteriovenous malformation (AVM) resection. Grade = (size) + (eloquence) + (venous drainage). Higher grades are associated with greater surgical morbidity and mortality.

Clinical presentation

Hemorrhage is the initial presenting symptom in 42%–53% of patients. This is followed, in decreasing order of frequency, by seizure (33%–46%), headache (14%–34%), or a progressive neurological deficit (21%–23%) [112]. Patients with AVMs >7 cm^3 are more likely to present with a seizure (72%) than with a hemorrhage (28%). In contrast, those with smaller AVMs are more likely to present with a hemorrhage (75%) than a seizure (25%). However, larger AVMs have a higher risk of rebleeding [112,113].

Hemorrhage is the most devastating complication of AVMs, and may be secondary to rupture of the AVM itself, an associated aneurysm, or both. The hemorrhage may be intraparenchymal or subarachnoid in location. The annual risk of hemorrhage is 3%–4% [112,113,115]. Annual mortality is 0.9%–1%, but decreases after 15 years from the last hemorrhage [112]. With each episode of hemorrhage there is a 20% risk of a major neurological deficit and a 10% risk of mortality [112,113,115].

Diagnosis

Cranial CT is the mainstay of AVM diagnosis, whether ruptured or unruptured. CT readily detects hemorrhage and is also very sensitive for calcification, which is frequently associated with AVMs [112]. MRI is more sensitive than CT for detecting unruptured AVMs and allows for the accurate delineation of normal and abnormal brain tissue. This is essential for the adequate determination of eloquence, as defined in the Spetzler–Martin scale [114]. Conventional four-vessel cerebral angiography is the gold standard test for preoperative and pre-embolization assessment. MRA is not an adequate substitute for conventional angiography.

Therapy

There are several treatment options for AVMs, including observation, embolization, stereotactic radiosurgery, microsurgery, or combinations of the above [116,117]. Most patients should be considered for some form of therapeutic intervention because of the poor natural history of AVMs. The goal of AVM therapy is the complete removal or obliteration of the AVM; although partial therapy may offer a palliative effect for headaches, seizures, and progressive neurological deficits, it does not decrease the risk of re-hemorrhage [117,118].

AVMs of Spetzler–Martin grades I–III can be successfully treated with microsurgical excision with a low morbidity (0%–4.2%) [119]. Surgery often results in a cure and should be considered the treatment of choice in this patient group [117,119]. On the other hand, Spetzler–Martin grade IV and V lesions are high surgical risk lesions because of their large size and deep venous drainage, or because they are located in an eloquent location. Endovascular therapy is the treatment of choice for these lesions, either alone or in combination with microsurgery or stereotactic radiosurgery [117,120–122]. The long-term morbidity of microsurgical excision alone is 21.9% and 16.7% in grade IV and V AVMs, respectively [119].

Treatment technique

Biplanar fluoroscopy is particularly useful in AVM embolizations. As with other intracranial procedures, the margin of safety can be greatly increased if the patient is awake for the intervention, facilitating intraoperative neurological assessment. Vascular access should be obtained through a femoral route with insertion of a 6- to 8-Fr guide catheter into the ICA or VA. Superselective catheterization of the feeding arterial pedicles is then performed.

Full radiographic evaluation is required for the planning of embolization (see **Figure 6**). MRI is essential to detail the proximity of the lesion to eloquent brain, the appropriate operative corridor needed to access the lesion surgically, and the feasibility of preoperative (surgical or radiosurgical) reductive or ablative embolization. High-resolution four-vessel catheter angiography with selective injections of feeding pedicles and high-speed filming rates (≥4 frames/s) is critical in the planning of surgical and endovascular approaches. The studies are performed to define the number and type of arterial pedicles, their relationship to the supply of surrounding normal brain, the size of the nidus, the presence of associated fistulae and aneurysms (both intranidal and remote), and the type of venous drainage (superficial or deep). Higher risks of hemorrhage have been associated with lesions that have deep venous drainage (especially if a venous stenosis is present) or a periventricular location, and intranidal aneurysms [123,124].

The angiographic anatomy of AVMs is quite complex. A variable number of arteries may feed the nidus, with two patterns of supply: the supplying artery either directly terminates in the nidus, or sends feeders (or twigs) to the nidus while the main trunk continues on to supply normal brain distal to the branch point. These latter vessels are known as *en passage* (or vessel in passage) feeders. The presence of an *en passage* arterial supply carries a higher risk of posttreatment (surgical or endovascular treatment) ischemic neurological deficits. This is because of the risk of injury or embolization to the parent vessel. Superselective angiography of single pedicles of AVMs with multiple feeders is very helpful. With this technique, it is possible to demonstrate whether a single feeder supplies one portion or compartment of the AVM or if it receives blood supply from multiple feeders. The presence of single-feeding pedicles increases the probability of successful occlusion of that portion of the AVM.

Equipment

More so than with other neuroendovascular procedures, small size is a requisite for access to the often diminutive arteries of an AVM. Catheters capable of reaching the distal cerebral arteries range in size from 1.8- to 2.3-Fr. Two types of catheters are available: over-the-wire and flow-directed. Both types have a hydrophilic coating.

Over-the-wire catheter vessel access is performed with a steerable 0.014- or 0.010-inch microguidewire. The AVMs are characterized by high flow rates into feeding pedicles, and this affords the use of flow-directed catheters. The high flow rate is a result of the lack of intervening capillaries and arterioles, which greatly decreases vascular resistance. As a consequence, catheters that have an extremely floppy, low-mass, bulb-shaped tip are preferentially directed into the AVM by the high flow, rather than into the normal branches of a feeding artery, which have much lower flow rates. Flow-directed catheters work best for accessing the nidus in the early stages of embolization when the high-flow state is maintained. As embolization proceeds and the arteriovenous shunt decreases, the ease with which these catheters "sail" to the nidus diminishes.

Embolic agents

There are two broad categories of embolic agents: liquids and particles. Cyanoacrylates ("glue") are the prototypical liquid agents and are the only agents that can lead to a permanent endovascular cure. The most widely used cyanoacrylate, n-butyl cyanoacrylate (NBCA), is a liquid that polymerizes immediately upon contact with an ionic solution containing free hydrogen ions. This characteristic of NBCA permits its use, but also makes its use very complicated, as will be discussed shortly. The low viscosity of cyanoacrylates permits their injection through the smallest of microcatheters, while particulate agents often require the use of larger microcatheters. The prototypical particulate agent is polyvinyl alcohol (PVA).

Embolization technique

The entire AVM nidus, including the components nearest the venous side, must be occluded for an endovascular cure or else the nidus will recruit a new arterial supply. Where surgery is indicated, embolization may be performed to reduce both the rate of blood flow and the size of the AVM in order to lessen operative morbidity and to increase the probability of successful treatment with radiosurgery. This is not always straightforward, and to achieve a cure without complications the interventionalist must have a thorough understanding of the polymerization characteristics of the embolic agent, the rate of blood flow through the nidus, the degree of pedicle occlusion by the microcatheter, and the rate of material delivery through any given microcatheter.

Before delivering embolic material to an AVM, the risk of causing focal ischemia and stroke by unintentional embolization of a normal vessel must be assessed by angiography through the microcatheter after it has been placed in its final position. This will show if any normal brain is being irrigated distal to the tip of the microcatheter. When there is doubt as to whether functional brain will be embolized, a provocative challenge can be performed by injecting amobarbital through the microcatheter. This short-acting barbiturate effectively shuts down neuronal activity – therefore, if no clinical deficits develop, embolization of that particular pedicle will be unlikely to cause a significant neurological deficit.

After access is obtained to the appropriate vessel, angiography is performed. The goal of the interventionalist is to determine the following:

• exactly which vessels supply the AVM

• how many feeding pedicles are present

• the relative flow rates in each pedicle

• the number and location of draining veins or nidal aneurysms

The largest pedicles and those feeding aneurysms and large draining veins should be selected as the initial targets for embolization. The location and size of the AVM also plays a role in determining the appropriate treatment strategy. AVMs that are superficially located usually have arterial supply from only one or a few cortical arteries. Large supratentorial AVMs are frequently wedge- or pyramidal-shaped, with their bases at the cortical surface and their apices extending down to the lateral ventricle. These AVMs, and those located entirely in a deep location, often have supply from the choroidal and lenticulostriate systems. Such a deep arterial supply increases the complexity of surgical excision, and the risk of blood loss and surgical complications. Therefore, deep-feeding vessels are ideal targets for embolization.

In deciding on the strategy for embolization, the interventionalist must also consider whether it will be necessary to re-access the feeding pedicles, in which case it will be important to ensure that gluing one pedicle does not prevent access to other pedicles. With a strategy in mind, the flow-directed microcatheter, usually with a tip shaped appropriately for the task at hand, is advanced into the feeding artery and directed into the appropriate pedicle. Selective angiography is then performed through the microcatheter, focusing on forward flow through the pedicle, retrograde flow (if any) into the feeding artery, and the opacification of any normal brain tissue. Once the microcatheter is appropriately positioned and the decision to treat that pedicle is made, the glue mixture is made.

NBCA polymerizes rapidly. For a slower and more controlled polymerization, NBCA is mixed with lipiodol, an oily contrast medium. An advantage of lipiodol is that it also opacifies the glue mixture for fluoroscopic visualization. With experience, the interventionalist can vary the ratios of the components of the cocktail to facilitate penetration of the entire nidus with glue before polymerization. The mixture must also be prepared so that polymerization occurs before the glue reaches the draining vein(s). If the draining veins are occluded, AVM rupture can occur due to increased back-pressure within the nidus. Finally, glue injection must be timed perfectly with withdrawal of the microcatheter to avoid both gluing the microcatheter to the nidus (usually an irrevocable situation) and embolization into normal vessels.

When handling the completed mixture, care must be taken to avoid contact with ionic fluids (eg, normal saline and blood), which could cause premature polymerization. The microcatheter is therefore flushed thoroughly with pure water. The injection of glue is then performed, keeping in mind the shape of the pedicle and the portion of the AVM that it feeds. Once opacification of the nidus and pedicle occurs, the injection is terminated and the microcatheter is quickly withdrawn into the guide catheter in one smooth motion. This is best performed by an experienced assistant at the command of the interventionalist performing the injection. The microcatheter is then removed and the guide aspirated to remove any glue particles before a repeat angiography is performed. This process is repeated as needed (see **Figure 6**).

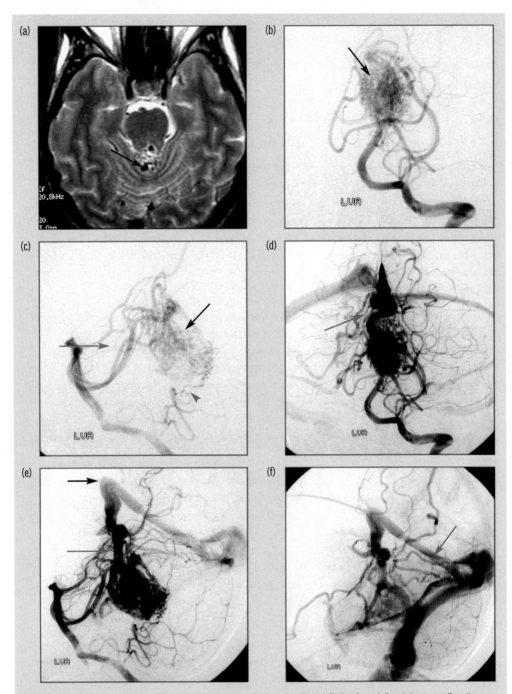

Figure 6. A 38-year-old woman with a history of cerebellar hemorrhage presented for preoperative embolization of a cerebellar arteriovenous malformation (AVM). A magnetic resonance imaging scan of the brain (**a**) showed several large flow voids within the fourth ventricle and cerebellar vermis (arrow). A cranial anteroposterior (AP) view (**b**) and a lateral view (**c**) of a selective left vertebral angiogram performed at a high frame rate (early arterial phase) showed the AVM nidus (black arrow) and the major arterial supply from the posterior inferior cerebellar artery (PICA) (arrowhead in **c**) and the superior cerebellar arteries (SCAs) (orange arrow in **c**). A late arterial phase image ([**d**] AP view, [**e**] lateral view) showed the large draining vein (orange arrow in **d** and **e**), which drains into the vein of Galen (black arrow in **e**). A venous phase lateral angiogram (**f**) showed venous drainage of the AVM, mainly via the straight sinus (arrow) into the torcular herophili. Following embolization of an SCA feeder and a PICA feeder, the nidus of the AVM was noticeably smaller (black arrow in **g**) and there was less flow

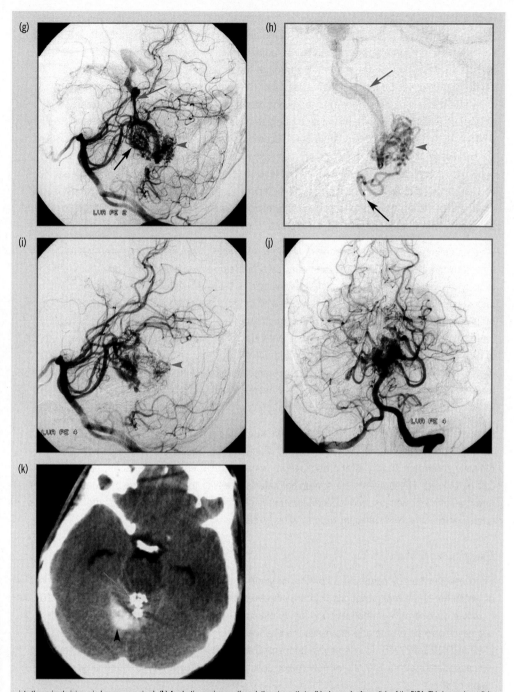

into the major draining vein (orange arrow in **g**). (**h**) A selective angiogram, through the microcatheter (black arrow), of a pedicle of the PICA. This is a major pedicle feeding the inferior pole of the nidus (arrowhead in **h**), which corresponds to the portion seen on nonselective injection (arrowhead in **g**). Note the major contribution of the selected pedicle to the draining vein (orange arrow in **h**). After embolization of the pedicle, the inferior pole of the nidus was nearly completely embolized (arrowhead in **i**); most importantly, the major draining vein no longer filled (compare with **g**). A final AP angiogram (**j**) showed the markedly reduced size of the AVM nidus and the lack of filling of the major vein. An immediate postembolization computed tomography scan (**k**) showed the glue cast (orange arrow) and stagnant blood and contrast in the draining vein (arrowhead). The patient underwent successful surgical excision of the AVM 2 days postembolization.

Particulate embolic agents are composed of a variety of materials and come in a range of sizes. The smallest are PVA particles, which are manufactured in sizes ranging from 50 to 1,500 µM. For injection, the particles are suspended in radiographic contrast media. The exact size of particle used depends on the rate of flow through the nidus and the presence of intranidal shunts and fistulae. If a large enough quantity of PVA particles pass through the nidus and cross into the venous circulation then transient pneumonitis can develop. To decrease the risk of this complication, intranidal shunts can be partially occluded by mixing the PVA with fibrillary collagen or by using Berenstein liquid coils (Boston Scientific/Target Therapeutics). These coils are composed of fine injectable platinum threads, which promote thrombus formation. When delivered to small feeding pedicles, they will lead to thrombosis and occlusion of the vessel. For very large feeding vessels (3–5 mm diameter), embolization with vortex or "tornado" shaped platinum coils can be performed through the microcatheter. Like the liquid coils, these coils are coated with fibered threads, which promote thrombosis and occlusion.

When a definitive cure is not needed or feasible, AVM embolization can be performed as a palliative treatment – or, more commonly, as a pretreatment prior to radiosurgery or open excision. Preoperative treatment decreases the size of the AVM nidus, which facilitates both radiosurgery and surgical excision. In the case of radiosurgery, embolization decreases the radiation dose required and the size of the treatment field, minimizing the exposure of healthy brain tissue to radiation and increasing the potential for a cure. Despite the complexities inherent in their use and their potential for serious complications, cyanoacrylates are particularly useful in reducing the size of selected AVMs before stereotactic radiosurgery. Their adhesive properties result in permanent occlusion, which is ideal before radiosurgery because the clinical benefit following radiation treatment (in terms of reduction of ICH risk) is delayed for at least 6 months.

Preoperative embolization also facilitates open surgical excision by decreasing the size of the AVM and decreasing intraoperative bleeding, which can be significant. Since open excision is typically performed shortly after embolization, nonpermanent embolic agents (ie, particulates) can be utilized. These agents are somewhat safer and easier to use than the cyanoacrylates and are sufficient because nidus recanalization is often delayed for a few weeks after particulate embolization, which is sufficient time to allow excision.

Results overview

Endovascular therapy results in a cure or complete obliteration in only 5%–20% of AVMs, most of which are small malformations that are also treatable with surgical excision [118,125,126]. However, preoperative embolization is highly effective in decreasing surgical bleeding, which decreases operative time and increases the chance of surgical success in high-grade lesions [117,120,121,127–9]. In one series, endovascular embolization followed by microsurgery was associated with a 5% rate of new major deficits compared with 31% in the surgery-only group [130].

The best results are obtained when surgery is performed within 2–14 days of embolization. Such a short interval decreases the probability of AVM recanalization via new leptomeningeal or deep collaterals [117,118]. Since AVM recanalization occurs with all embolic agents except cyanoacrylate glue, endovascular therapy should be followed by early microsurgery in lesions treated with these nonpermanent agents [117,118]. Large AVMs should be treated with staged embolization to decrease the risk of perfusion pressure breakthrough and ICH [118,119]. The combination of endovascular embolization and radiosurgery has not been adequately studied and is controversial [118,131–4].

Complications of endovascular therapy include embolic stroke, ICH, pulmonary embolism, and microcatheter retention [117,118]. The reported complication rates vary from 3% to 25%, but serious neurological events or death occur in only 3%–8% of cases [117,120]. Staged embolization of large AVMs, meticulous technique, and rapid withdrawal of the microcatheter after injection greatly reduce the risk of complications [117,118].

Cerebral aneurysms

With the advances in microsurgical techniques, clipping via craniotomy remains the most widely accepted method of treating cerebral aneurysms. Concurrently, advances have been made in the endovascular treatment of a variety of vascular diseases, including cerebral aneurysms. Initially, endovascular treatments utilized balloons to occlude the parent vessel, but the techniques were refined to the point where packing and occlusion of the aneurysm itself with detachable balloons was possible [135–138]. However, these techniques were not very durable [137,139].

The most significant advance in endovascular therapy was the development of the Guglielmi detachable coil (GDC) (Boston Scientific/Target Therapeutics) [140]. These coils of soft platinum are delivered within an aneurysm by a microcatheter, resulting in occlusion. Multiple trials and reports have confirmed the efficacy and safety of this technique in carefully selected patients, leading in 1995 to FDA approval for the treatment of patients at high risk of surgical morbidity. This treatment has emerged as a safe and effective alternative to surgical clipping.

Epidemiology of subarachnoid hemorrhage and cerebral aneurysms

SAH due to aneurysm rupture is one of the most dramatic and devastating stroke disorders. Intracranial aneurysms are common and have a prevalence of 0.3%–8% in the general population [141,142]. Aneurysmal rupture and SAH affect 25,000 individuals annually in the USA with an incidence of 1 in 10,000, and account for 5% of all strokes. As a result, 18,000 of these individuals will die or have severe disability.

Cerebral aneurysms are located at the base of the brain and involve the arteries of the Circle of Willis. The most common location is the anterior communicating artery, followed (in order of decreasing frequency) by the ICA, MCA, and VB circulation. Multiple aneurysms occur in 20% of individuals, and approximately 80% of intracranial aneurysms are "congenital" or saccular. Aneurysms develop from defects of the arterial wall at bifurcations. Other etiologies include atherosclerosis (fusiform), infection (mycotic), trauma, or arterial dissection.

Clinical presentation

SAH classically presents with a sudden ("thunderclap") onset of severe headache accompanied by loss of consciousness, nausea, and vomiting. A total of 25% of patients die immediately; if a patient does survive the initial event then nuchal rigidity, focal neurological deficits, seizures, fever, and a depressed level of consciousness often develop. Onset is not so catastrophic in 20%–50% of cases; instead, patients develop a sudden, but less severe, headache, which is not associated with neurological deficits other than mild signs of meningeal irritation. These are called "sentinel" bleeds [143]. Some aneurysms, particularly larger ones, manifest with symptoms of mass effect, such as headache, cranial nerve dysfunction (especially occulomotor and abducens nerve palsies), or hydrocephalus. Rarely, a direct carotid–cavernous sinus fistula is the presenting sign of a cavernous ICA aneurysm.

Patients with aneurysmal SAH are graded with the Hunt and Hess scale, which is a predictor of overall outcome and surgical morbidity [144,145]. The scale ranges from a score of 0 (asymptomatic) to 5 (moribund and comatose). Patients who present with a high Hunt and Hess grade (grades 4–5) have the worst prognosis: they have a 2-fold higher risk of death than those with a lower score. Treatment for unruptured aneurysms carries a better prognosis than for ruptured aneurysms. The rate of aneurysm rupture is 0.05%–2.3% per year, depending on the size and location of the aneurysm [146,147]. Aneurysms >7 mm in size that are in the VB circulation have the highest risk of rupture.

The natural history of untreated ruptured cerebral aneurysms is grim. There is an 81% mortality rate in the first 3 months following SAH, mostly due to rebleeding if an aneurysm is not secured [148]. The risk of rebleeding is 6%–9% in the first week, but this increases to >20% at 30 days. The mortality rate with rebleeding is nearly 70% [148,149].

Diagnosis

SAH should be suspected in all patients who develop a sudden severe headache, particularly if there are other neurological signs. The diagnosis is confirmed with a CT scan, which has a sensitivity of 92% and a specificity of nearly 100% [150]. If there is a strong clinical suspicion of SAH but the CT scan is not diagnostic, a lumbar puncture should be performed. Cerebral angiography is the gold standard for appropriate diagnosis and therapeutic decision-making after SAH, and four-vessel digital subtraction cerebral angiography must be performed emergently in all patients with an SAH, except for those with a high Hunt and Hess grade who would not be considered for emergent surgical or endovascular treatment. The aim of angiography is to identify the location, size, and shape of the aneurysm(s), the presence and size of the neck, and the relationship of the aneurysm to the parent vessel and its adjacent branches.

Therapy

The therapy for intracranial aneurysms remains controversial. There are controversies not only over the durability of endovascular therapy versus surgical therapy, but also over the timing of aneurysm surgery. The International Cooperative Study on the Timing of Aneurysm Surgery was conducted to address the timing of aneurysm surgery [145,149]. The investigators found equivalent results in patients treated with clipping in the first few days after SAH compared with those treated after 10 days. The best outcomes were found in patients who had a low Hunt and Hess grade at presentation and who had surgery within 3 days. The general approach is to clip ruptured aneurysms as soon as practical, especially in patients with a Hunt and Hess grade ≤3.

In addition, the indications for intervention for unruptured aneurysms are controversial. The current indications for endovascular therapy include [151]:

• failure of surgery due to anatomical or technical factors

• aneurysms with a high surgical risk (eg, basilar-tip or ICA aneurysms)

• incomplete surgical clipping

• high patient surgical risks secondary to the SAH or underlying medical conditions

Treatment techniques

In contrast to the complex planning needed for the endovascular treatment of AVMs, the endovascular options for the treatment of cerebral aneurysms are more simple. Surgical clipping via craniotomy is a well-established and effective treatment, but endovascular treatment is emerging as a safe alternative in most patients and the only safe treatment for some. Unlike endovascular embolization of AVMs, the goal of endovascular treatment of aneurysms is the complete obliteration of the aneurysm dome and its neck. In some cases even partial occlusion is acceptable – for example, near complete occlusion of a symptomatic aneurysm at the basilar apex in a debilitated 80-year-old patient may be a more appropriate option than 100% occlusion via craniotomy.

Successful obliteration of an aneurysm requires the development of permanent thrombosis of the aneurysm sac. Two general approaches can be used to achieve this: *constructive* embolization or *deconstructive* embolization. Constructive treatment is designed to recreate the parent vessel's normal lumen, preserving the patient's normal vascular anatomy and flow patterns. Deconstructive treatment involves the planned sacrifice of the parent vessel with subsequent antegrade thrombosis of the aneurysm as thrombus propagates beyond the point of iatrogenic occlusion. This latter approach can only be performed in patients with an adequate collateral blood supply to the distal territory, otherwise cerebral infarction will develop.

Endovascular tools

Constructive treatment

The most commonly used endovascular device for the treatment of intracranial aneurysms is the GDC. This coil is available in several different forms (small coil, large coil, 2D, 3D). Occlusion of the aneurysm (ie, isolation of the aneurysmal dome from the systemic circulation) is accomplished by placing the GDC coils into the sac of the aneurysm through a microcatheter. As in the treatment of AVMs, the microcatheter is advanced through a previously positioned guiding catheter in the cervical ICA or VA using the techniques discussed previously, in particular those techniques that ensure stable vessel access and support. With the microcatheter in the appropriate position, the coils are pushed through it into the aneurysm. After insertion of the full length of the coil into the aneurysm, angiography is performed to ensure that there is no prolapse of the coil mass or individual loops into the arterial lumen. If there is prolapse, the coil can be withdrawn and then repositioned, or, alternatively, a different coil of another size and configuration can be used. When a satisfactory position is obtained, the GDC coil is detached from the delivery wire via a low-amplitude electrical current, which dissolves a solder joint between the coil and the delivery wire. The goal of the first coil placement is to create a "basket" that will act as a scaffold, permitting

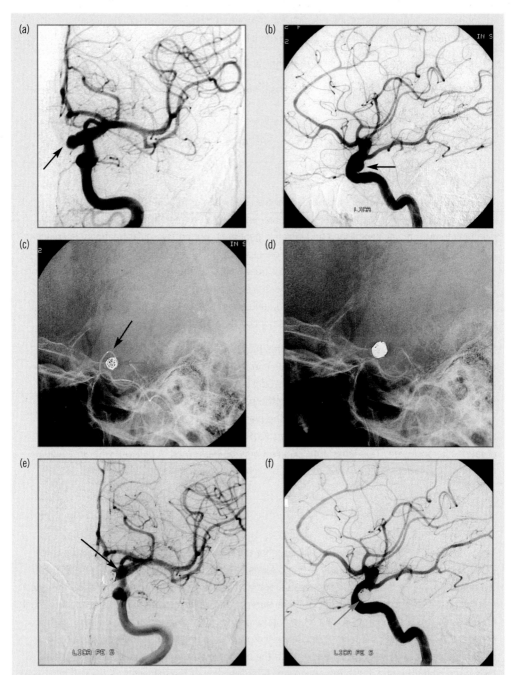

Figure 7. (a) A selective left internal carotid artery (ICA) angiogram, anteroposterior (AP) cranial view, in a patient with new-onset headaches discovered to have an ICA aneurysm by magnetic resonance angiography. The arrow points to the dome of the aneurysm, which was pointing inferiomedially from the supraclinoid ICA and measured 6.8×4 mm. Note the very wide neck of the aneurysm, which is tubular in configuration. The lateral view (b) does not show the aneurysm well, but careful inspection shows an extra density pointing posteriorly (arrow). ICA aneurysms in this location and of this size can cause SAH and are difficult to access surgically. Endovascular treatment was performed (c; lateral view) with placement of a microcatheter into the aneurysm (black arrow). The first coil is the most crucial coil to place as it forms a scaffold (orange arrow) within which the other coils will be trapped. In this case, five GDC coils were placed (d; lateral view). The broad base of the aneurysm, however, did not permit tight packing of the neck without prolapse of the coils into the ICA lumen; therefore, some residual neck was present on the final AP angiogram (arrow in e; AP cranial view). On the lateral angiogram, the location of the aneurysm is now better appreciated by noting the densely packed coil mass (arrow in f).

filling of the basket with progressively smaller and shorter coils until dense packing is achieved (see **Figure 7**). This dense packing results in the formation of a thrombus within the interstices of the coil mass. The stability of the thrombus is proportional to the amount of metal (thrombus nidus) that can be placed.

The major obstacle to the successful occlusion of all aneurysms is the width of the aneurysm neck. A dome-to-neck ratio of <2 is difficult to treat with standard coil embolization techniques [152]. Several new devices and techniques have been developed to overcome this limitation. The balloon-remodeling method has been successful in many cases [153]. In this technique, a soft distensible balloon is inflated within the parent vessel lumen across the aneurysm neck, trapping the microcatheter and therefore the coils within the aneurysm. Once the full length of the coil has been deployed, the balloon is deflated and angiography is performed to assess the stability of the coil in relation to the parent vessel before coil detachment. The sequence is repeated until the entire aneurysm has been densely packed.

Special "three-dimensional" GDC coil shapes have been developed (Boston Scientific/Target Therapeutics), which are more stable when deployed in wide-necked aneurysms. The three-dimensional coil is a variant of the original circular coil design that assumes a spherical, cage-like configuration when deployed. Another development is the "Tri-Span" coil (Boston Scientific/Target Therapeutics), which is specifically designed for use in wide-necked aneurysms. The device assumes a "flower petal" configuration that is designed to mechanically recreate a small neck out of the wide-necked aneurysm. Conventional GDC coils are then deployed to stabilize the "petals" against the aneurysm's walls. After the sac has been filled, the petal is detached by electrolysis. A new and very promising device is the Neuroform stent (Boston Scientific/Smart Therapeutics, San Leandro, CA, USA). This self-expanding stent is made of very thin struts and as a result is very trackable and can be delivered via a microcatheter. The stent is placed within the lumen of the parent vessel across the neck of the aneurysm. Coils are then deployed through a microcatheter placed through the stent struts, which act as a scaffold. This technique is particularly effective for ultra-wide neck and fusiform aneurysms.

Deconstructive treatment

Although it is preferable to preserve the parent vessel, some aneurysms, because of their location and the pattern of available collateral circulation, are best treated by sacrificing the parent vessel. The most common locations for such aneurysms are the cavernous segment of the ICA and the distal branches of the cerebellar arteries. Surgical treatment of these aneurysms is technically challenging. They often have a wide neck, or they arise from or incorporate the anterior loop of the carotid artery as it emerges from the cavernous sinus. Hunterian occlusion (planned carotid sacrifice) should be preceded by a functional test to measure the adequacy of collateral circulation. This test is best performed with a test balloon occlusion (TBO) [154].

If the patient passes the TBO then carotid occlusion may be performed with one of two devices. The safest and most rapid method is to use detachable silicone balloons (DSBs) [155]. The balloons are delivered on a microcatheter to the site of occlusion, where they are rapidly inflated with an iso-osmolar concentration of contrast. They are detached by mechanical traction. Two or three balloons should be serially deployed to decrease the likelihood of balloon deflation and migration. A plain skull radiograph should be obtained following the procedure and is a convenient means of following the position of the balloons over time to monitor for migration, which can occur. The alternative to DSBs is to use large, fiber-coated coils, which rapidly induce thrombus formation [156,157]. Anticoagulation with warfarin sodium is necessary for a period of 6 months following either of the above techniques.

The desirable approach is to trap the aneurysm between two occlusive devices, one proximal and one distal to the neck of the aneurysm. This technique prevents retrograde blood flow to the aneurysm. Unfortunately, aneurysms of the cavernous carotid often have such broad necks that distal device placement compromises the origin of the ophthalmic artery, resulting in retinal ischemia. However, since the occlusion of an artery often causes thrombus formation up to the next branch point, proximal carotid artery occlusion will typically result in thrombosis of the ICA and occlusion of the aneurysm up to the ophthalmic artery.

Results of endovascular therapy

Viñuela et al. reported on the first 403 patients treated in the USA [158]. The technical success rate, defined as complete aneurysm occlusion, was 70.8% in small aneurysms with small necks, but only 31.2% in small aneurysms with large necks. Large aneurysms and giant aneurysms were successfully completely occluded 35% and 50% of the time, respectively. A total of 23 patients (5.7% overall) had treatment failure due to the inability to achieve even partial occlusion. Patients with better clinical grades prior to therapy had better clinical outcomes: 93% of Hunt and Hess grade 1 patients improved or were unchanged compared with only 54% of grade 5 patients. Early rebleeding was decreased with endovascular treatment, and the associated morbidity and mortality were 8.9% and 6.2%, respectively. Complications included aneurysm perforation (2.7%), parent artery occlusion (3%), and distal embolization (2.5%). Aneurysmal perforation occurred almost exclusively in patients with small aneurysms. Follow-up was limited to 36 months; in that period, nine aneurysms (2.2%) re-bled, all of which were incompletely occluded aneurysms. Other, smaller series have also reported complete occlusion rates of approximately 80% [159].

With increasing clinical experience, morbidity, mortality, and technical success rates have improved, and are now approaching the results achieved with surgery [152,159–164]. Factors associated with an increased likelihood of complete angiographic occlusion include the presence of a small neck (≤4 mm), a small aneurysm, indirect inflow of the blood stream into the aneurysm, and the technical experience of the interventionalist [163,165]. Immediate technical success is the best predictor of the likelihood of persistent occlusion [163,165]. Complications of endovascular therapy, including macro- and microembolization with resultant ischemia, parent artery occlusion, and aneurysm perforation, have been reported to occur in 2.8%–28% of patients, depending on the series [158–160,162,166,167].

In comparing the results of endovascular therapy with surgical clipping, it must be kept in mind that, until recently, most of the available data on endovascular therapy were from small series of patients who were poor surgical candidates, many of whom had a poor neurological grade (Hunt and Hess grades 4 and 5). The major reasons for exclusion from surgery were poor clinical condition or a high risk and complexity of surgery [159,162]. Although the risk for early rebleeding is decreased with successful endovascular therapy, there are few available data on the durability of endovascular occlusion and hemorrhage recurrence risks. Studies of patients with follow-up angiography performed 0–72 months after embolization have shown that 61%–86% of aneurysms are unchanged [161,165]. The risk of recanalization and rebleeding does increase with time. The risk of rebleeding over 1–72 months is as low as 0%–3.2% in small aneurysms, but as high as 4% for large aneurysms and 33% for giant aneurysms [161,165,168].

Results for the endovascular treatment of asymptomatic and unruptured aneurysms are better than for acutely ruptured aneurysms because of the better clinical condition of the patients. In a series of 120 aneurysms, 91% of incidental aneurysms were successfully treated (complete or near-complete occlusion), with a morbidity of 4.3% [169]. Endovascular treatment has also been used to successfully treat the consequences of mass effect produced by large and giant unruptured aneurysms (eg, cranial neuropathies) [170]. As with ruptured aneurysms, long-term follow-up is lacking and the durability of endovascular occlusions remains unknown.

References

1. Furlan A, Higashida R, Wechsler L, et al. Intra-arterial prourokinase for acute ischemic stroke. The PROACT II study: a randomized controlled trial. Prolyse in Acute Cerebral Thromboembolism. *JAMA* 1999;282:2003–11.
2. Adams HP Jr, Brott TG, Furlan AJ, et al. Guidelines for thrombolytic therapy for acute stroke: a supplement to the guidelines for the management of patients with acute ischemic stroke. A statement for healthcare professionals from a Special Writing Group of the Stroke Council, American Heart Association. *Circulation* 1996;94:1167–74.
3. Moskowitz M, Caplan LR, editors. Thrombolytic treatment in acute stroke: review and update of selective topics. In: *Cerebrovascular Diseases: Nineteenth Princeton Stroke Conference*. Boston: Butterworth-Heinemann, 1995.
4. del Zoppo GJ, Ferbert A, Otis S, et al. Local intra-arterial fibrinolytic therapy in acute carotid territory stroke. A pilot study. *Stroke* 1988;19:307–13.
5. del Zoppo GJ, Poeck K, Pessin MS, et al. Recombinant tissue plasminogen activator in acute thrombotic and embolic stroke. *Ann Neurol* 1992;32:78–86.
6. The National Institute of Neurological Disorders and Stroke rt-PA Stroke Study Group. Tissue plasminogen activator for acute ischemic stroke. *N Engl J Med* 1995;333:1581–7.
7. del Zoppo G, Higashida R, Furlan A, et al. PROACT: A phase II randomized trial of recombinant pro-urokinase by direct arterial delivery in acute middle cerebral artery stroke. PROACT Investigators. Prolyse in Acute Cerebral Thromboembolism. *Stroke* 1998;29:4–11.
8. Hacke W, Kaste M, Fieschi C, et al. Intravenous thrombolysis with recombinant tissue plasminogen activator for acute hemispheric stroke. The European Cooperative Acute Stroke Study (ECASS). *JAMA* 1995;274:1017–25.
9. Albers GW, Clark WM, Madden KP, et al. ATLANTIS trial: results for patients treated within 3 hours of stroke onset. Alteplase Thrombolysis for Acute Noninterventional Therapy in Ischemic Stroke. *Stroke* 2002;33:493–5.
10. Hacke W, Kaste M, Fieschi C, et al. Randomised double-blind placebo-controlled trial of thrombolytic therapy with intravenous alteplase in acute ischaemic stroke (ECASS II). Second European–Australasian Acute Stroke Study Investigators. *Lancet* 1998;352:1245–51.
11. Hacke W, Zeumer H, Ferbert A, et al. Intra-arterial thrombolytic therapy improves outcome in patients with acute vertebrobasilar occlusive disease. *Stroke* 1988;19:1216–22.
12. del Zoppo GJ, Sasahara AA. Interventional use of plasminogen activators in central nervous system diseases. *Med Clin North Am* 1998;82:545–68.
13. Hoffman AI, Lambiase RE, Haas RA, et al. Acute vertebrobasilar occlusion: treatment with high-dose intraarterial urokinase. *AJR Am J Roentgenol* 1999;172:709–12.
14. Cross DT 3rd, Moran CJ, Akins PT, et al. Collateral circulation and outcome after basilar artery thrombolysis. *AJNR Am J Neuroradiol* 1998;19:1557–63.
15. von Kummer R, Hacke W. Safety and efficacy of intravenous tissue plasminogen activator and heparin in acute middle cerebral artery stroke. *Stroke* 1992;23:646–52.
16. Brandt T, von Kummer R, Muller-Kuppers M, et al. Thrombolytic therapy of acute basilar artery occlusion. Variables affecting recanalization and outcome. *Stroke* 1996;27:875–81.
17. Katzan IL, Masaryk TJ, Furlan AJ, et al. Intra-arterial thrombolysis for perioperative stroke after open heart surgery. *Neurology* 1999;52:1081–4.
18. Lee DH, Jo KD, Kim HG, et al. Local intraarterial urokinase thrombolysis of acute ischemic stroke with or without intravenous abciximab: a pilot study. *J Vasc Interv Radiol* 2002;13:769–74.

19. Lanzino G, Fessler RD, Wakhloo AK, et al. Successful intracranial thrombolysis for cerebral thromboembolic complications resulting from cardiovascular diagnostic and interventional procedures. *J Invasive Cardiol* 1999;11:439–43.

20. Hacke W, Brott T, Caplan L, et al. Thrombolysis in acute ischemic stroke: controlled trials and clinical experience. *Neurology* 1999;53(7 Suppl. 4):S3–14.

21. Callahan AS 3rd, Berger BL. Intra-arterial thrombolysis in acute ischemic stroke. *Tenn Med* 1997;90:61–4.

22. The Multicenter Acute Stroke Trial–Europe Study Group. Thrombolytic therapy with streptokinase in acute ischemic stroke. *N Engl J Med* 1996;335:145–50.

23. Yokogami K, Nakano S, Ohta H, et al. Prediction of hemorrhagic complications after thrombolytic therapy for middle cerebral artery occlusion: value of pre- and post-therapeutic computed tomographic findings and angiographic occlusive site. *Neurosurgery* 1996;39:1102–7.

24. Ringer AJ, Qureshi AI, Fessler RD, et al. Angioplasty of intracranial occlusion resistant to thrombolysis in acute ischemic stroke. *Neurosurgery* 2001;48:1282–8; discussion 1288–90.

25. Nakano S, Iseda T, Yoneyama T, et al. Direct percutaneous transluminal angioplasty for acute middle cerebral artery trunk occlusion: an alternative option to intra-arterial thrombolysis. *Stroke* 2002;33:2872–6.

26. Qureshi AI, Siddiqui AM, Suri MF, et al. Aggressive mechanical clot disruption and low-dose intra-arterial third-generation thrombolytic agent for ischemic stroke: a prospective study. *Neurosurgery* 2002;51:1319–27; discussion 1327–9..

27. Abou-Chebl A, Krieger D, Bajzer C, et al. Multimodal therapy for the treatment of severe ischemic stroke combining GPIIb/IIIa antagonists and angioplasty after failure of thrombolysis. *Stroke* 2003;34:312.

28. Alexandrov AV, Grotta JC. Arterial reocclusion in stroke patients treated with intravenous tissue plasminogen activator. *Neurology* 2002;59:862–7.

29. Doggrell SA. Alteplase: descendancy in myocardial infarction, ascendancy in stroke. *Expert Opin Investig Drugs* 2001;10:2013–29.

30. International Stroke Trial Collaborative Group. The International Stroke Trial (IST): a randomised trial of aspirin, subcutaneous heparin, both, or neither among 19435 patients with acute ischaemic stroke. *Lancet* 1997;349:1569–81.

31. The Abciximab in Ischemic Stroke Investigators. Abciximab in acute ischemic stroke: a randomized, double-blind, placebo-controlled, dose-escalation study. *Stroke* 2000;31:601–9.

32. Collet J, Montalescot G, Lesty C, et al. Disaggregation of in vitro preformed platelet-rich clots by abciximab increases fibrin exposure and promotes fibrinolysis. *Areterioscler Thromb Vasc Biol* 2001;21:142–8.

33. Wikholm G. Mechanical intracranial embolectomy: A report of two cases. *Interventional Neuroradiology* 1998;4:159–64.

34. Chopko BW, Kerber C, Wong W, et al. Transcatheter snare removal of acute middle cerebral artery thromboembolism: technical case report. *Neurosurgery* 2000;46:1529–31.

35. Adams HP Jr, Brott TG, Crowell RM, et al. Guidelines for the management of patients with acute ischemic stroke. A statement for healthcare professionals from a special writing group of the Stroke Council, American Heart Association. *Circulation* 1994;90:1588–601.

36. Ahmed N, Nasman P, Wahlgren N. Effect of intravenous nimodipine on blood pressure and outcome after acute stroke. *Stroke* 2000;31:1250–5.

37. Juvela S, Heiskanen O, Poranen A, et al. The treatment of spontaneous intracerebral hemorrhage. A prospective randomized trial of surgical and conservative treatment. *J Neurosurg* 1989;70:755–8.

38. Auer LM, Deinsberger W, Niederkorn K, et al. Endoscopic surgery versus medical treatment for spontaneous intracerebral hematoma: a randomized study. *J Neurosurg* 1989;70:530–5.

39. Batjer HH, Reisch JS, Allen BC, et al. Failure of surgery to improve outcome in hypertensive putaminal hemorrhage. A prospective randomized trial. *Arch Neurol* 1990;47:1103–6.

40. Sacco RL, Kargman DE, Gu Q, et al. Race-ethnicity and determinants of intracranial atherosclerotic cerebral infarction. The Northern Manhattan Stroke Study. *Stroke* 1995;26:14–20.

41. Hass WK, Fields WS, North RR, et al. Joint study of extracranial arterial occlusion. II. Arteriography, techniques, sites, and complications. *JAMA* 1968;203:961–8.

42. Moufarrij NA, Little JR, Furlan AJ, et al. Vertebral artery stenosis: long-term follow-up. *Stroke* 1984;15:260–3.

43. Moufarrij NA, Little JR, Furlan AJ, et al. Basilar and distal vertebral artery stenosis: long-term follow-up. *Stroke* 1986;17:938–42.

44. Chimowitz MI, Kokkinos J, Strong J, et al. The Warfarin–Aspirin Symptomatic Intracranial Disease Study. *Neurology* 1995;45:1488–93.

45. The EC/IC Bypass Study Group. Failure of extracranial–intracranial arterial bypass to reduce the risk of ischemic stroke. Results of an international randomized trial. *N Engl J Med* 1985;313:1191–200.

46. Marzewski DJ, Furlan AJ, St Louis P, et al. Intracranial internal carotid artery stenosis: longterm prognosis. *Stroke* 1982;13:821–4.

47. Craig DR, Meguro K, Watridge C, et al. Intracranial internal carotid artery stenosis. *Stroke* 1982;13:825–8.

48. Caplan LR, Babikian V, Helgason C, et al. Occlusive disease of the middle cerebral artery. *Neurology* 1985;35:975–82.

49. Abou-Chebl A, Rensel M, Krieger D, et al. Long-term outcome in symptomatic intracranial vertebrobasilar occlusive disease. Oral presentation at the 25th International Stroke Conference, Feb 12, 2000; New Orleans, LA.

50. Caplan LR. Large-vessel occlusive disease of the anterior circulation. In: *Caplan's Stroke: A Clinical Approach.* Boston: Butterworth-Heinemann, 1993:195–236.

51. Caplan LR. Large-vessel occlusive disease of the posterior circulation. In: *Caplan's Stroke: A Clinical Approach.* Boston: Butterworth-Heinemann, 1993:237–272.

52. Chimowitz MI. Angioplasty or stenting is not appropriate as first-line treatment of intracranial stenosis. *Arch Neurol* 2001;58:1690–2.

53. Gomez CR, Orr SC. Angioplasty and stenting for primary treatment of intracranial arterial stenoses. *Arch Neurol* 2001;58:1687–90.

54. Caplan LR. Intracranial branch atheromatous disease: a neglected, understudied, and underused concept. *Neurology* 1989;39:1246–50.

55. Caplan LR. Penetrating and branch artery disease. In: *Caplan's Stroke: A Clinical Approach.* Boston: Butterworth-Heinemann, 1993: 273–97.

56. Sundt TM Jr, Smith HC, Campbell JK, et al. Transluminal angioplasty for basilar artery stenosis. *Mayo Clin Proc* 1980;55:673–80.

57. Mori T, Arisawa M, Honda S, et al. Percutaneous transluminal angioplasty of supra-aortic arterial stenoses in patients with concomitant cerebrovascular and coronary artery diseases – report of two cases. *Neurol Med Chir (Tokyo)* 1993;33:368–72.

58. Mori T, Mori K, Fukuoka M, et al. Percutaneous transluminal cerebral angioplasty: serial angiographic follow-up after successful dilatation. *Neuroradiology* 1997;39:111–6.

59. Mori T, Mori K, Fukuoka M, et al. Percutaneous transluminal angioplasty for total occlusion of middle cerebral arteries. *Neuroradiology* 1997;39:71–4.

60. Mori T, Fukuoka M, Kazita K, et al. Follow-up study after intracranial percutaneous transluminal cerebral balloon angioplasty. *AJNR Am J Neuroradiol* 1998;19:1525–33.

61. Mori T, Fukuoka M, Kazita K, et al. Follow-up study after percutaneous transluminal cerebral angioplasty. *Eur Radiol* 1998;8:403–8.

62. Mori T, Kazita K, Mori K. Cerebral angioplasty and stenting for intracranial vertebral atherosclerotic stenosis. *AJNR Am J Neuroradiol* 1999;20:787–9.

63. Lanzino G, Wakhloo AK, Fessler RD, et al. Efficacy and current limitations of intravascular stents for intracranial internal carotid, vertebral, and basilar artery aneurysms. *J Neurosurg* 1999;91:538–46.

64. Lanzino G, Fessler RD, Miletich RS, et al. Angioplasty and stenting of basilar artery stenosis: technical case report. *Neurosurgery* 1999;45:404–7; discussion 407–8.

65. Rasmussen PA, Perl J, Barr JD, et al. Stent-assisted angioplasty of intracranial vertebrobasilar atherosclerosis: an initial experience. *J Neurosurg* 2000;92:771–8.

66. Higashida RT, Hieshima GB, Tsai FY, et al. Transluminal angioplasty of the vertebral and basilar artery. *AJNR Am J Neuroradiol* 1987;8:745–9.

67. Higashida RT, Tsai FY, Halbach VV, et al. Cerebral percutaneous transluminal angioplasty. *Heart Dis Stroke* 1993;2:497–502.

68. Higashida RT, Tsai FY, Halbach VV, et al. Transluminal angioplasty for atherosclerotic disease of the vertebral and basilar arteries. *J Neurosurg* 1993;78:192–8.

69. Al-Mubarak N, Gomez CR, Vitek JJ, et al. Stenting of symptomatic stenosis of the intracranial internal carotid artery. *AJNR Am J Neuroradiol* 1998;19:1949–51.

70. Connors JJ 3rd, Wojak JC. Percutaneous transluminal angioplasty for intracranial atherosclerotic lesions: evolution of technique and short-term results. *J Neurosurg* 1999;91:415–23.

71. Ramee SR, Dawson R, McKinley KL, et al. Provisional stenting for symptomatic intracranial stenosis using a multidisciplinary approach: acute results, unexpected benefit, and one-year outcome. *Catheter Cardiovasc Interv* 2001;52:457–67.

72. Uchiyama N, Kida S, Watanabe T, et al. Improved cerebral perfusion and metabolism after stenting for basilar artery stenosis: technical case report. *Neurosurgery* 2001;48:1386–91; discussion 1391–2.

73. Levy EI, Horowitz MB, Koebbe CJ, et al. Transluminal stent-assisted angiplasty of the intracranial vertebrobasilar system for medically refractory, posterior circulation ischemia: early results. *Neurosurgery* 2001;48:1215–21; discussion 1221–3.

74. Malek AM, Higashida RT, Phatouros CC, et al. Treatment of posterior circulation ischemia with extracranial percutaneous balloon angioplasty and stent placement. *Stroke* 1999;30:2073–85.

75. Phatouros CC, Lefler JE, Higashida RT, et al. Primary stenting for high-grade basilar artery stenosis. *AJNR Am J Neuroradiol* 2000;21:1744–9.

76. Meyers PM, Higashida RT, Phatouros CC, et al. Cerebral hyperperfusion syndrome after percutaneous transluminal stenting of the craniocervical arteries. *Neurosurgery* 2000;47:335–43; discussion 343–5.

77. Bando K, Satoh K, Matsubara S, et al. Hyperperfusion phenomenon after percutaneous transluminal angioplasty for atherosclerotic stenosis of the intracranial vertebral artery. Case report. *J Neurosurg* 2001;94:826–30.

78. Samuels OB, Joseph GJ, Lynn MJ, et al. A standardized method for measuring intracranial arterial stenosis. *AJNR Am J Neuroradiol* 2000;21:643–6.

79. Groves HM, Kinlough-Rathbone RL, Richardson M, et al. Platelet interaction with damaged rabbit aorta. *Lab Invest* 1979;40:194–200.

80. Wilentz JR, Sanborn TA, Haudenschild CC, et al. Platelet accumulation in experimental angioplasty: time course and relation to vascular injury. *Circulation* 1987;75:636–42.

81. The EPIC Investigation. Use of a monoclonal antibody directed against the platelet glycoprotein IIb/IIIa receptor in high-risk coronary angioplasty. *N Engl J Med* 1994;330:956–61.

82. Bhatt DL, Kapadia SR, Bajzer CT, et al. Dual antiplatelet therapy with clopidogrel and aspirin after carotid artery stenting. *J Invasive Cardiol* 2001;13:767–71.

83. Chastain HD 2nd, Gomez CR, Iyer S, et al. Influence of age upon complications of carotid artery stenting. UAB Neurovascular Angioplasty Team. *J Endovasc Surg* 1999;6:217–22.

84. Gomez CR, Misra VK, Liu MW, et al. Elective stenting of symptomatic basilar artery stenosis. *Stroke* 2000;31:95–9.

85. Qureshi AI, Suri MF, Khan J, et al. Abciximab as an adjunct to high-risk carotid or vertebrobasilar angioplasty: preliminary experience. *Neurosurgery* 2000;46:1316–24; discussion 1324–5.

86. Qureshi AI, Saad M, Zaidat OO, et al. Intracerebral hemorrhages associated with neurointerventional procedures using a combination of antithrombotic agents including abciximab. *Stroke* 2002;33:1916–9.

87. Callahan AS 3rd, Berger BL. Balloon angioplasty of intracranial arteries for stroke prevention. *J Neuroimaging* 1997;7:232–5.

88. Suh DC, Sung KB, Cho YS, et al. Transluminal angioplasty for middle cerebral artery stenosis in patients with acute ischemic stroke. *AJNR Am J Neuroradiol* 1999;20:553–8.

89. Takis C, Kwan ES, Pessin MS, et al. Intracranial angioplasty: experience and complications. *AJNR Am J Neuroradiol* 1997;18:1661–8.

90. Higashida RT, Halbach VV, Tsai FY, et al. Interventional neurovascular techniques for cerebral revascularization in the treatment of stroke. *AJR Am J Roentgenol* 1994;163:793–800.

91. Mori T, Kazita K, Chokyu K, et al. Short-term arteriographic and clinical outcome after cerebral angioplasty and stenting for intracranial vertebrobasilar and carotid atherosclerotic occlusive disease. *AJNR Am J Neuroradiol* 2000;21:249–54.

92. Clark WM, Barnwell SL, Nesbit G, et al. Safety and efficacy of percutaneous transluminal angioplasty for intracranial atherosclerotic stenosis. *Stroke* 1995;26:1200–4.

93. Marks MP, Marcellus M, Norbash AM, et al. Outcome of angioplasty for atherosclerotic intracranial stenosis. *Stroke* 1999;30:1065–9.

94. Malek AM, Higashida RT, Halbach VV, et al. Tandem intracranial stent deployment for treatment of an iatrogenic, flow-limiting, basilar artery dissection: technical case report. *Neurosurgery* 1999;45:919–24.

95. Piotin M, Blanc R, Kothimbakam R, et al. Primary basilar artery stenting: immediate and long-term results in one patient. *AJR Am J Roentgenol* 2000;175:1367–9.

96. Gomez CR, Misra VK, Campbell MS, et al. Elective stenting of symptomatic middle cerebral artery stenosis. *AJNR Am J Neuroradiol* 2000;21:971–3.

97. Callahan AS 3rd, Berger BL. Basilar artery endoprosthesis placement: rescue therapy for recurrent thrombosis. *J Neuroimaging* 2000;10:47–8.

98. Dorros G, Cohn JM, Palmer LE. Stent deployment resolves a petrous carotid artery angioplasty dissection. *AJNR Am J Neuroradiol* 1998;19:392–4.

99. Fessler RD, Lanzino G, Guterman LR, et al. Improved cerebral perfusion after stenting of a petrous carotid stenosis: technical case report. *Neurosurgery* 1999;45:638–42.

100. Horowitz MB, Pride GL, Graybeal DF, et al. Percutaneous transluminal angioplasty and stenting of midbasilar stenoses: three technical case reports and literature review. *Neurosurgery* 1999;45:925–30.

101. Morris PP, Martin EM, Regan J, et al. Intracranial deployment of coronary stents for symptomatic atherosclerotic disease. *AJNR Am J Neuroradiol* 1999;20:1688–94.

102. Abou-Chebl A, Krieger D, Bajzer C, et al. Intracranial angioplasty and stenting in the awake patient. *Stroke* 2003;34:312 (Abstr.).

103. Fischman DL, Leon MB, Baim DS, et al. A randomized comparison of coronary-stent placement and balloon angioplasty in the treatment of coronary artery disease. Stent Restenosis Study Investigators. *N Engl J Med* 1994;331:496–501.

104. Altmann DB, Racz M, Battleman DS, et al. Reduction in angioplasty complications after the introduction of coronary stents: results from a consecutive series of 2242 patients. *Am Heart J* 1996;132:503–7.

105. Ohman EM, Marquis JF, Ricci DR, et al. A randomized comparison of the effects of gradual prolonged versus standard primary balloon inflation on early and late outcome. Results of a multicenter clinical trial. Perfusion Balloon Catheter Study Group. *Circulation* 1994;89:1118–25.

106. Masuo O, Terada T, Walker G, et al. Study of the patency of small arterial branches after stent placement with an experimental in vivo model. *AJNR Am J Neuroradiol* 2002;23:706–10.

107. Lylyk P, Cohen JE, Ceratto R, et al. Endovascular reconstruction of intracranial arteries by stent placement and combined techniques. *J Neurosurg* 2002;97:1306–13.

108. Lylyk P, Cohen JE, Ceratto R, et al. Angioplasty and stent placement in intracranial atherosclerotic stenoses and dissections. *AJNR Am J Neuroradiol* 2002;23:430–6.

109. Callahan AS 3rd, Berger BL. Balloon angioplasty of intracranial arteries for stroke prevention. *J Neuroimaging* 1997;7:232–5.

110. Alazzaz A, Thornton J, Aletich VA, et al. Intracranial percutaneous transluminal angioplasty for arteriosclerotic stenosis. *Arch Neurol* 2000;57:1625–30.

111. Nahser HC, Henkes H, Weber W, et al. Intracranial vertebrobasilar stenosis: angioplasty and follow-up. *AJNR Am J Neuroradiol* 2000;21:1293–301.

112. Wilkins RH. Natural history of intracranial vascular malformations: a review. *Neurosurgery* 1985;16:421–30.

113. Perret G, Nishioka H. Report on the cooperative study of intracranial aneurysms and subarachnoid hemorrhage. Section VI. Arteriovenous malformations. An analysis of 545 cases of cranio-cerebral arteriovenous malformations and fistulae reported to the cooperative study. *J Neurosurg* 1966;25:467–90.

114. Spetzler RF, Martin NA. A proposed grading system for arteriovenous malformations. *J Neurosurg* 1986;65:476–83.

115. Ondra SL, Troupp H, George ED, et al. The natural history of symptomatic arteriovenous malformations of the brain: a 24-year follow-up assessment. *J Neurosurg* 1990;73:387–91.

116. Lewis AI, Rosenblatt SS, Tew JM Jr. Surgical management of deep-seated dural arteriovenous malformations. *J Neurosurg* 1997;87:198–206.

117. Rosenblatt S, Lewis AI, Tew JM. Combined interventional and surgical treatment of arteriovenous malformations. *Neuroimaging Clin N Am* 1998;8:469–82.

118. Deveikis JP. Endovascular therapy of intracranial arteriovenous malformations. Materials and techniques. *Neuroimaging Clin N Am* 1998;8:401–24.

119. Hamilton MG, Spetzler RF. The prospective application of a grading system for arteriovenous malformations. *Neurosurgery* 1994;34:2–6; discussion 6–7.

120. Fox AJ, Pelz DM, Lee DH. Arteriovenous malformations of the brain: recent results of endovascular therapy. *Radiology* 1990;177:51–7.

121. Lawton MT, Hamilton MG, Spetzler RF. Multimodality treatment of deep arteriovenous malformations: thalamus, basal ganglia, and brain stem. *Neurosurgery* 1995;37:29–35; discussion 35–6.

122. Sasaki T, Kurita H, Saito I, et al. Arteriovenous malformations in the basal ganglia and thalamus: management and results in 101 cases. *J Neurosurg* 1998;88:285–92.

123. Marks MP, Lane B, Steinberg G, et al. Vascular characteristics of intracerebral arteriovenous malformations in patients with clinical steal. *AJNR Am J Neuroradiol* 1991;12:489–96.

124. Marks MP, Lane B, Steinberg GK, et al. Hemorrhage in intracerebral arteriovenous malformations: angiographic determinants. *Radiology* 1990;176:807–13.

125. Wikholm G, Lundqvist C, Svendsen P. Transarterial embolization of cerebral arteriovenous malformations: improvement of results with experience. *AJNR Am J Neuroradiol* 1995;16:1811–7.

126. Wikholm G. Occlusion of cerebral arteriovenous malformations with N-butyl cyano-acrylate is permanent. *AJNR Am J Neuroradiol* 1995;16:479–82.

127. DeMeritt JS, Pile-Spellman J, Mast H, et al. Outcome analysis of preoperative embolization with N-butyl cyanoacrylate in cerebral arteriovenous malformations. *AJNR Am J Neuroradiol* 1995;16:1801–7.

128. Grzyska U, Westphal M, Zanella F, et al. A joint protocol for the neurosurgical and neuroradiologic treatment of cerebral arteriovenous malformations: indications, technique, and results in 76 cases. *Surg Neurol* 1993;40:476–84.

129. Vinuela F, Dion JE, Duckwiler G, et al. Combined endovascular embolization and surgery in the management of cerebral arteriovenous malformations: experience with 101 cases. *J Neurosurg* 1991;75:856–64.

130. Pasqualin A, Scienza R, Cioffi F, et al. Treatment of cerebral arteriovenous malformations with a combination of preoperative embolization and surgery. *Neurosurgery* 1991;29:358–68.

131. Dawson RC 3rd, Tarr RW, Hecht ST, et al. Treatment of arteriovenous malformations of the brain with combined embolization and stereotactic radiosurgery: results after 1 and 2 years. *AJNR Am J Neuroradiol* 1990;11:857–64.

132. Mathis JA, Barr JD, Horton JA, et al. The efficacy of particulate embolization combined with stereotactic radiosurgery for treatment of large arteriovenous malformations of the brain. *AJNR Am J Neuroradiol* 1995;16:299–306.

133. Flickinger JC, Kondziolka D, Pollock BE, et al. Radiosurgical management of intracranial vascular malformations. *Neuroimaging Clin N Am* 1998;8:483–92.

134. Flickinger JC, Kondziolka D, Maitz AH, et al. Analysis of neurological sequelae from radiosurgery of arteriovenous malformations: how location affects outcome. *Int J Radiat Oncol Biol Phys* 1998;40:273–8.

135. Serbinenko FA. [Balloon occlusion of saccular aneurysms of the cerebral arteries]. *Vopr Neirokhir* 1974;Jul–Aug:8–15 (In Russian).

136. Debrun G, Fox A, Drake C, et al. Giant unclippable aneurysms: treatment with detachable balloons. *AJNR Am J Neuroradiol* 1981;2:167–73.

137. Higashida RT, Halbach VV, Barnwell SL, et al. Treatment of intracranial aneurysms with preservation of the parent vessel: results of percutaneous balloon embolization in 84 patients. *AJNR Am J Neuroradiol* 1990;11:633–40.

138. Higashida RT, Halbach VV, Dowd C, et al. Endovascular detachable balloon embolization therapy of cavernous carotid artery aneurysms: results in 87 cases. *J Neurosurg* 1990;72:857–63.

139. Higashida RT, Halbach VV, Dowd CF, et al. Intracranial aneurysms: interventional neurovascular treatment with detachable balloons – results in 215 cases. *Radiology* 1991;178:663–70.

140. Guglielmi G, Vinuela F, Dion J, et al. Electrothrombosis of saccular aneurysms via endovascular approach. Part 2: Preliminary clinical experience. *J Neurosurg* 1991;75:8–14.

141. Jellinger K. Pathology of intracerebral hemorrhage. *Zentralbl Neurochir* 1977;38:29–42.

142. Kassell NF, Iorner JC. Epidemiology of intracranial aneurysms. *Int Anesthesiol Clin* 1982;20:13–7.

143. Edlow JA, Caplan LR. Avoiding pitfalls in the diagnosis of subarachnoid hemorrhage. *N Engl J Med* 2000;342:29–36.

144. Hunt WE, Hess RM. Surgical risk as related to time of intervention in the repair of intracranial aneurysms. *J Neurosurg* 1968;28:14–20.

145. Kassell NF, Torner JC, Jane JA, et al. The International Cooperative Study on the Timing of Aneurysm Surgery. Part 2: Surgical results. *J Neurosurg* 1990;73:37–47.

146. Kassell NF, Boarini DJ, Adams HP Jr, et al. Overall management of ruptured aneurysm: comparison of early and late operation. *Neurosurgery* 1981;9:120–8.

147. International Study of Unruptured Intracranial Aneurysms Investigators. Unruptured intracranial aneurysms – risk of rupture and risks of surgical intervention. *N Engl J Med* 1998;339:1725–33.

148. Graf CJ. Prognosis for patients with nonsurgically-treated aneurysms. Analysis of the Cooperative Study of Intracranial Aneurysms and Subarachnoid Hemorrhage. *J Neurosurg* 1971;35:438–43.

149. Kassell NF, Torner JC, Haley EC Jr, et al. The International Cooperative Study on the Timing of Aneurysm Surgery. Part 1: Overall management results. *J Neurosurg* 1990;73:18–36.

150. Vespa PM, Gobin YP. Endovascular treatment and neurointensive care of ruptured aneurysms. *Crit Care Clin* 1999;15:667–84.

151. Pruvo JP, Leclerc X, Ares GS, et al. Endovascular treatment of ruptured intracranial aneurysms. *J Neurol* 1999;246:244–9.

152. Debrun GM, Aletich VA, Kehrli P, et al. Aneurysm geometry: an important criterion in selecting patients for Guglielmi detachable coiling. *Neurol Med Chir (Tokyo)*. 1998;38(Suppl.):1–20.

153. Moret J, Cognard C, Weill A, et al. [Reconstruction technic in the treatment of wide-neck intracranial aneurysms. Long-term angiographic and clinical results. Apropos of 56 cases]. *J Neuroradiol* 1997;24:30–44 (In French).

154. van Rooij WJ, Sluzewski M, Metz NH, et al. Carotid balloon occlusion for large and giant aneurysms: evaluation of a new test occlusion protocol. *Neurosurgery* 2000;47:116–21.

155. Vazquez Anon V, Aymard A, Gobin YP, et al. Balloon occlusion of the internal carotid artery in 40 cases of giant intracavernous aneurysm: technical aspects, cerebral monitoring, and results. *Neuroradiology* 1992;34:245–51.

156. Graves VB, Perl J, Strother CM, et al. Endovascular occlusion of the carotid or vertebral artery with temporary proximal flow arrest and microcoils: clinical results. *AJNR Am J Neuroradiol* 1997;18:1201–6.

157. Barr JD, Lemley TJ. Endovascular arterial occlusion accomplished using microcoils deployed with and without proximal flow arrest: results in 19 patients. *AJNR Am J Neuroradiol* 1999;20:1452–6.

158. Vinuela F, Duckwiler G, Mawad M. Guglielmi detachable coil embolization of acute intracranial aneurysm: perioperative anatomical and clinical outcome in 403 patients. *J Neurosurg* 1997;86:475–82.

159. Bryan RN, Rigamonti D, Mathis JM. The treatment of acutely ruptured cerebral aneurysms: endovascular therapy versus surgery. *AJNR Am J Neuroradiol* 1997;18:1826–30.

160. Eskridge JM, Song JK. Endovascular embolization of 150 basilar tip aneurysms with Guglielmi detachable coils: results of the Food and Drug Administration multicenter clinical trial. *J Neurosurg* 1998;89:81–6.

161. Bavinzski G, Killer M, Gruber A, et al. Treatment of basilar artery bifurcation aneurysms by using Guglielmi detachable coils: a 6–year experience. *J Neurosurg* 1999;90:843–52.

162. Lempert TE, Malek AM, Halbach VV, et al. Endovascular treatment of ruptured posterior circulation cerebral aneurysms. Clinical and angiographic outcomes. *Stroke* 2000;31:100–10.

163. Turjman F, Massoud TF, Sayre J, et al. Predictors of aneurismal occlusion in the period immediately after endovascular treatment with detachable coils: a multivariate analysis. *AJNR Am J Neuroradiol* 1998;19:1645–51.

164. Bavinzski G, Killer M, Ferraz-Leite H, et al. Endovascular therapy of idiopathic cavernous aneurysms over 11 years. *AJNR Am J Neuroradiol* 1998;19:559–65.

165. Hope JK, Byrne JV, Molyneux AJ. Factors influencing successful angiographic occlusion of aneurysms treated by coil embolization. *AJNR Am J Neuroradiol* 1999;20:391–9.

166. Kremer C, Groden C, Hansen HC, et al. Outcome after endovascular treatment of Hunt and Hess grade IV or V aneurysms: comparison of anterior versus posterior circulation. *Stroke* 1999;30:2617–22.

167. Kremer C, Groden C, Lammers G, et al. Outcome after endovascular therapy of ruptured intracranial aneurysms: morbidity and impact of rebleeding. *Neuroradiology* 2002;44:942–5.

168. Malisch TW, Guglielmi G, Vinuela F, et al. Intracranial aneurysms treated with the Guglielmi detachable coil: midterm clinical results in a consecutive series of 100 patients. *J Neurosurg* 1997;87:176–83.

169. Murayama Y, Vinuela F, Duckwiler GR, et al. Embolization of incidental cerebral aneurysms by using the Guglielmi detachable coil system. *J Neurosurg* 1999;90:207–14.

170. Birchall D, Khangure MS, Mcauliffe W. Resolution of third nerve paresis after endovascular management of aneurysms of the posterior communicating artery. *AJNR Am J Neuroradiol* 1999;20:411–3.

11 Dialysis access intervention

Walter A Tan and Charles T Burke

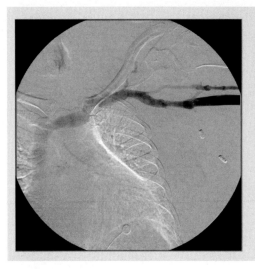
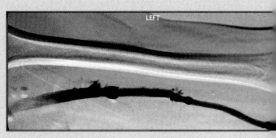

Figure 1. Native (or autogenous) arteriovenous fistula (radial artery to basilic vein).

Introduction

In 2001, more than 400,000 Americans required renal replacement therapy for end-stage renal disease (ESRD). Based on the United States Renal Data System (USRDS) statistical projections, 1.3 million diabetics and 945,000 nondiabetics, or more than 2.2 million people in total, will require ESRD treatment by the year 2030. Medicare ESRD costs alone in 2001 were approximately $15.4 billion (6.4% of the entire Medicare budget), a 33% increase from the previous decade.

The acceptance, ease, and standardization of hemodialysis have come a long way since the 1950s, when Willem J Kolff first adapted an ordinary Maytag washing machine at the Cleveland Clinic. Unfortunately, the limited durability of long-term vascular access for hemodialysis continues to be a major restriction of this therapy [1]. The morbidity from hemodialysis access issues alone has been estimated to account for almost 25% of the cost of ESRD programs, or more than $8,000 per patient per year at risk. Since dialysis is a central and persistent health issue for the lifetime of ESRD patients, expert panels have published guidelines regarding planning and patient selection for optimal long-term preservation of permanent vascular access (see **Table 1**) [2].

Types of arteriovenous dialysis access

An arteriovenous (AV) fistula for hemodialysis can be created using native (primary or autogenous) vessels, or with a synthetic bridge conduit, typically a polytetrafluoroethylene (PTFE) graft.

Native fistulae

For long-term dialysis, a native or autogenous AV fistula (see **Figure 1**) is the recommended choice for several reasons [2]:

• it has the longest patency rates among the access options

• it has low rates of local or systemic infection

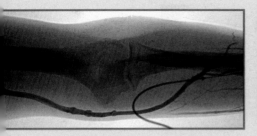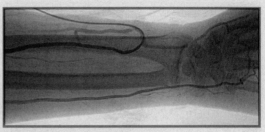

I.	Efforts should be made to preserve the veins in patients with chronic kidney disease for future AV access. Venipuncture or trauma to the cephalic veins of the nondominant arm and other upper extremity veins should be avoided.
II.	The recommended order of preference for permanent hemodialysis access is as follows:
	1. radiocephalic (wrist) primary AV fistula in the nondominant arm
	2. brachiocephalic (elbow) primary AV fistula
	3. PTFE graft versus transposed brachiobasilic vein AV fistula

Table 1. The National Kidney Foundation Kidney Disease Outcomes Quality Initiative (K/DOQI) abridged access planning recommendations. AV: arteriovenous; PTFE: polytetrafluoroethylene.

- it has low rates of thrombosis

- the delivered dialysis dose is superior to tunneled cuffed dual lumen catheters and comparable with grafts

These fistulae are typically fashioned to connect the radial artery to the cephalic vein, the brachial artery to the cephalic vein, or the brachial artery to a basilic vein.

Grafts

The preponderance of hemodialysis access in the US consists of synthetic AV fistulae, primarily PTFE grafts (see **Figure 2**) [3]. Reasons for this practice include the following:

- bridge grafts are technically easier to create and manipulate than native fistulae

- grafts have lower initial nonfunction rates than autogenous fistulae (see the **Failure to mature** section)

- grafts can be used earlier postoperatively compared with native fistulae, which require 1–4 months to mature

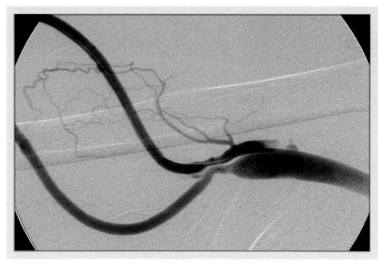

Figure 2. Upper-arm polytetrafluoroethylene loop graft (brachial artery to basilic vein).

	Reported rates (%)	Suggested quality assurance thresholds (%)
Procedural success	85–98	85
Cumulative primary patency		
6 months	38–63[a]	40[a]
12 months	23–44[a]	–
Cumulative secondary patency		
6 months	81	–

Table 2. Patency rates with balloon angioplasty for graft stenosis without thrombosis [10]. [a]Higher primary patency rates are typically attained with autogenous AV fistulae compared with grafts.

Even with contemporary graft materials such as PTFE, however, the 3–4 year occlusion or failure rate is still ~50%, and multiple secondary procedures are required to maintain patency (see **Figure 3** and **Table 2**). This compares with a failure rate of 20%–40% in autogenous fistulae.

When there is a paucity of remaining viable sites, bridge grafting between the superficial femoral artery and the femoral vein, or from an axillary artery to the jugular or contralateral axillary vein, can be performed (see **Figure 4**).

Assessment

Pertinent history-taking includes the following information:

- reason for referral: difficult access, prolonged bleeding at cannulation sites, poor dialysis flows, etc.

- type, location, and age of dialysis access

- any prior venous access: dialysis or central catheters, peripherally inserted central catheter (PICC) lines, or transvenous pacemaker

- previous trauma or surgery, or multiple previous accesses along the course of venous drainage

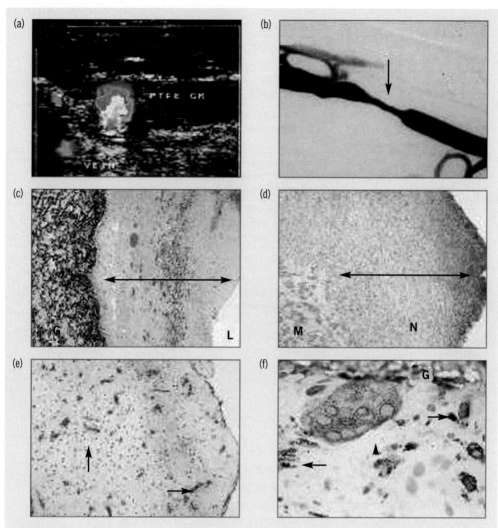

Figure 3. Dialysis graft intimal hyperplasia. (a) Color-flow Doppler ultrasound indicating turbulence at the graft–vein anastomosis. (b) Venography revealing significant stenosis at the graft–vein anastomosis. (c) Histopathologic section showing graft venous neointimal hyperplasia (arrow). G: graft; L: lumen. This region is characterized by: (d) smooth muscle cells (M) and myofibroblasts (N) that have migrated and proliferated; (e) microvessel formation or angiogenesis (arrows show immunohistochemical staining); and (f) inflammatory cells consisting of a macrophage layer adjacent to the graft (arrows) with macrophage giant cells (arrowhead). Adapted with permission from the National Kidney Foundation (Roy-Chaudhury P, Kelly BS, Narayana A, et al. Hemodialysis vascular access dysfunction from basic biology to clinical intervention. *Adv Ren Replace Ther* 2002;9:74–84).

Inspection, palpation, and auscultation form the cornerstone of the physical examination. Scars from prior trauma or procedures should be noted. Normally, a reasonably long segment of the graft or mature venous outflow should be visible for easy cannulation for dialysis. A palpable thrill should be strongest near the arterial anastomosis, and followed along most or even the entire length of the graft or venous outflow. Occasionally, it is difficult to clinically differentiate the arterial from the venous anastomosis of a loop graft. The segment that remains pulsatile when the midgraft is compressed should be the arterial limb. **Table 3** summarizes potentially pathologic findings that may indicate dialysis access malfunction.

Sign or symptom	Pathophysiology	Differential diagnoses
New swelling of the ipsilateral extremity	Elevated venous pressures	Venous outflow or central venous stenosis
Visible superficial veins over the shoulder and upper chest	Collateral venous circulation bypassing an occluded segment	Central venous occlusion or severe stenosis
Bulbous segments along the graft or vein	Degeneration and pseudoaneurysm due to repeated needle trauma	Graft degeneration or puncture-site pseudoaneurysms, with or without mural thrombus
Arterial limb pulse with an abrupt transition to a thrill in the venous limb or outflow	Pressure gradient across a stenosis – higher pressure upstream, pressure drop-off downstream from a stenosis	Stenosis of the venous anastomosis of the graft, or sometimes of the venous outflow
Focal, harsh, high-pitched bruit	Pressure gradient across a stenosis – higher pressure upstream, pressure drop-off downstream from a stenosis	Stenosis of the venous anastomosis of the graft, or sometimes of the venous outflow of an AV fistula
Poor thrill and pulse along the entire dialysis access, including near the arterial anastomosis	Low arterial inflow pressure	Arterial stenosis typically at the anastomosis, but rarely more proximally
No thrill or pulse even with compression of the venous anastomosis or outflow	No blood flow across the dialysis access	Thrombosed graft
Thrill, pulse, or distension of the dorsal hand veins	Blood flow into side-branch veins and distally to the hands	Stenosis near anastomosis of a radiocephalic fistula; failure of arteriovenous fistula to mature due to multiple outflow veins; unligated distal cephalic vein

Table 3. Common physical findings and corresponding pathophysiologic and clinical implications.

Knowledge of the location of the anastomotic site(s) and preprocedural diagnosis of the likely location of pathology will save the interventionalist's time and effort and decrease patient discomfort. For instance, if stenosis of the venous anastomosis of a graft is suspected, the introducer sheath can be inserted in the direction of the stenosis, with a few centimeters margin to allow unconstrained balloon inflation or thrombectomy device use.

Conditions and treatment options

Stenosis

There is a trend towards increased and more aggressive graft surveillance and pre-emptive angioplasty in an effort to prolong the limited lifespan of hemodialysis access (see **Table 4**). There are no randomized trial data, but several observational studies suggest that these proactive strategies are associated with a decreased access thrombosis rate (by 38%–77%) and referral for urgent salvage procedures, less need for hemodialysis catheter placement (from 29% to 7% per patient-year), and lower access-related hospital length of stay (from 1.8 to 0.4 days per patient-year) [4–6].

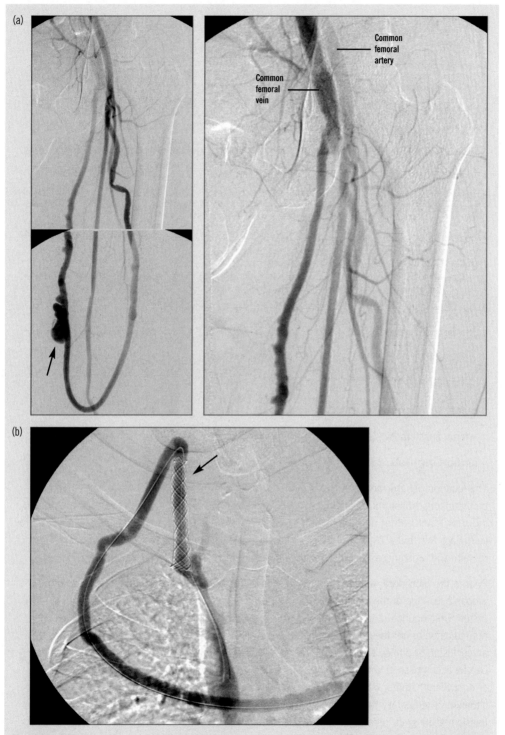

Figure 4. Hemodialysis access of last resort: (**a**) left superficial femoral artery to common femoral vein loop graft. Pseudoaneurysms (arrow) related to repeated cannulation for hemodialysis are noted on the venous limb of the graft. (**b**) Left axillary artery to right jugular vein loop graft. Note a prior self-expandable stent in the right jugular.

Grafts

- intra-access flow

- static venous dialysis pressure

- dynamic venous pressures

- measures of access recirculation

- unexplained decreases in hemodialysis dose

- physical findings such as persistent swelling, prolonged bleeding after dialysis needle withdrawal, or altered pulse or thrill

- elevated negative arterial prepump pressures with diminished blood flow

- Doppler ultrasound evidence of stenosis or occlusion

AV fistulae

- static and dynamic venous pressures used for AV grafts are not as accurate when applied to primary AV fistulae. Direct flow measurements are generally preferred over indirect measures

Table 4. Surveillance of hemodialysis access: parameters for the early detection of flow-limiting stenosis. AV: arteriovenous.

A representative distribution of lesions in AV grafts is as follows [7]:

- venous anastomosis: 60%

- intragraft: 38%

- peripheral vein: 37%

- central vein (proximal to the axillary vein): 3%

- arterial anastomosis: 2%–5%

- multiple segments: 31%

The location, length, and number of stenotic segments are important in deciding whether percutaneous transluminal angioplasty (PTA) is likely to be worthwhile or futile. The patency rates for lesions other than those at the venous anastomosis (ie, peripheral/outflow and central veins) are low, but PTA may still be indicated in patients in whom a few viable access sites remain. Circumstances that require more complex therapies are listed in **Table 5**.

Prior to the procedure, a baseline physical examination should be performed to ascertain the probable location of the stenosis. Initial diagnostic venography can be performed with a smaller system (micropuncture kit and a 4-Fr dilator, catheter, or sheath) since PTA is sometimes either not indicated or not feasible. It is often futile to proceed with an intervention in the presence of an occlusion or diffuse stenosis of the outflow or central veins. More selective central venography can be accomplished with the tip of a short Berenstein, Cobra (Cardean, Cupertino, CA, USA), or equivalent catheter (sheathless technique) positioned across the venous anastomosis. In this situation, a temporary hemodialysis catheter should be placed and arrangements for surgical revision of the graft initiated. Visualization of the arterial anastomosis may also require external manual compression of the graft or outflow vein just beyond the tip of the catheter or sheath. Injected contrast is therefore forced to flow retrogradely to fill the feeding artery.

I. Although not first-line therapy, stenting can be considered when:

- there are few remaining access sites

- the lesion is surgically inaccessible

- PTA fails and surgery is contraindicated

- restenosis occurs in a central vein within 3 months (however, stenting across contralateral central access should be avoided, eg, brachiocephalic vein, as this may compromise future access options)

II. Patients should be referred for surgery when:

A. Puncture sites for hemodialysis are severely limited or the risk of graft rupture is increased:

- large or multiple pseudoaneurysms exceeding twice the graft diameter or rapidly expanding

- poor eschar formation, or skin overlying graft is severely degenerated

- spontaneous bleeding

B. Infection

- Grafts:

  - extensive infection should prompt total resection

  - infection of a new graft (within 1 month) regardless of extent of infection

- AV fistula:

  - while infection of autogenous fistulae is rare, it is treated with prolonged antibiotics in a similar manner to subacute bacterial endocarditis. Take-down (ligation and excision) of the fistula when there is septic embolization

C. Complex or diffuse stenosis with exceedingly high restenosis rates anticipated (futile percutaneous intervention)

D. Select cases of occluded or thrombosed AV access

E. Aneurysms of primary AV fistula that involve the anastomosis

Table 5. Indications for more complex treatment (stenting or surgical revision) for hemodialysis access. AV: arteriovenous; PTA: percutaneous transluminal angioplasty.

If percutaneous intervention is indicated, a sheath that will accept up to an 8-mm diameter balloon is typically used. The cannulation site is selected accordingly, with the needle aimed in the direction of the likely culprit lesion segment. In grafts, this is commonly towards the venous anastomosis or central veins, unless inflow stenosis is suspected or discovered. In native fistulae, this is typically towards the AV anastomosis.

A floppy, straight-tipped, 0.035-inch wire (eg, Bentson wire [Cook, Bloomington, IN, USA]) may be less liable to cause spasm than the J-tipped wires used in larger-caliber vessels. The estimation of the "normal" target-vessel diameter is often subjective, and the balloon diameter is typically oversized by ~10%–20% relative to the segment just distal to the lesion. Alternatively, initial predilation and sizing with a smaller balloon is a safe strategy. The balloon is usually inflated to at least 10 atm of pressure; manual inflations can achieve pressures between 10 and 30 atm (using a 10- and 3-cc syringe, respectively). Some refractory lesions may require very high pressures of 18 atm or more to break, and a metered inflator coupled to a smaller diameter but longer balloon may be optimal and less prone to "watermelon seed" (balloon squeezing forward of backwash).

The desired endpoint is to achieve a residual stenosis <30%, and perhaps to improve flow by >20% [2,6]. Unfortunately, acute vessel recoil is not uncommon, despite multiple aggressive and prolonged balloon dilations. Furthermore, stents are not recommended within grafts since they may impair or even be damaged by repeated access cannulation for hemodialysis. Therefore, the guidewire is not withdrawn until the final postprocedural venography is completed. This is ideally done through the sheath not less than 10 minutes after the final balloon inflation. It is sobering to note that repeat procedures will be necessary for most of these patients; the mean time interval to reintervention is 6 months for grafts and 11 months for fistulae (see **Figure 5** and **Table 2**).

Although some operators do not use heparin, particularly if the procedure is anticipated to be short, we typically administer 3,000–5,000 U of heparin empirically. A nurse should be available to monitor the patient and administer conscious sedation and analgesia, since severe pain often accompanies PTA and occasionally accompanies access manipulation.

Occlusion and thrombosis

With proper surveillance, the rate of graft thrombosis is not expected to exceed 0.5 episodes per patient-year (0.25 for AV fistulae). Unfortunately, thrombosis portends failure and loss of hemodialysis access. Modern interventional techniques can offer acute salvage rates of >85%, and in 40% of these patients, patency and functionality would be expected to be maintained for a further 3 months (see **Table 6**). Perhaps more importantly, endovascular recanalization allows immediate reuse of the access site and avoids placement of a temporary dialysis catheter. This conserves other venous sites for future access, and helps to avoid the necessity for permanent hemodialysis catheters, which have many disadvantages.

Site selection for cannulation can be very difficult, and sonographic visual guidance may be required if a pulse or thrill are absent. Once thrombosis is confirmed, numerous treatment strategies are employed in various combinations (see **Figure 6**). The broad categories include:

- localized fibrinolytic therapy
- mechanical clot disruption
- maceration or suction
- percutaneous embolectomy
- balloon angioplasty

Nonlytic or predominantly mechanical therapies are quicker, but some pulmonary embolism occurs. It is interesting that, except for rare reports in the literature regarding patients with very poor cardiopulmonary reserve, clinically significant pulmonary embolism is almost never encountered, even after multiple declotting procedures [8]. Contemporary strategies therefore employ various combinations of the above therapies to achieve a balance between efficacy, safety, and procedural complexity and length. Adjunctive medications should include heparin and aspirin.

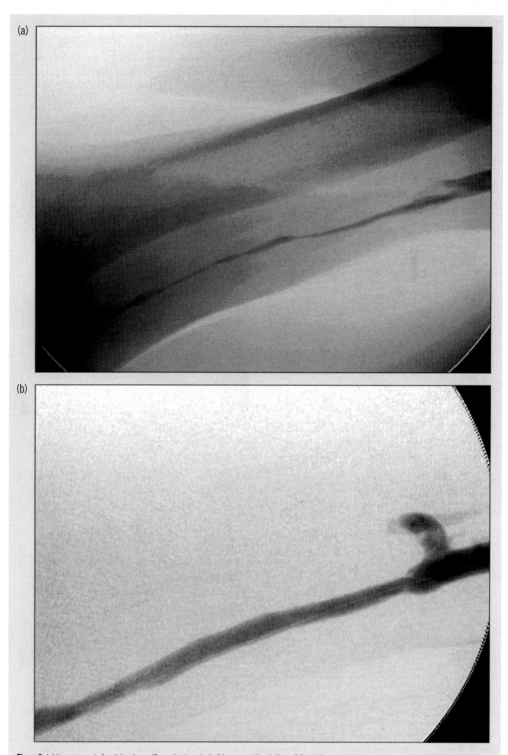

(a)

(b)

Figure 5. (**a**) Long segment of peripheral or outflow vein stenosis. In this case, cutting balloons followed by conventional percutaneous transluminal angioplasty with prolonged inflations achieved a good anatomic and hemodynamic result (**b**). However, this segment reoccluded within 3 months of the procedure (not shown).

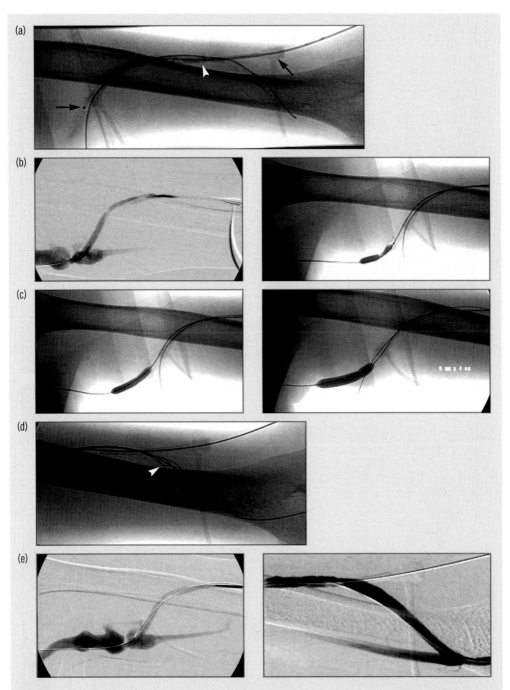

Figure 6. Pharmacomechanical treatment of a thrombosed graft. (**a**) A very small amount of contrast was gently injected through the infusion catheter to illustrate the residual clot (arrowhead) along the graft after an initial pulse spray (not shown) with a total of 4 mg of tissue plasminogen activator. Crisscrossing sheaths (arrows) are seen. (**b**) The outflow is improved by treating the underlying stenosis in the venous anastomosis of the graft. Note the indentation that the focal lesion makes on the angioplasty balloon. (**c**) A suboptimal initial result required repeated and prolonged percutaneous transluminal angioplasty using high pressure, as well as subsequent balloon upsizing. (**d**) Passage of the percutaneous thrombectomy device (rotating basket, arrow) allowed further clearance of clots and mural thrombi. Following this, a Fogarty embolectomy balloon was passed into the brachial artery to pull back the platelet plug at the arterial anastomosis of the graft (not shown). (**e**) A typical procedural result for graft venous intimal hyperplasia, with re-establishment of good graft flow.

	Reported rates (%)	Suggested quality assurance thresholds (%)
Procedural success	75–94	85
Cumulative primary patency		
3 months	37–58	40
6 months	18–39	20
Cumulative secondary patency		
6 months	62–80[a]	65
12 months	57–69[a]	–

Table 6. Patency rates with strategies that incorporate thrombolysis or mechanical thrombectomy for the treatment of graft stenosis with thrombosis. [a]Reflects results for thrombolytic and not mechanical devices (insufficient data exist for the latter). Reproduced with permission from the Society of Interventional Radiology Standards of Practice Committee [10].

The pharmacomechanical approach begins with a small dose (<10% of the dose used for myocardial infarction) of a lytic agent being infused into the clot, either via a small angiocatheter (eg, 22 gauge) or pulse-sprayed across the thrombosed segment using an infusion catheter once the catheter position(s) is confirmed [9]. The length of lytic dwell-time allowed (from minutes to hours) determines the amount of residual clot, which varies widely from center to center. In general, the venous limb is treated first to re-establish outflow, and the arterial limb is addressed later. Two sheaths are therefore employed in a crisscrossing, but preferably nonoverlapping, fashion. Specifically, one sheath is located near the arterial anastomosis and aimed towards the venous anastomosis or outflow veins, while the other sheath is located near the venous anastomosis and directed towards the arterial anastomosis. This enables the operator to pass embolectomy devices or a Fogarty balloon through the sheath located near the venous anastomosis to suction, macerate, and pull thrombi into the venous outflow (see **Figure 7**). This is followed by device or balloon insertion through the other sheath to make further passes to macerate or push residual clots towards the central veins. An underlying stenosis is seen in almost 90% of thrombosed grafts and should therefore be sought for [2]. Any significant stenosis should be resolved with PTA.

Finally, the sheath removal protocol avoids acute rethrombosis by allowing blood flow into the newly treated graft or fistula. This is accomplished with either nonocclusive light manual compression or with temporary ("woggle technique" [11]) or temporary purse-string suturing. **Table 7** summarizes the outcome benchmarks for stenosed versus thrombosed grafts.

Failure of autogenous fistulae to mature

Access maturation (venous enlargement and wall thickening ["arterialization"] to allow for regular and repeated cannulation for hemodialysis) is expected by the third or fourth postoperative month. Venography is indicated if the access surface area for needle punctures remains small, or if bleeding and hematomas occur frequently. Poor quality of the arm veins is often the culprit, especially in elderly diabetics or in the context of previous trauma or usage of these veins. Occasionally, selective surgical obliteration of major venous side branches can facilitate increased flow and hence maturation. Percutaneous techniques such as embolization of venous branches or sequential dilatation have been described, but are not well-validated approaches [7].

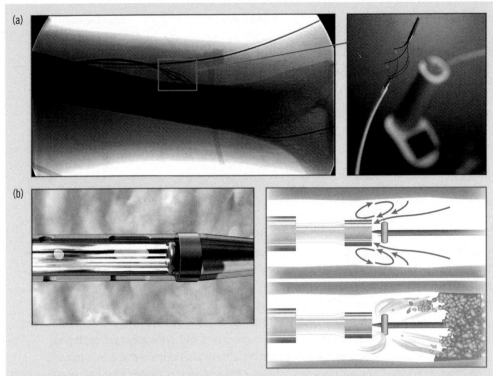

Figure 7. Representative mechanical thrombectomy devices used for arteriovenous shunt declotting. (**a**) The Arrow-Trerotola Percutaneous Thrombolytic Device (PTD) (Arrow International, Reading, PA, USA) is a battery-operated fragmentation wire basket that rotates at up to 3000 rounds/min and is passed across the graft. Older clot adherent to the vessel or graft wall can also be scraped off. (**b**) The AngioJet (Possis, Minneapolis, MN, USA) shoots high-velocity saline jets backwards into the center of the catheter. This creates a low-pressure zone, which suctions thrombus into the catheter (Bernoulli effect) where it is fragmented by the jets and evacuated from the body.

The benchmark 30-day primary access failure rates for virgin grafts are 15% for forearm straight grafts, 10% for forearm loop grafts, and 5% for upper-arm grafts [2].

Complications

The complication rate for percutaneous access interventions is highly dependent on the center-specific case mix. However, the quality assurance threshold rates suggested by the Society of Interventional Radiology Standards of Practice Committee include not more than 2% for symptomatic embolic occlusion of ipsilateral hand arteries, <1% for puncture site complications, and not greater than 0.5% each for symptomatic pulmonary embolism, major vascular perforation or rupture, and nonaccess site bleeding in association with thrombolysis [10].

I. Stenosis without thrombosis

A. The outcome benchmarks are:

- residual stenosis of ≤30% and resolution of symptoms or dialysis limitation

- 50% 6-month unassisted patency rate (ie, did not require repeat PTA or surgery to keep open) for balloon angioplasty (PTA)

- 50% unassisted patency at 12 months after surgical revision

II. Thrombosis and associated stenosis

The choice of pharmacologic, mechanical, or surgical thrombectomy should be based on local expertise.

A. Grafts

- The outcome benchmarks are:

  - 85% acute success rate for both PTA and surgery

  - 40% 3-month unassisted patency rate for PTA

  - 50% and 40% unassisted patency at 6 and 12 months, respectively, after surgical revision

B. AV fistula thrombosis is less frequent, but salvage and patency rates are even poorer

Table 7. The National Kidney Foundation Kidney Disease Outcomes Quality Initiative (K/DOQI) outcome benchmarks for dialysis access interventions. AV: arteriovenous; PTA: percutaneous transluminal angioplasty.

Acknowledgments

The authors are grateful to Bob Dixon, MD, and Mr James Ferson for their assistance with this manuscript. Walter A Tan, MD, MS, is also partly supported by the American College of Cardiology Foundation/William F Keating Career Development Award.

References

1. Kolff W. First clinical experience with the artificial kidney. *Ann Intern Med* 1965;62:609–19.
2. NKF-K/DOQI. Clinical Practice Guidelines for Vascular Access: update 2000. *Am J Kidney Dis* 2001;37(1 Suppl. 1): S137–81.
3. Reddan D, Klassen P, Frankenfield DL, et al. National profile of practice patterns for hemodialysis vascular access in the United States. *J Am Soc Nephrol* 2002;13:2117–24.
4. Martin LG, MacDonald MJ, Kikeri D, et al. Prophylactic angioplasty reduces thrombosis in virgin ePTFE arteriovenous dialysis grafts with greater than 50% stenosis: subset analysis of a prospectively randomized study. *J Vasc Interv Radiol* 1999;10:389–96.
5. McCarley P, Wingard RL, Shyr Y, et al. Vascular access blood flow monitoring reduces access morbidity and costs. *Kidney Int* 2001;60:1164–72.
6. Schwab SJ, Oliver MJ, Suhocki P, et al. Hemodialysis arteriovenous access: detection of stenosis and response to treatment by vascular access blood flow. *Kidney Int* 2001;59:358–62.
7. Beathard GA. Angioplasty for arteriovenous grafts and fistulae. *Semin Nephrol* 2002;22:202–10.
8. Swan TL, Smyth SH, Ruffenach SJ, et al. Pulmonary embolism following hemodialysis access thrombolysis/thrombectomy. *J Vasc Interv Radiol* 1995;6:683–6.
9. Cynamon J, Pierpont CE, Vogel PM, et al. Multicenter prospective randomized comparison of "lyse and wait" versus pulse-spray pharmacomechanical thrombolysis for treating thrombosed hemodialysis access grafts. *J Vasc Interv Radiol* 2000;11:253(Abstr.).
10. Aruny JE, Lewis CA, Cardella JF, et al.; Society of Interventional Radiology Standards of Practice Committee. Quality improvement guidelines for percutaneous management of the thrombosed or dysfunctional dialysis access. *J Vasc Interv Radiol* 2003;14:S247–53.
11. Simons ME, Rajan DK, Clark TW. The Woggle technique for suture closure of hemodialysis access catheterization sites. *J Vasc Interv Radiol* 2003;14:485–8.

12

Stent grafting for abdominal aortic aneurysms

Gregory S Domer, Brendan P Girschek, and Frank J Criado

Introduction

The first surgical repair of an abdominal aortic aneurysm (AAA) was performed by Charles Dubost in 1952 [1]. Morbidity and mortality were quite high in the early days. However, with refined operative techniques and improved patient care, the mortality rate dropped to a relatively low 3%–5%, where it stands today. These advances notwithstanding, surgical treatment continues to cause major disability and requires a prolonged recovery period. Additionally, a significant number of patients are deemed high-risk candidates or truly inoperable because of medical comorbidities and/or anatomical factors. Together, these issues provided a major incentive for the development of less invasive approaches. In 1991, Juan Parodi was the first to report endovascular AAA repair (EVAR) [2]. This publication and many presentations around the world signaled the beginning of a new era in vascular surgery and aneurysm management. Since then, more than 25,000 stent-graft devices have been implanted and many technologies created, leaving no doubt that EVAR is feasible and of clear benefit to many patients. Experienced endovascular teams are reporting that 60% (or more) of patients with AAA can be treated with the currently available devices [3]. EVAR has become a critical treatment tool, especially in the management of high-risk individuals who may not have another option.

There are currently three commercially available, Food and Drug Administration-approved devices in the USA. They are the AneuRx (Medtronic Vascular, Santa Rosa, CA, USA), Excluder (WL Gore and Associates, Sunnyvale, CA, USA), and Zenith (Cook, Bloomington, IN, USA) stent grafts (see **Figures 1** and **2**). The fabric composition of each stent graft is composed of Dacron, with the exception of the Excluder device, which is composed of polytetrafluroethylene (PTFE). The Ancure device (Guidant, Indianapolis, IN, USA) was also approved, but has since been withdrawn from the market. In Europe and other countries the choices are far wider, with the Talent stent graft (Medtronic Vascular) used in the largest number of implants worldwide (see **Figure 3**).

Anatomic and clinical considerations

The inclusion and exclusion criteria for endovascular therapy are influenced by device type, but are mostly determined by anatomy. In general, candidates should have an infrarenal neck of at least 10–15 mm in length and a diameter that does not exceed 26 mm. Other components of the "ideal neck" (see **Figure 4**) are listed in **Table 1**. Neck angulation and configuration are particularly important, as is a combination of two or more unfavorable features. The distal aorta should be large enough to allow placement of a bifurcated device with the passage of two limbs side-by-side across the region of the bifurcation [4].

Iliac artery anatomy and disease is the second most common limitation to this therapy. At least one external iliac artery of ≥7.5 mm is necessary for successful access and delivery of the device. The common iliac arteries should be free of aneurysmal dilatation or marked ectasia (<20 mm diameter), and there should be a landing zone of 10–15 mm or more for distal endograft limb fixation. Focal iliac stenoses are best managed with angioplasty at the time of stent-graft intervention; in such situations, it may become necessary to place a self-expanding stent within the endograft limb at the site of narrowing. Persistent stenosis of the limb from extrinsic

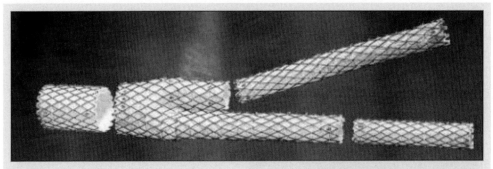

Figure 1. AneuRx stent graft (Medtronic Vascular, Santa Rosa, CA, USA).

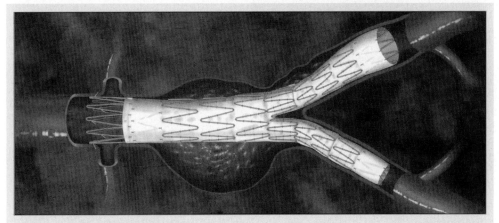

Figure 2. Zenith stent graft (Cook, Bloomington, IN, USA).

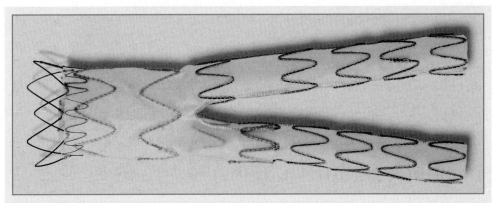

Figure 3. Talent stent graft (Medtronic Vascular, Santa Rosa, CA, USA).

compression or angulation must be treated aggressively to avoid limb thrombosis and the need for secondary procedures. Performing angioplasty and stenting ahead of time, before the stent-graft procedure, should generally be avoided because the stent might interfere with transluminal

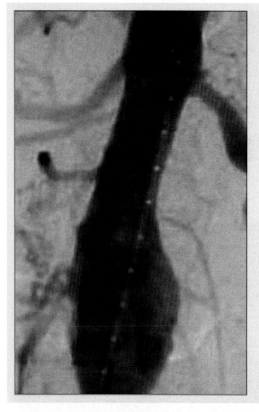

Figure 4. Angiographic example of "ideal" abdominal aortic aneurysm neck.

>15-mm length	<45° angulation
<26-mm diameter	Little or no calcification
Cylindrical	Little or no mural thrombus

Table 1. The "ideal" abdominal aortic aneurysm neck.

passage of the endograft delivery system. We have found it very useful to probe questionable (borderline small) access iliac arteries with Coons dilators (Cook). Iliac artery tortuosity, in the absence of significant calcification, is no longer a major technical issue as stiff guidewires (such as the Lunderquist wire [Cook]) can straighten such pathways relatively easily [5,6].

Planning endovascular AAA repair

Assessment of morphology

Axial and three-dimensional contrast-enhanced computed tomography (CT) images constitute the most common and useful means of assessing the relevant anatomy and determining suitability for EVAR [7]. Preoperative angiography (with a calibrated diagnostic catheter) continues to be used, but less frequently. Our group finds it helpful, especially in combination with intravascular ultrasound imaging and measurements. The importance of, and difficulties with, length measurements have been underestimated in the past; length measurement is a crucially important feature with a potentially large impact on device choice and design, as well as on outcome. Magnetic resonance angiography has not yet achieved the diagnostic "stature" of CT for this assessment, but it can be useful. Its main limitation is that it is contraindicated in the presence of steel-based devices (ie, the Zenith stent graft), where it cannot be used for postimplantation follow-up.

Device choice and implantation: general principles

In most cases, the choice will be for a modular bifurcated device, such as one of the three endografts that are currently approved and available in the USA. The distinguishing feature of the Zenith (and Talent) stent graft is that it incorporates suprarenal fixation and anchoring barbs at the top end. Aneurysm exclusion requires secure anchoring and a hemostatic seal at all fixation sites. The selection of a particular device for a given case is dependent on several factors, including – perhaps most powerfully – operator choice and personal experience. Some degree of diameter oversizing (<20%) is necessary with all endografts, and is especially important to achieve adequate fixation and a seal at the proximal neck. However, it must be made clear that excessive oversizing can be counterproductive and lead to poor apposition and endoleak [8].

Complications

Endoleaks

Endoleaks, or continued arterial flow within the aneurysm sac but outside of the endograft, are complications unique to EVAR. They imply "failure" to attain complete circulatory isolation of the sac. Type 1 (proximal or distal attachments) and type 3 (modular disconnections or graft defects) endoleaks are directly related to device or implantation issues, whereas type 2 (branch back flow) endoleaks are perhaps only partially influenced by endograft type, but are mostly dependent on anatomical characteristics. Type 4 endoleaks reflect transgraft flow and porosity; they tend to only occur during the procedure, especially while the patient is anticoagulated.

Overall, endoleak rates vary widely (10%–30%), and management guidelines continue to evolve. A definitive diagnosis of the endoleak type is paramount, usually requiring a combination of CT and angiographic techniques. Ultrasound can also be helpful. Most leading investigators agree that a type 2 endoleak requires careful follow-up and observation only, but would consider intervention in the case of sac growth. On the other hand, type 1 and 3 leaks signify that the sac is still pressurized and at risk of rupture. They must be repaired; this usually involves placement of cuff extensions, but surgical conversion may have to be considered, depending on the individual case [9,10]. Type 4 endoleaks are not clinically significant and typically resolve spontaneously.

Device migration

Device migration has been reported to occur in 3%–45% of patients. It was found in 96 of 3,251 EUROSTAR patients (2.95%) [10]. Data analysis showed migration to be an independent predictor of late rupture, with a risk ratio of 5.3 [11]. The reasons attributed to migration were inadequate anchorage, deterioration of stent-graft integrity, and proximal neck dilatation. Morphological studies have shown a progressive increase in the cross-sectional area of the infrarenal neck after endovascular repair: by >10% at 6 months and by >15% at 1 year. Suprarenal fixation and active anchoring with barbs and hooks are felt to enhance stability and minimize or prevent migration, but there is no scientific proof that this is the case [12].

Conclusion

Endovascular treatment of AAA represents a significant advance in our procedural capabilities, enabling vascular specialists to offer patients a less invasive approach that compares favorably with standard surgical repair in terms of morbidity, length of hospitalization, and recovery time [13]. Present-day stent-graft technology provides the tools for the possible repair of >50% of patients with AAA. On the "downside", long-term durability and device integrity, costs, need for life-long surveillance, and a 10% rate of secondary interventions over time remain significant concerns. Patients who are poor candidates for surgery or who are truly inoperable clearly benefit the most from stent-graft intervention. Continued technological evolution will undoubtedly result in further improvements in devices and techniques. In the future, the role of surgical treatment is likely to be limited to those situations where anatomy and disease preclude successful endovascular repair.

References

1. Dubost C, Allary M, Oeconomos N. Resection of an aneurysm of the abdominal aorta: establishment of the continuity by a preserved human arterial graft, with result after five months. *Arch Surg* 1952;64:405–8.
2. Parodi JC, Palmaz JC, Barone HD. Transfemoral intraluminal graft implantation for abdominal aortic aneurysms. *Ann Vasc Surg* 1991;5:491–9.
3. Tanquilut EM, Ouriel K. Current outcomes in endovascular repair of abdominal aortic aneurysms. *J Cardiovasc Surg (Torino)* 2003;44:503–9.
4. Sternbergh WC 3rd, Carter G, York JW, et al. Aortic neck angulation predicts adverse outcome with endovascular abdominal aortic aneurysm repair. *J Vasc Surg* 2002;35:482–6.
5. Criado FJ, Barnatan MF, Lingelbach JM, et al. Abdominal aortic aneurysm: overview of stent-graft devices. *J Am Coll Surg* 2002;194(1 Suppl.):S88–97.
6. Amesur NB, Zajko AB, Orons PD, et al. Endovascular treatment of iliac limb stenosis or occlusions in 31 patients treated with the ancure endograft. *J Vasc Interv Radiol* 2000;11:421–8.
7. White RA, Donayre CE, Walot I, et al. Computed tomography assessment of abdominal aortic aneurysm morphology after endograft exclusion. *J Vasc Surg* 2001;33(2 Suppl.):S1–10.
8. Prinssen M, Wever JJ, Mali WP, et al. Concerns for the durability of the proximal abdominal aortic aneurysm endograft fixation from a 2-year and 3-year longitudinal computed tomography angiography study. *J Vasc Surg* 2001;33(2 Suppl.):S64–9.
9. Chaikof EL, Blankensteijn JD, Harris PL, et al. Reporting standards for endovascular aortic aneurysm repair. *J Vasc Surg* 2002;35:1048–60.
10. Mohan IV, Laheij RJ, Harris PL; EUROSTAR Collaborators. Risk factors for endoleak and the evidence for stent-graft oversizing in patients undergoing endovascular aneurysm repair. *Eur J Vasc Endovasc Surg* 2001;21:344–9.
11. Wever JJ, de Nie AJ, Blankensteijn JD, et al. Dilatation of the proximal neck of infrarenal aortic aneurysms after endovascular AAA repair. *Eur J Vasc Endovasc Surg* 2000;19:197–201.
12. Conners MS 3rd, Sternbergh WC, Carter G, et al. Endograft migration one to four years after endovascular abdominal aortic aneurysm repair with the AneuRx device: a cautionary note. *J Vasc Surg* 2002;36:476–84.
13. Zarins CK, White RA, Schwarten D, et al. AneuRx stent graft versus open surgical repair of abdominal aortic aneurysms: multicenter prospective clinical trial. *J Vasc Surg* 1999;29:292–305.

13

Stent grafting for thoracic aortic aneurysms

Gregory S Domer, Brendan P Girschek, and Frank J Criado

Introduction

Surgical repair of thoracic aortic aneurysms (TAAs) is associated with considerable serious morbidity and mortality, which has led to a growing reluctance to offer treatment to many patients. In addition, some cases are truly inoperable because of comorbid conditions that make the risk of major transthoracic aortic surgery prohibitive. The need for a less invasive treatment alternative is being addressed with amazing rapidity at this time, with the current evolution of endovascular stent-graft techniques. Such interventions can offer TAA patients hope where none existed before. They promise to revolutionize the field of thoracic aortic surgery, and will have a major impact on management paradigms and therapeutic indications in a number of pathologic conditions affecting the aortic arch and descending thoracic aorta.

Incidence and nature

The incidence of TAA is estimated to be 8 per 100,000 people per year [1]. The incidence in men is 3 times that in women, and most present at a younger age (62 years vs 76 years for women). The risk factors associated with the development of TAA are the same as those for atheromatous disease – namely age, gender, smoking, hypertension, and hypercholesterolemia. The incidence of TAA appears to have doubled over the last two decades, which is probably related to the aging of the population combined with a significant increase in the rate of discovery through the more common use of better imaging – in particular, computed tomography, chest x-rays, and fluoroscopy.

Most TAAs are considered to represent atherosclerotic lesions; they tend to be fusiform and are more common in older males with multiple comorbidities, such as hypertension, coronary artery disease, and chronic obstructive pulmonary disease. Most importantly, they often (>30%) coexist with an infra-abdominal aortic aneurysm (AAA) [2]. Chronic type B dissection is the second most common cause of TAA ("dissecting aneurysm"). Posttraumatic aneurysms associated with deceleration injuries are most often located at the isthmic portion of the aorta. Other, less common, etiologies include dystrophic aneurysms (eg, Marfan's disease, Ehlers–Danlos disease, tuberous sclerosis), false aneurysms (found at points of surgical anastomosis), congenital aneurysms, and inflammatory aneurysms secondary to aortitis (Takayasu's, Beçhet's, and Horton's diseases).

Natural history

The natural history of TAAs is less well understood than that of AAAs, but represents a clear and gradually increasing threat to life. Like AAAs, TAAs tend to enlarge progressively and eventually rupture. The risk of rupture grows with aneurysm size. The 5-year life expectancy of a patient with an untreated TAA is <20% [3,4]. The most common cause of death associated with TAA is rupture with exsanguinating hemorrhage that tends to be rapid and beyond repair, even when it occurs in the hospital. TAA size >6 cm is generally regarded as particularly ominous in this regard. Other potential morbid consequences include fistulization into and compression of neighboring organs, and distal embolization to visceral and lower extremity vascular beds.

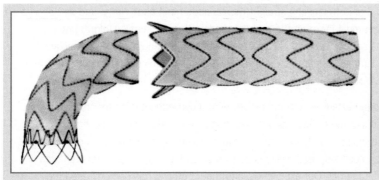

Figure 1. Talent thoracic stent graft.

Surgical intervention

Surgical repair involves segmental graft replacement of the aneurysmal aorta through a thoracotomy or thoracoabdominal incision. It is attended by a multitude of risks and technical difficulties. The in-hospital surgical mortality ranges from 3% to 15% for elective procedures. Prolonged respiratory support is required by at least 15% of all patients and up to 20% develop renal failure [5–7]. Nearly 20% of patients will rupture from an aneurysm developing at a different site from that which was previously repaired. In addition, the need for re-do operations for the correction of residual or recurring aneurysms is relatively common. Nonetheless, a 5-year survival of 70% has been reported.

Endovascular stent-graft intervention

Benefits

The avoidance of a thoracotomy incision and of aortic cross-clamping are the most obvious advantages of the endovascular approach, making it a safer and much more appealing form of therapy. Moreover, the occurrence of spinal cord ischemia and paraplegia, renal failure, and myocardial infarction is low in comparison with surgery. As a result, the need for intensive care and the length of hospitalization and recovery can be significantly reduced. All of these factors make it possible to offer treatment to many more TAA patients, even those who are considered at high surgical risk.

Only a few devices are available for endovascular intervention in the thoracic aorta. The largest experiences have been accumulated with the Talent (Medtronic Vascular, Santa Rosa, CA, USA) (see **Figure 1**) and Zenith (Cook, Bloomington, IN, USA) stent grafts. Newer designs and further refinements of existing thoracic endografts are likely to emerge in the near future.

Anatomy and case-selection strategies

Stent-graft intervention is designed to segmentally exclude the aneurysm-bearing portion of the aorta. This requires the availability of proximal and distal fixation and seal zones that should be >20 mm in length. Optimal results and technical ease can be anticipated when favorable anatomy is present, such as a (relatively) straight thoracoabdominal aorta, large and soft access iliac arteries, and a target focal lesion in the mid descending thoracic aorta. Unfortunately, in real-life practice, the majority of patients offer more challenging situations. Some physicians have advocated the use of a simple guideline for optimal anatomical suitability: the length (for fixation and seal) of the proximal and distal neck should match the aortic diameter at that segment.

Aneurysmal disease is often extensive and multifocal, with a consequent need for endograft coverage of long segments of the thoracic and thoracoabdominal aorta. Frequently, the proximal fixation site is within the distal or mid aortic arch. Coverage (occlusion) of the origin of the left subclavian artery is often necessary to achieve good fixation and a seal in the distal arch area, which is more likely to be normal. Our experience, and that of others, has demonstrated the safety of this technique. Although about one third of these patients develop left arm claudication, this tends to be self-limited and nonincapacitating, and improves or spontaneously resolves in approximately 70% of cases. However, the potential for serious complications (eg, stroke) exists when the contralateral vertebral artery is occluded, or when a prior left internal mammary artery procedure has been performed. Such conditions would demand preliminary left subclavian transposition or bypass to avert serious adverse events. In all other situations, we have found endograft coverage/occlusion of the vessel to be safe and very well tolerated. The need for more proximal graft attachment (ie, to the innominate artery origin), however, would dictate the performance of left carotid artery transposition-bypass, typically in the form of a retropharyngeal carotid–carotid crossover bypass with proximal ligation of the left common carotid artery. At the distal end, the celiac artery signals the caudad boundary of present-day endovascular grafting techniques. Crossing of this vessel with a naked stent is considered safe, but coverage/occlusion of the celiac artery should be avoided where possible because of numerous anecdotal reports of serious ischemic consequences to the liver and gastrointestinal tract.

As with endovascular treatment of AAA, TAA patients need to be tested and undergo life-long evaluation following stent-graft repair. Long-term device failures and metal frame and stent fractures have been reported, but clinical consequences have been few, if any [8–10]. Imperatives for reintervention would include a type 1 attachment site endoleak, device migration with loss of fixation, a progressively enlarging aneurysm sac (in spite of stent-graft "exclusion"), and some persistent type 2 back-flow endoleaks. Both computed tomography scans and plain chest x-rays constitute excellent imaging tools in this regard.

Unresolved issues and complications

The long-term durability of stent-graft devices and endovascular aneurysm repair are a continuing concern. Unlike surgical replacement, endovascular aneurysm exclusion does not "cure" the disease. The aneurysm sac remains and can be re-pressurized or "recur" in the face of device failure or migration. These considerations apply to both AAAs and TAAs. Although short-term and even mid-term results are quite encouraging, serious complications – such as paraplegia and strokes – have been described [8]. The risk of spinal cord ischemia seems to be considerably lower than in conventional surgical repair [11]. Patients at increased risk for spinal cord ischemia have been identified, and include those with a history of prior infrarenal AAA repair. Prophylactic use of a cerebrospinal fluid drainage catheter (kept in place for 2–3 days postoperatively), empiric use of steroids, and the prevention of hypotension have been shown to be helpful [9].

Other potential procedure- and device-related complications include visceral artery and lower extremity embolization, renal failure, aortic rupture – especially of the false lumen in acute dissection cases – and "postimplant syndrome". This last is relatively frequent after stent-graft repair in the thoracic aorta, and often causes low-grade fever, back pain, and leukocytosis [10,12]. It tends to be self-limited, however, resolving spontaneously in several days without sequelae.

Conclusion

Endovascular repair of thoracic aortic pathology has emerged as the most promising and perhaps best clinical application of stent-graft technology. Such patients are often treated with "benign neglect", and these newer techniques may represent their only hope of survival. Early and mid-term results are encouraging, but longer follow-up of a larger group of patients is necessary before more definitive statements on durability and clinical efficacy can be made. Technological refinements and new devices are an almost certain development in the near future. Clinical indications will probably expand and the standards of care and various treatment paradigms regarding thoracic aortic lesions are likely to change significantly as these endovascular options continue to evolve.

References

1. Bickerstaff LK, Pairolero PC, Hollier LH, et al. Thoracic aortic aneurysms: a population-based study. *Surgery* 1982;92:1103–8.
2. Pressler V, McNamara JJ. Thoracic aortic aneurysm: natural history and treatment. *J Thorac Cardiovasc Surg* 1980;79:489–98.
3. Perko MJ, Norgaard M, Herzog TM, et al. Unoperated aortic aneurysm: a survey of 170 patients. *Ann Thorac Surg* 1995;59:1204–9.
4. Coady MA, Rizzo JA, Hammond GL, et al. What is the appropriate size criterion for resection of thoracic aortic aneurysms? *J Thorac Cardiovasc Surg* 1997;113:476–91.
5. Verdant A, Cossette R, Page A, et al. Aneurysms of descending thoracic aorta: three hundred sixty-six consecutive cases resected without paraplegia. *J Vasc Surg* 1995;21:385–90; discussion 390–1.
6. Coselli JS, Plestis KA, La Francesca S, et al. Results of contemporary surgical treatment of descending thoracic aortic aneurysms: experience in 198 patients. *Ann Vasc Surg* 1996;10:131–7.
7. Hayashi J et al. Operation for non-dissecting aneurysm in the descending thoracic aorta. *Ann Thorac Surg* 1997;63:93–7.
8. Dake MD, Miller DC, Mitchell RS, et al. The "first generation" of endovascular stent-graft for patients with aneurysms of the descending thoracic aorta. *J Thorac Cardiovasc Surg* 1998;116:689–703; discussion 703–4.
9. Gowda RM, Misra D, Tranbaugh RF, et al. Endovascular stent grafting of descending thoracic aortic aneurysms. *Chest* 2003;124:714–9.
10. Ohki T, Veith FJ. Endovascular grafts and other image-guided catheter-based adjuncts to improve the treatment of ruptured aortoiliac aneurysm. *Ann Surg* 2000;232:466–79.
11. Gravereaux EC, Faries PL, Burks JA, et al. Risk of spinal cord ischemia after endograft repair of thoracic aortic aneurysms. *J Vasc Surg* 2001;34:997–1003.
12. Criado FJ, Barnatan MF, Rizk Y, et al. Technical strategies to expand stent-graft applicability in the aortic arch and proximal descending thoracic aorta. *J Endovasc Ther* 2002;9(Suppl. 2):I132–8.

14

Deep vein thrombosis, pulmonary embolism, lytic therapy, and venous intervention

Albert W Chan and Yung-Wei Chi

Introduction

The venous system occupies 50% of the human circulatory system. Diseases associated with venous circulation are one of the most common admitting diagnoses among patients who require hospitalization in North America. These include:

• venous thrombosis and postthrombotic syndrome (PTS)

• pulmonary embolism (PE)

• venous valvular insufficiency

• venous stenosis

Many patients have suffered from chronic morbidity as a result of undiagnosed, under-treated, or delayed treatment of venous diseases. Prompt diagnosis and intervention play an important role in improving clinical outcome in these disease entities. This chapter is organized so as to be particularly relevant to interventional practice.

Anatomy

The venous systems of the upper and lower extremities are composed of deep and superficial venous networks (see **Figure 1**). The two networks are connected by perforator branches. One-way valves are present within the superficial and the deep veins, as well as in the perforators, so that blood flow is allowed in only one direction from the superficial veins to the deep veins and to the heart.

Lower extremity system

Blood flows from the digital veins to the plantar arch veins, which then drain into the calf veins. In the deep venous system, two calf veins accompany each of the calf arteries, such that there are two anterior tibial veins, two posterior tibial veins, and two peroneal veins. Blood flow continues into the popliteal vein and then the superficial femoral vein, which joins the profundus femoris vein to form the common femoral vein. Once it passes the inguinal ligament, the common femoral vein continues as the external iliac vein, which then joins the internal iliac vein to become the common iliac vein. The iliac veins on each side join together and form the inferior vena cava (IVC).

The superficial venous system consists of greater and lesser saphenous veins running in the superficial fascia. The greater saphenous vein originates from the foot and courses anterior to the medial malleolus and on the medial aspect of the lower extremity until it meets the common femoral vein. The lesser saphenous vein originates behind the lateral malleolus and runs along the lateral aspect of the calf until it joins the popliteal vein above the knee. Bicuspid valves are present throughout the superficial, perforating, and deep venous system and direct blood from the superficial into the deep venous system. Blood is emptied into the deep veins with the aid of muscular contraction.

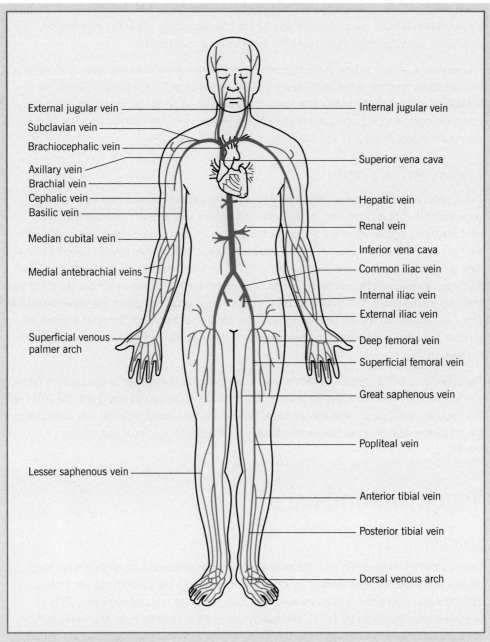

External jugular vein

Subclavian vein

Brachiocephalic vein

Axillary vein

Brachial vein

Cephalic vein

Basilic vein

Median cubital vein

Medial antebrachial veins

Superficial venous palmer arch

Lesser saphenous vein

Internal jugular vein

Superior vena cava

Hepatic vein

Renal vein

Inferior vena cava

Common iliac vein

Internal iliac vein

External iliac vein

Deep femoral vein

Superficial femoral vein

Great saphenous vein

Popliteal vein

Anterior tibial vein

Posterior tibial vein

Dorsal venous arch

Figure 1. Anatomy of the human venous circulation.

Upper extremity system

Blood drains from the digital vein to the palmar arch vein. Similarly to in the lower extremities, the deep vein system of the forearm is composed of two veins for each artery with the same name, such that there are two radial veins, two ulnar veins, and two interosseus veins. The deep veins then form a brachial vein, which often exists in duplicate, and continues as an axillary vein in the axilla, and then drains into the subclavian vein in the thorax. This is joined by the internal jugular vein to become the innominate vein (or the brachiocephalic vein). The right and left innominate veins join together and form the superior vena cava (SVC).

The superficial venous system of the forearm consists of cephalic and basilic veins. The cephalic vein originates from the radial head, courses on the lateral aspect of the forearm, and forms the antecubital vein within the antecubital fossa. It then continues on the lateral aspect of the arm, enters the deltopectoral groove, and drains into the axillary vein. The basilic vein arises from the medial aspect of the arm and enters the axillary vein in the axilla.

Azygous venous system

The azygous and hemiazygous veins drain the ascending lumbar veins and the intercostal veins from the right and left side, respectively. The azygous vein receives drainage from the right ascending lumbar veins and the right intercostal veins, and it communicates caudally with the infrarenal IVC. It then ascends on the posterior thoracic wall, arches forward superior to the right pulmonary bronchus, and enters into the SVC. The inferior division of the hemiazygous vein connects caudally with the left renal vein and also drains the left ascending lumbar veins and the lower intercostal space. The superior division of the hemiazygous vein drains the upper intercostal space and enters into the left brachiocephalic vein. Usually, at the eighth thoracic vertebra, the superior and inferior divisions of the hemiazygous veins cross the midline and communicate with the azygous vein.

The importance of the azygous system is that, in the presence of blockage to the proximal IVC due to pathologic conditions (eg, metastasis, IVC thrombosis), blood can empty into the SVC via the azygous, hemiazygous, and lumbar veins. Similarly, in the case of proximal SVC obstruction, the azygous system offers an alternative pathway for blood from the upper body to drain into the IVC.

Venous thrombosis

Statistics

Venous thromboembolism (VTE) is the third most common cardiovascular disease (after heart disease and stroke) with an average annual incidence of over 1 per 1,000. In North America, 200,000–300,000 cases of deep venous thrombosis (DVT) are reported each year, 25% of which are associated with PE [1–3]. The fatality rate of PE is close to 15%, and nearly 90% of PE are secondary to lower extremity DVT [4,5]. PTS is a chronic pathologic sequela of DVT and occurs in 25%–50% of patients after the first onset of DVT. Perioperative DVT has been found to occur in 50% of orthopedic surgeries of the lower extremities, but this figure has dropped to <15% with the administration of DVT prophylaxis.

Etiology and classification

In 1884, Rudolph Virchow proposed Virchow's triad (vascular endothelial damage, stasis of blood flow, and hypercoagulability) as the etiological factors behind thrombosis. Over the last

Specific for upper extremities	Common to upper or lower extremities, or IVC	Specific for lower extremities
Indwelling catheters or permanent pacemaker leads causing venous fibrosis and flow obstruction	Hypercoagulable state	Prolonged immobility
Radiation therapy	• inherited (protein C or S deficiency; antithrombin III deficiency; factor V Leiden; MTHFR, PT G20210A)	Orthopedic surgery of the lower extremity
Extrinsic compression	• acquired (tumor invasion or extension, myeloproliferative, autoimmune)	
Muscular impingement on the axillary or subclavian vein	• situational (surgery, trauma, oral contraceptives, hormone replacement)	

Table 1. Risk factors and etiologies associated with deep venous thrombosis. IVC: inferior vena cava; MTHFR: methylenetetrahydrofolate reductase; PT: prothrombin.

century, there has been increased recognition that all VTE risk factors reflect these underlying pathophysiological mechanisms (see **Table 1**). While hypercoagulable factors may trigger thrombosis in any venous segment, they predominately affect the lower extremities. Venous thrombosis of the upper extremities is often caused by direct vein injury (eg, from an indwelling catheter or pacemaker lead), extrinsic venous compression (eg, a mass encasing the great veins), or muscular impingement on the axillary or subclavian vein (eg, Paget–von Schroetter syndrome).

Since the lower extremity veins have a larger diameter than those of the upper extremities, the potential complications associated with DVT are different. Proximal lower extremity DVT (above the knee DVT) is associated with a higher risk of PE than upper extremity DVT [6].

Risk factors for venous thromboembolic disease can be divided into three categories [7–10]:

• inherited

• acquired

• situational

Inherited risk factors are characterized by genetic polymorphisms and mutations that result in deficiency of a natural anticoagulant (eg, antithrombin, protein S, protein C), procoagulant factor accumulation (eg, prothrombin G20210A, the thermolabile variant of methylenetetrahydrofolate reductase), or coagulation factor resistance to inactivation by a natural anticoagulant (eg, factor V Leiden) [11].

Acquired risk factors result from either medical conditions or coagulation abnormalities that disrupt normal hemostasis; examples include cancer, autoimmune diseases, nephrotic syndrome, antiphospholipid antibodies, and myeloproliferative and hyperviscosity syndrome [10]. These conditions interfere with the coagulation cascade and result in excess thrombin generation, thus increasing the risk of VTE. Limited age- and gender-appropriate cancer screening is recommended. This work-up consists of a comprehensive history and physical examination, basic laboratory screening, and a chest x-ray. In people with VTE, a pelvic exam, prostate exam, colon exam including colonoscopy, and breast exam including mammography should be pursued according to published guidelines. Elevated factor VIII functional activity and hyperhomocysteinemia are two examples of VTE risk factors that can be either acquired or inherited.

Situational risk factors are represented by transient clinical situations that are associated with a higher risk of VTE, such as surgery, prolonged immobilization, oral contraceptive pill (OCP) use, pregnancy, hormone replacement therapy, cancer, and chemotherapy.

Before 1993, 85% of idiopathic VTE was attributed to unknown etiology, but since the discovery of activated protein C resistance (APC-R) and the PT G20210A prothrombin gene mutation, along with more sensitive assays for various hypercoagulable states, only 32% of the total idiopathic VTE remains of unknown etiology [7].

Common hypercoagulable states

Anticoagulant deficiency

In unselected patients with VTE, the frequency of antithrombin III, protein S, or protein C deficiencies is low (see **Table 2**). However, the lifetime relative risk of VTE has been reported to be up to 40-, 31-, and 36-fold higher than in "normal" patients, respectively [12].

Activated protein C resistance

APC-R is defined as a decreased anticoagulant response to activated protein C. Between 10% and 64% of patients with recurrent VTE have APC-R (see **Table 2**) [13]. Factor V Leiden accounts for 90% of cases of APC-R [10]. About 4%–6% of the general population are heterozygous carriers of this trait, with the highest prevalence of the mutation found in northern and western Europe, the Americas, Australia, the Middle East, and the Indian subcontinent. The remaining causes of APC-R include pregnancy, OCP use, other factor V mutations, and antiphospholipid antibodies. Heterozygous carriers of factor V Leiden have a 2- to 10-fold increased lifetime relative risk of developing VTE; the risk is increased to 80-fold in homozygous carriers.

PT G20210A

The PT G20210A mutation has been associated with increased plasma prothrombin activity, thus leading to greater thrombin generation. The prevalence of the PT G20210A mutation is highest in white individuals, but, unlike factor V Leiden, whites from southern Europe are affected more often than those from the north or west [7]. A heterozygous PT G20210A mutation is associated with a 2- to 6-fold increased risk of VTE (see **Table 2**). Moreover, in heterozygous carriers who are pregnant or use OCP, the risks are further increased by nearly 16-fold. Among females who are and those who are not taking OCP, the incidence of cerebral vein thrombosis increases by 150- and 10-fold, respectively [13].

Hyperhomocysteinemia

Elevated plasma homocysteine can cause vascular damage via various mechanisms, including direct endothelial cell damage with enhanced macrophage binding, increased factor V activation, protein C inhibition, enhanced platelet aggregation and adhesiveness, and a mitogenic effect on vascular smooth muscle cells [14]. Hyperhomocysteinemia has been associated with a 2- to 4-fold increase in VTE risk, regardless of the etiology (see **Table 3**) [14].

Syndrome	General population (%)	Unselected patients with VTE (%)	Selected patients with VTE (%)
Antithrombin III deficiency	0.02–0.17	1.1	0.5–4.9
Protein C deficiency	0.14–0.50	3.2	1.4–8.6
Protein S deficiency	–	2.2	1.4–7.5
APC resistance	3.6–6.0	21.0	10.0–64.0
PT GT20210A	1.7–3.0	6.2	18.0

Table 2. Incidence of inherited thrombophilic syndromes in the general population and in patients with venous thrombosis. APC: activated protein C; PT: prothrombin; VTE: venous thromboembolism; –: unknown. Reproduced with permission from the American Heart Association (Anderson FA Jr, Spencer FA. Risk factors for venous thromboembolism. *Circulation* 2003;107[23 Suppl.1]:I9–16).

Hypercoagulable state	General population (%)	Patients with first VTE (%)
Hyperhomocysteinemia	5–10	10–25
Lupus anticoagulants	0–3	5–15
Anticardiolipin antibodies	2–7	14
Elevated factor VIII	11	25

Table 3. Prevalence of selected inherited and acquired hypercoagulable states in different patient populations. VTE: venous thromboembolism. Reproduced with permission from Arnold Journals (Deitcher SR, Gomes MP. Hypercoagulable state testing and malignancy screening following venous thromboembolism events. *Vasc Med* 2003;8:33–46).

Hyperhomocysteinemia may be inherited or acquired. Acquired hyperhomocysteinemia can be related to deficiencies in vitamins B6, B12, and folate, hypothyroidism, diabetes mellitus, pernicious anemia, inflammatory bowel disease, carcinoma, renal insufficiency, and medications such as methotrexate, theophylline, and phenytoin. Inherited hyperhomocysteinemia includes genetic polymorphisms and mutations such as the thermolabile variant of the enzyme methylenetetrahydrofolate reductase and cystathionine-β-synthase deficiency.

Antiphospholipid antibodies

Antiphospholipid antibodies consist of lupus anticoagulants and anticardiolipin antibodies [10,13]. The overall prevalence of antiphospholipid antibodies in the general population is estimated to be up to 7% (see **Table 3**); however, the prevalence is 60% in patients with systemic lupus erythematosus. There is a 10-fold increased risk of VTE in individuals with primary antiphospholipid antibodies. In addition, the presence of lupus anticoagulants or persistently elevated anticardiolipin immunoglobulin (Ig)G antibodies is associated with a high rate of VTE recurrence.

Elevated factor activity

Elevated factor VIII, IX, and XI activity levels are associated with a 2- to 11-fold increased risk of VTE [13]. Inherited elevation of factor activity levels is difficult to distinguish from increased factor levels in response to acute inflammation or infection (as an acute phase reactant).

Indications for hypercoagulability tests

Patients with VTE without obvious factors associated with stasis or trauma should undergo hypercoagulability tests. Other indications for testing include VTE in unusual sites, recurrent VTE, VTE at a young age (<45 years), VTE in the setting of a strong family history, and recurrent pregnancy loss [7]. Moreover, testing should also be considered in the close relatives of patients with known inherited hypercoagulable conditions. Testing should only be done if it may impact management by guiding the duration of anticoagulant therapy, the intensity of such therapy, or therapeutic monitoring strategies. Test results may also influence family screening, family planning, and the use of concomitant medications [10].

Lower extremity DVT

DVT in the lower extremities usually starts in the valve sinuses of the muscular calf veins. Clinical manifestations of lower extremity DVT include:

* unilateral or bilateral leg swelling or pain

* tenderness, cyanosis, erythema, palpable calf cord, or Homans' sign

* phlegmasia cerulea dolens

* phlegmasia alba dolens

* PE, paradoxical embolism

Color-flow duplex ultrasound is accurate in diagnosing acute thrombosis in common femoral, superficial femoral, popliteal, and tibial veins. It provides direct imaging of the venous contents. Factors that are evaluated during duplex ultrasonography include compressibility, augmentation, phasic variation with respiration, and echogenicity. An acute thrombus appears as an echolucent mass on duplex, while a chronic thrombus appears echodense. An inability of the transducer to compress the vessel suggests the presence of a thrombus (see **Figure 2**). Extrinsic causes of venous occlusion or leg pain can also be assessed by ultrasound (eg, Baker's cyst, popliteal artery aneurysm, hematoma). If this test is inconclusive, ascending venography is required. This can be achieved by inserting a 22- or 24-gauge angiocath in the dorsal vein and injecting nonionic contrast at 1 cc/s. A tourniquet can be applied at the ankle to force contrast into the deep venous system.

Treatment

Anticoagulation

The initial treatment of VTE consists of administration of unfractionated heparin (eg, 80 U/kg bolus followed by 18 U/kg/h; target activated partial thromboplastin time 1.5–2.0 of upper limit of normal) or low molecular weight heparin (eg, enoxaparin, 1 mg/kg subcutaneously twice daily), and overlap with oral warfarin for at least 4 days and until the international normalization ratio (INR) reaches 2. Overlapping the therapies is important for two reasons: (a) effective anticoagulation with warfarin will not be achieved within the first few days of the loading period; (b) the patient may be in a transient hypercoagulable state due to the rapid depletion of vitamin K-dependent anticoagulation factors protein C and protein S, which have shorter half-lives as compared with the other vitamin K-dependent coagulation factors (ie, factors II, VII, IX, and X).

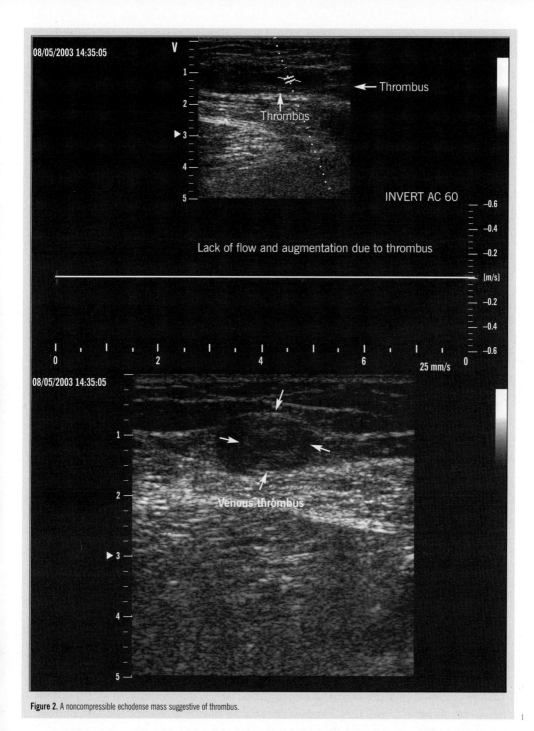

Figure 2. A noncompressible echodense mass suggestive of thrombus.

Warfarin is usually started between 5 and 10 mg once daily, depending on the patient's weight and general health. Conventionally, patients with idiopathic VTE would receive 6 months of warfarin with a target INR ranging from 2 to 3. Ridker and coworkers have suggested that prolonged warfarin administration beyond 6 months, with a target INR of 1.5–2.0, could further reduce the risk of recurrent VTE by >60% [15]. Another study by Kearon et al. confirms that prolonged warfarin therapy with maintenance of a target INR of 2–3 has a 65% lower risk of recurrent VTE as compared with a target INR of 1.5–1.9, without an increased risk of bleeding [16]. Long-term warfarin therapy should be given to patients with lupus anticoagulant, persistently elevated anticardiolipin IgG, antithrombin III deficiency, protein S and C deficiencies, and homozygous factor V Leiden [10]. In patients with VTE associated with temporary clinical conditions, oral warfarin therapy is typically indicated for at least 3 months or until the condition resolves, whichever is longer.

Oral direct antithrombin therapy, such as high-dose ximelagatran, is effective in the prophylaxis and treatment of thromboembolism [17]. Compared with warfarin, it eliminates the need for monitoring the therapeutic level, but may be associated with a higher incidence of liver enzyme elevation in the blood. Among patients with VTE associated with cancer, dalteparin 200 IU/kg/day for 1 month followed by 150 IU/kg/day for 5 months may be more effective than warfarin in preventing recurrent thromboembolism [18].

Filters

IVC filter placement may prevent large PE from lower extremity DVT, but it does not reduce the risk of minor PE or the risk of thrombus propagation. The indications for an IVC filter are listed in **Table 4**. More recently, newer retrievable IVC filters (eg, Günther Tulip [Cook, Bloomington, IN, USA] retrievable vena cava filter; Optease [Cordis, Miami Lakes, FL, USA]) have been made available. These may prove to be useful when patients require temporary IVC filter protection (eg, patients at high risk for DVT who are undergoing surgery in which anticoagulation is contraindicated) [19–21].

Factors that determine the choice of IVC filter are listed in **Table 5**. No studies have demonstrated the superiority of one filter type over the others in preventing PE. The incidence of symptomatic PE can be reduced to 2%–5%, but asymptomatic PE can still occur. While most filters can fit into an IVC <30 mm in diameter, the Bird's Nest (Cook) filter may be more suitable for an IVC >40 mm in diameter. However, this filter is relatively long and may not be suitable if the infrarenal IVC segment is short (ie, <70 mm). Venous access should be gained in the common femoral vein contralateral to the side with DVT. If an IVC thrombus is present, the filter needs to be placed cephalad to the thrombus via the right internal jugular vein. The uppermost part of the filter should be placed immediately below the level of the renal veins, such that, if a thrombus is formed in the filter or if it is filled by emboli, the rapid renal vein flow may stop a thrombus from forming above the filter.

Complications resulting from IVC filter placement are listed in **Table 6**. Filter thrombosis is a serious complication, and is the result of either thrombus formation within the filter or embolization. Cephalad propagation of the thrombus can cause PE. IVC occlusion may occur, but it is often well-tolerated because of the gradual course of development and sufficient venous collaterals. IVC filter placement without concomitant anticoagulation therapy is associated with a 21% DVT recurrence rate within 2 years [22]. Excessive tilt of conical filters may be associated with a higher rate of recurrent PE, but appears to be relatively more important in vessels with a large diameter rather than a small diameter. Filter migration is another serious complication, but, fortunately, rarely occurs. Transvenous retrieval or repositioning of the retrievable IVC filter can be safely performed within the first 15 days of implantation using a looped guidewire or snare [20,21].

Absolute	Relative
Contraindication to anticoagulation (active bleeding, surgery)	Massive, life-threatening pulmonary embolism with residual DVT
Failure of anticoagulation (eg, recurrent DVT or pulmonary embolism despite therapeutic INR level)	High risk for DVT in a patient undergoing surgery and in whom anticoagulation is prohibited
	Pulmonary thrombectomy
	Poor cardiopulmonary reserve

Table 4. Indications for inferior vena cava filter placement. DVT: deep venous thrombosis; INR: international normalization ratio.

Clot-trapping efficiency	Ease of placement
Risk of filter migration or embolization	Vessel–filter size-matching
Risk of thrombosis of the filter	Permanent or temporary filter

Table 5. Factors determining the selection of an inferior vena cava filter.

IVC thrombosis	Filter fracture
Pulmonary embolism	Filter dislodgement or entrapment during catheterization
IVC perforation	Filter thrombosis
IVC penetration	Venous access-site thrombosis
Filter malposition	Infection
Filter migration	Deep venous thrombosis

Table 6. Potential complications from inferior vena cava (IVC) filter placement.

Limb-threatening DVT and endovascular thrombolysis

DVT involving multiple lower extremity vein segments may result in ineffective blood drainage, causing massive leg swelling, severe pain, and cyanosis. It can lead to phlegmasia cerulea dolens then phlegmasia alba dolens or arterial ischemia. Computed tomography (CT) or magnetic resonance imaging (MRI) are usually required to confirm the level of occlusion. When limb-threatening ischemia occurs, or when swelling does not respond to anticoagulation alone, endovascular thrombolysis should be considered. Thrombolysis is particularly effective if performed within 2 weeks.

The rationale for aggressive antithrombolytic therapy is provided in **Table 7**. Various modalities of interventional therapy are listed in **Table 8**. Randomized studies have suggested that systemic thrombolysis results in a 2- to 4-fold increase in partial or complete clot lysis and that it reduces the incidence of late PTS as compared with systemic heparin alone. Both flow-directed thrombolytic infusion and catheter-directed thrombolytic therapy improve the efficiency of thrombolysis by increasing the local concentration of the fibrinolytic while minimizing the risk of systemic hemorrhage (see **Table 9**).

Indications
Extensive thrombus burden (eg, iliofemoral DVT) in a highly active patient
Extension of lower extremity DVT to IVC
Phlegmasia cerulea dolens or phlegmasia alba dolens
High risk of fatal pulmonary embolism
Propagation of DVT despite anticoagulation

Objectives
Short-term
• rapid reduction of pain and swelling of the extremity involved
• management of phlegmasia cerulea dolens or venous gangrene
• prevention of pulmonary embolism
Long-term
• prevention of postthrombotic syndrome by preventing organization of a thrombus, which can lead to venous hypertension
• preservation of venous valvular function

Table 7. Indications and objectives of interventional therapy during acute deep venous thrombosis (DVT). IVC: inferior vena cava.

Surgical thrombectomy
Systemic thrombolysis
Flow-directed thrombolytic infusion (especially for infrapopliteal DVT)
Catheter-directed regional thrombolytic therapy
• drug infusion
• pulse-spray infusion
• cycled infusion (eg, daily t-PA plus heparin infusion between cycles)
Percutaneous mechanical thrombectomy
Balloon dilation and stent placement for residual stenosis after a trial of thrombolysis

Table 8. Techniques of interventional thromboablative therapy for acute lower extremity deep venous thrombosis (DVT). t-PA: tissue plasminogen activator.

Flow-directed regional infusion of a concentrated thrombolytic agent is administered through the ipsilateral dorsal foot vein into the deep venous system (see **Table 10**). Compared with catheter-directed thrombolysis, the flow-directed approach requires a longer period of infusion and a larger dose of thrombolysis. When extensive iliofemoral and infrageniculate venous thrombosis is present, flow-directed and catheter-directed approaches can be used simultaneously.

The National Venous Thrombolysis Registry enrolled a total of 287 patients to catheter-directed thrombolysis. They reported complete thrombolysis in 31% of cases, whereas partial thrombolysis with restoration of forward flow was achieved in 52% of patients. Predictors of success included acute DVT and no history of DVT [23]. Complications of catheter-directed

Flow-directed thrombolysis
Infusion (tourniquet-assisted) via superficial dorsalis pedis vein

Catheter-directed thrombolysis	
Iliocaval DVT	Infrapopliteal DVT
• right internal jugular vein (upstream)	• single popliteal vein (upstream)
• common femoral vein (downstream)	• posterior tibial vein (downstream)
Iliofemoral DVT	Concomitant iliofemoral and infrapopliteal DVT
• single popliteal vein (downstream)	• dual popliteal vein (upstream and downstream)

Table 9. Various approaches for access during regional thrombolytic therapy for lower extremity deep venous thrombosis (DVT).

1. Insert a 22-gauge intercath into the dorsalis vein of the affected limb. Inject contrast under fluoroscopy to confirm no extravasation of contrast. Connect the catheter with the extension tube and 3-way stopcock to facilitate infusion. Cover the insertion site with an op-site dressing.

2. Place a velcro tourniquet at the malleolar level in order to compress the saphenous vein and to improve the contrast flow in the deep system. A baseline venogram is obtained with a total of 50–200 mL of low osmolar contrast, depending on the renal function.

3. Urokinase (1,000–2,000 U/mL of normal saline or D5W) can be given at 100,000–200,000 U/h via the pedal catheter. When catheter-directed infusion is used simultaneously, the divided doses can be given through each catheter.

4. Unfractionated heparin should be given as a bolus and infusion in the urokinase line (eg, 5,000 U bolus plus 500–1,000 U/h), rather than systemically. PTT should be maintained between 50 and 90 seconds.

5. A venogram should be repeated every 12–24 hours. Thrombolysis is considered successful and should be terminated if there is significant improvement on the venogram or symptomatic improvement. This may occur after 24–48 hours of infusion. A decrease in edema can be monitored with tape measurement of the leg circumference.

6. The patient should be placed on an iris mattress and IM injections should be avoided. The patient should be kept NPO or clear liquid only during the infusion. Reglan (10 mg q4h) can be given for nausea during urokinase infusion.

7. After termination of urokinase, the patient should be maintained on heparin until an INR of 2–3 is reached with warfarin administration.

Table 10. Flow-directed and catheter-directed thrombolysis for deep venous thrombosis (DVT). DSW: 5% dextrose in water; INR: international normalization ratio; IM: intramuscular; NPO: nothing by mouth; PTT: partial thromboplastin time.

thrombolysis included an 11% transfusion rate and a 16% incidence of minor bleeding. The intracranial hemorrhage rate was 0.2%. At 1 year, the primary patency rate was 80% and valvular reflux occurred in 28% of patients in whom complete thrombolysis was achieved. Thrombolytic therapy was most effective for acute thrombosis (<3 days); its effectiveness decreased markedly when the thrombus was old (>4 weeks).

The incidence of hemorrhage depends on the dosing regimen, type of thrombolytic used, duration of therapy, and dosing of concomitant anticoagulation. Other complications associated with thrombolysis include PE, infections, and valvular incompetence during catheter manipulation. IVC filter placement may be considered in patients with limited cardiopulmonary reserve; however, anticoagulation is still the first treatment of choice. Mechanical thrombectomy (eg, AngioJet, Possis, Minneapolis, MN, USA) offers rapid relief of clot burden and can improve the efficacy of thrombolysis. It may be considered when thrombolytic therapy is contraindicated.

The main advantages of catheter-directed thrombolysis include the following:

- it allows angiographic assessment of the effectiveness of thrombolytic therapy (eg, transpopliteal venography to assess deep venous blood flow and their collaterals)

- it facilitates the use of adjunctive mechanical devices if pharmacologic treatment gives a suboptimal result

Angioplasty and stent placement may be useful in treating mechanical venous obstruction or extrinsic compression. In particular, endovascular interventions are particularly useful in the management of postthrombotic venous stenosis, which is the result of failed recanalization, leading to subsequent fibrotic organization of occlusive thrombus and fixed stenosis. Self-expanding elgiloy or nitinol stents are useful because: (a) they allow passive over-sizing without a major risk of perforation while ensuring proper apposition and a lower risk of migration; and (b) they conform better to the irregular and diseased vessel wall as compared with conventional self-expanding stents, even within segments of vessels that are under frequent stretching and compression. Nevertheless, stent placement at the common femoral or popliteal veins is best avoided unless flow-limiting dissection or significant residual stenosis is present. After endovascular interventions, anticoagulation with warfarin should be given as scheduled for DVT treatment, and duplex ultrasound should be performed at 3, 6, and 12 months. Surgical reconstruction is indicated if endovascular recanalization fails amongst patients with highly symptomatic iliocaval obstruction.

Acute IVC thrombosis

This is most commonly due to extension of iliofemoral thrombosis, but other considerations include a hypercoagulable state, thrombosis of the IVC filter, abdominal or pelvic malignancy, abdominal aortic aneurysm, retroperitoneal fibrosis, or multiple catheterizations. Major sequelae of IVC thrombosis include lethal PE, venous gangrene, nephrotic syndrome, and acute renal failure secondary to renal vein thrombosis. Catheter-directed thrombolytic therapy with or without percutaneous mechanical thrombectomy is the treatment of choice.

Infrapopliteal DVT

Infrapopliteal thrombosis alone rarely causes PE unless proximal extension occurs. Thrombophlebitis can be treated conservatively with anticoagulation, leg elevation, and anti-inflammatory agents for pain.

Upper extremity DVT

Upper extremity venous thrombosis is much less common than lower extremity thrombosis. Patients who first experience DVT in the upper extremities have prior or chronic catheter or pacemaker lead placement, are in a hypercoagulable state (eg, malignancy), or have extrinsic compression due to an abnormal mass (eg, lymphoma). Ultrasonography can accurately diagnose DVT in the axillary, subclavian, brachiocephalic, and jugular veins. Color Doppler and waveform analysis can also identify more central obstructions, but CT of the chest is the imaging modality of choice in central venous obstruction. MRI and venography can also be used for diagnosis, but the availability of ultrasonography makes them rarely needed.

Treatment of upper extremity DVT should begin with removal of the precipitating factors (eg, indwelling catheters, pacemaker leads, venous stenosis). If a central venous catheter is causing venous obstruction, removal of the catheter followed by anticoagulation is usually all that is required for complete resolution of the signs and symptoms; a venogram or angioplasty is rarely indicated (see **Venous stenosis** section). Acute DVT without mechanical obstruction should be treated conservatively with anticoagulation alone, and thrombolysis should be reserved for extreme cases.

Pulmonary embolism

About 25% of symptomatic DVT cases are complicated by PE. Depending on the size of the embolus, the presentation of acute PE can vary from no symptoms to pleuritic chest pain, dyspnea, palpitations, syncope, or circulatory arrest. Details of the standard investigational approach have been described elsewhere [24]. In many institutions, this includes a ventilation–perfusion scan and ultrasound Doppler of the leg veins, while some institutions use spiral CT angiography as the initial approach. Measurement of serum D-dimer is highly sensitive for thrombotic events and a negative test is useful in ruling out DVT/PE in the emergency room [25].

Pulmonary angiography remains the gold standard when the results of these tests are inconclusive. Because clots may dissolve rapidly, the procedure should be undertaken without unnecessary delay. In the largest PE study to date, which involved 1,111 patients undergoing pulmonary angiography (PIOPED [Prospective Investigation of Pulmonary Embolism Diagnosis]), old age was the sole predictor for complications (eg, renal dysfunction) after pulmonary angiography – pulmonary arterial pressures and the volume of contrast used did not predict adverse outcomes, in contrast to conventional belief [26]. However, adequate hydration and use of the minimal volume of contrast necessary for performing a pulmonary angiogram are still key to performing the procedure safely.

Before performing a pulmonary angiogram, ultrasound duplex should be reviewed in order to avoid entering a vein that could potentially mobilize a thrombus. Venous access can be established in the common femoral, internal jugular, or antecubital veins, using a 5- to 7-Fr catheter (eg, angulated pigtail, Grollman catheter, or Berman catheter). Selective angiography can be started from each of the right and the left main pulmonary arteries in the anteroposterior view using power-injection of low osmolar contrast (20 cc/s for a total of 40 cc). Digital subtraction arteriography with breath-holding is preferred. Selective lobar or segmental pulmonary angiography can be performed by exchanging the pigtail catheter with a multipurpose or hockey-stick catheter through a 0.035-inch exchange guidewire. Various projections (often assisted by ipsilateral angulation) and magnified views may be needed to adequately exclude a thrombus. Acute PE may appear as an intraluminal filling defect that is partially surrounded with contrast material, abrupt vessel cut-off, lobar or segmental hypoperfusion, or pruning of the vessels, associated with pulmonary oligemia. Pulmonary emboli are usually present bilaterally, and more often involve the lower than the upper lobes.

Once the diagnosis of PE is established, the patient can be anticoagulated using unfractionated heparin or low molecular weight heparin, until an INR of 2–3 is achieved with warfarin (see **Treatment of DVT** section). Fondaparinux, a factor Xa inhibitor, given subcutaneously once a day (5–10 mg, depending on body weight) without the need for monitoring, is as effective as unfractionated heparin during the initial treatment for PE [27].

Hemodynamically significant PE is evidenced by profound hypoxemia, hypotension, circulatory arrest or electromechanical dissociation, right ventricular dysfunction, or pulmonary hypertension. Therefore, transthoracic echocardiography is a useful tool for risk stratification for PE with normal arterial pressure. The elevation of some serum biochemical markers (eg, troponin, b-type natriuretic peptides) is a predictor for adverse outcomes after PE, and these biochemical markers may become important for risk stratification [28–34]. Thrombolytic therapy, either systemic or catheter-based, should be considered in case of massive or submassive PE [35–49]. Patients should first be assessed for contraindications to thrombolytic administration. During administration of lytic therapy, either systemic or catheter directed, continuous monitoring for signs of bleeding (headaches, acute mental status change, gastrointestinal bleeding, and cutaneous enlargement of hematoma or hemarthrosis) is crucial to the success of the treatment.

Previous randomized studies have not detected any significant clinical differences between bolus (50 mg over 10 minutes) and infusion (100 mg over 2 hours) of alteplase (recombinant tissue plasminogen activator [rt-PA]) [38–50]; between rt-PA and streptokinase [51]; or between rt-PA and urokinase [52]. In patients with massive or submassive PE, concomitant systemic infusion of alteplase (rt-PA, 100 mg given over 2 hours) plus unfractionated heparin can rapidly reduce pulmonary arterial pressure and right ventricular dysfunction, and can lower the incidence of clinical deterioration by 60% during index hospitalization as compared with heparin alone [43,44,46,49]. In contrast to myocardial infarction, a 2-week time window is available for the treatment of PE [53,54].

When a catheter-directed thrombolytic is used, the pigtail catheter with side-holes should be positioned within the proximal segment of the clot. If bilateral PE is present, the catheter can be positioned in the main pulmonary artery, or two catheters can be used with one in each of the right and left pulmonary arteries (see **Figure 3** and **Table 11**) [48,55]. Pulmonary arterial pressure and arterial oxygen saturation should be monitored continuously to detect clinical improvement. Pulmonary angiography should be repeated within the first 4–8 hours of thrombolytic administration. Thrombolysis should be terminated when clinical or angiographic improvement is evident, or if clinically significant bleeding occurs. Balloon angioplasty may achieve rapid fragmentation and distal dispersion of clots, and may complement the use of thrombolysis [55]. Thrombectomy (eg, AngioJet [Possis, Minneapolis, MN, USA], HYDROLYSER [Cordis]) is technically feasible and may reduce thrombus burden, particularly when done within 3 weeks [56]; however, because of the large diameter of the pulmonary arteries and the extensive thrombus load and distribution, there may be limited clinical benefit with thrombectomy when the pulmonary embolus is located in the proximal artery.

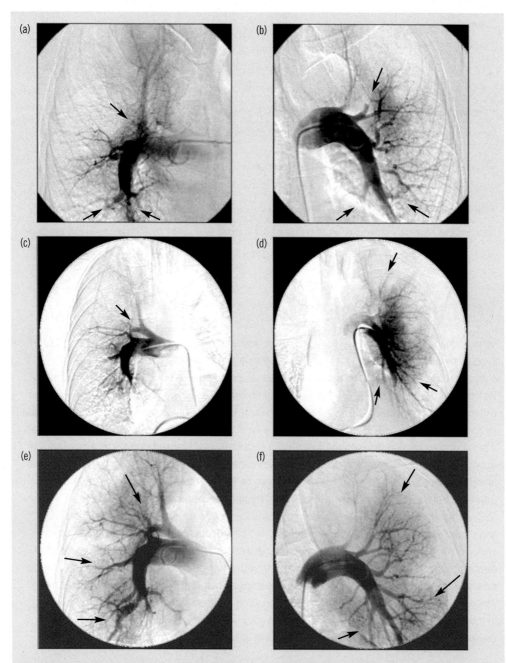

Figure 3. Catheter-directed thrombolysis for pulmonary embolism (PE). A 78-year-old female was put on warfarin after her first presentation with PE. She was diagnosed with antiphospholipid antibody syndrome. Three months later, she presented with acute flank pain and hypotension, secondary to spontaneous bleeding of one of the renal arterioles (international normalization ratio [INR] 1.6); this was successfully treated with microembolization using detachable coils. Warfarin was stopped for 4 days and then restarted. Nine days later, she presented with syncope and hypotension (INR 1.7). Right heart catheterization confirmed a pulmonary arterial pressure of 60/36 mm Hg and a pulmonary capillary wedge pressure of 8 mm Hg. Pulmonary angiography revealed the presence of clots in the right upper, mid, and lower lobes, as well as in the left upper lobes (arrows, **Figures a** and **b**). A urokinase infusion of 1,500 U/h was given through a 6-Fr pigtail catheter. The patient tolerated this well, without bleeding complications. During the subsequent 12 hours, her systemic pressure increased from 90 to 120 mm Hg and her arterial saturation returned to normal. A repeat angiogram showed improvement in the angiographic appearance of the pulmonary arteries (arrows, **Figures c** and **d**). Afterwards, she was kept on warfarin, and her INR was maintained at 3–4. **Figures e** and **f** show the pulmonary angiograms 9 months later.

Systemic infusion:

- alteplase 100 mg over 2 hours, **or**

- urokinase 4,400 U/kg bolus over 10 minutes followed by 4,400 U/kg/h for 12–24 hours, **or**

- streptokinase 250,000 U over 30 minutes followed by 100,000 U/h for 24 hours

- **plus** unfractionated heparin (eg, 5,000 U bolus and 1,000 U/h) to maintain PTT 50–90 seconds

Catheter-directed infusion through one catheter positioned in the main pulmonary artery or a divided dose through one catheter in each of the right and left pulmonary arteries:

- urokinase 250,000 U/h for 2 hours followed by 100,000 U/h for 12–24 hours, **or**

- alteplase 10 mg bolus followed by 20 mg/h for 2 hours

- **plus** unfractionated heparin infusion in the thrombolytic line to maintain PTT at 50–90 seconds

Fibrinogen level should be monitored q4–6h; thrombolytic infusion should be stopped if the fibrinogen level drops by >60%.

Table 11. Recommended thrombolytic regimens for the treatment of pulmonary embolism. PTT: partial thromboplastin time. Adapted from references [35–46,48,49].

Venous stenosis

Venous stenosis can manifest with swelling, pain, and superficial varicosities. Clinically significant venous stenosis is much more common in the upper than in the lower extremities. The most commonly affected sites include the axillary, brachial, cephalic, or brachiocephalic veins, or the SVC. Venous stenosis is due to intimal hyperplasia and fibrosis secondary to placement of central venous catheters, pacemaker leads, hemodialysis catheters, prior radiation, trauma, or extrinsic compression by musculoskeletal structures. Chronic intimal injury of the subclavian or axillary veins can occur as a result of compression between the first rib and costoclavicular ligament during strenuous shoulder activity, resulting in venous thrombosis (Paget–Schroetter disease, "effort" thrombosis, or the venous form of thoracic outlet syndrome) [57]. SVC syndrome is a life-threatening condition secondary to extrinsic compression or intrinsic obstruction (eg, thrombotic occlusion) of the SVC. Patients with SVC syndrome usually complain of a rapidly progressive headache and swelling in the head, neck, and upper extremities; jugular venous distention and plethora in the affected parts of the body are obvious. If left untreated, the patient may further develop confusion and obtundation as a result of cerebral hypoperfusion. Nearly half of the patients with a hemodialysis arteriovenous fistula develop subclavian vein stenosis due to prior temporary hemolysis catheter insertion and subsequent high venous outflow that propagates intimal hyperplasia and exaggerates the pressure gradient even in moderate stenosis. Iliofemoral venous stenosis may be due to extrinsic compression (eg, pelvic malignancy, retroperitoneal fibrosis), fibrotic healing after surgery, or irradiation (see **Figure 4**).

Treatment for upper extremity venous stenosis

Balloon angioplasty is the therapy of choice for symptomatic venous stenosis. Venous access can be established via the antecubital vein, dialysis fistula, or common femoral vein. Conservative balloon sizing should be adopted at the start because these vessels have less muscular tissue than the arterial system. Fibrotic stenosis that fails to yield to balloon angioplasty may be treated with cutting balloons or directional atherectomy. Stents should be used when significant residual

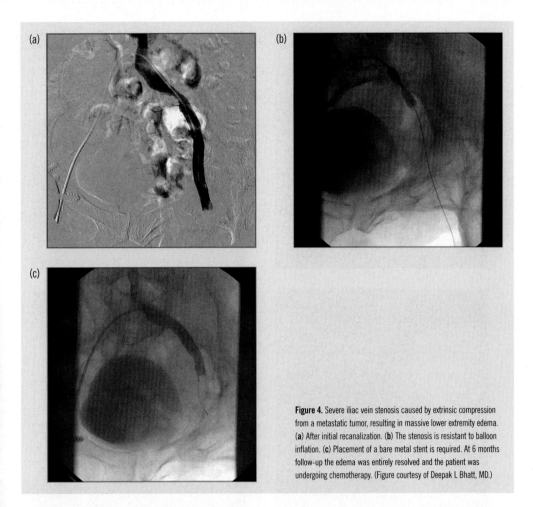

Figure 4. Severe iliac vein stenosis caused by extrinsic compression from a metastatic tumor, resulting in massive lower extremity edema. (**a**) After initial recanalization. (**b**) The stenosis is resistant to balloon inflation. (**c**) Placement of a bare metal stent is required. At 6 months follow-up the edema was entirely resolved and the patient was undergoing chemotherapy. (Figure courtesy of Deepak L Bhatt, MD.)

angiographic stenosis or flow-limiting stenosis is present. Self-expanding stents (eg, WALLSTENT [Boston Scientific, Natick, MA, USA] or SMART [Cordis]) may be used for lesions located in highly mobile sites. The nominal size of the self-expanding stent should be 1–2 mm above the estimated reference diameter of the vein to ensure proper apposition and to minimize the risk of stent migration (8–12 mm for subclavian or axillary veins, 14–20 mm for SVC). Resolution of symptoms (eg, cyanosis, swelling, pain) begins almost instantaneously after successful revascularization. Stent placement across the ostia of other venous drainage should be avoided if possible. Stents are relatively contraindicated when the lesion is due to thoracic outlet syndrome.

Fibrotic adhesion of permanent pacemaker or defibrillator leads can occasionally result in venous obstruction (causing swelling and pain in the arm) or SVC syndrome, depending on the location of the obstruction. Traditionally, treatment involves surgical explantation of the device and the leads and replacement of the vessel with an artificial conduit. The feasibility of an endovascular strategy has been demonstrated [58]. First, a percutaneous telescoping excimer laser sheath with countering force is used to remove the leads (see **Figure 5**). The lumen can then be enlarged with standard balloon angioplasty and stent placement procedures. A new set of permanent

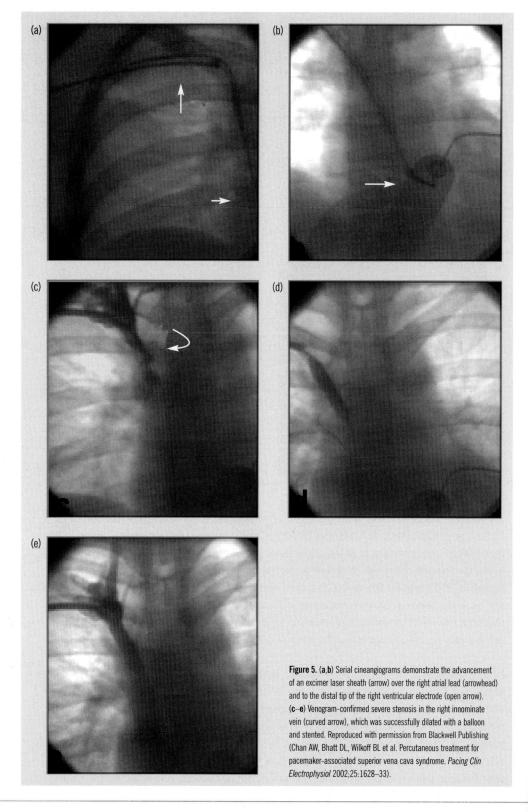

Figure 5. (a,b) Serial cineangiograms demonstrate the advancement of an excimer laser sheath (arrow) over the right atrial lead (arrowhead) and to the distal tip of the right ventricular electrode (open arrow). **(c–e)** Venogram-confirmed severe stenosis in the right innominate vein (curved arrow), which was successfully dilated with a balloon and stented. Reproduced with permission from Blackwell Publishing (Chan AW, Bhatt DL, Wilkoff BL et al. Percutaneous treatment for pacemaker-associated superior vena cava syndrome. *Pacing Clin Electrophysiol* 2002;25:1628–33).

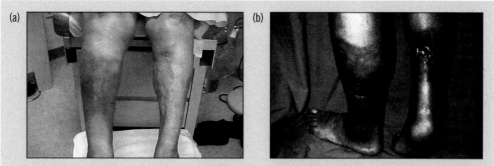

Figure 6. (a) Hyperpigmentation, chronic swelling, and varicose veins are common findings of postthrombotic syndrome. (b) Lipodermatosclerosis (trophic skin changes, hyperpigmentation, nonhealing ulceration, and fibrotic scarring) as a late sequela of postthrombotic syndrome.

pacemaker leads may then be implanted within the treated venous vessels. Most operators would favor anticoagulation with warfarin for a few weeks to a few months, with or without antiplatelet therapy (aspirin and clopidogrel).

Treatment for lower extremity venous stenosis

Symptomatic venous stenosis of the iliofemoral vein can be treated with endovascular techniques. Venous access can be established via the right internal jugular vein, ipsilateral popliteal vein, or contralateral femoral vein. Balloon predilation should be performed and self-expanding stents should be used, followed by optimal expansion of the stent by matching the diameter of the vein with a postdilating balloon catheter (usually 10–14 mm diameter). Similar to endovascular revascularization of the upper extremities, most physicians favor short-term warfarin, with or without dual antiplatelet therapy, after stent placement. Close surveillance with duplex ultrasound is recommended to assess patency within the first year.

Venous valvular insufficiency and PTS

PTS or postphlebitic syndrome, manifesting as pain, edema, hyperpigmentation, and ulceration, typically develops in 29%–79% of patients with lower extremity DVT. Erythema and cutaneous thickening that mimics cellulitis typically occurs on the medial malleolus of the lower leg. Later on, aching of the leg, venous varicosities, and chronic cutaneous lipodermatosclerosis (consisting of trophic skin changes, hyperpigmentation, nonhealing ulceration, and fibrotic scarring) ensue. At the end, the skin of the affected lower leg may become fibrosed and the ankle circumference becomes narrowed; the ankle may also become fixated (see **Figure 6**). These severe manifestations are usually the consequence of venous hypertension as a result of valvular reflux and persistent venous obstruction (see **Figure 7**). In fact, DVT is the main cause of venous valvular insufficiency. A number of studies have demonstrated that the rate of recanalization and recurrent thrombotic events are important determinants of valvular insufficiency. Although superficial, deep, or perforating veins, or combinations, can be involved in the development of postthrombotic valvular insufficiency, popliteal and posterior tibial vein valvular incompetence are particularly important in the delayed development of trophic skin changes and ulceration as part of PTS.

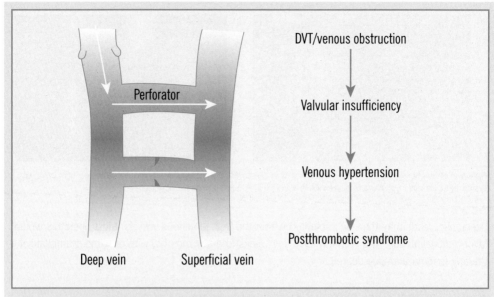

Figure 7. The mechanism of postthrombotic syndrome. Venous obstruction leads to valvular insufficiency, and subsequent venous hypertension and postthrombotic syndrome. DVT: deep venous thrombosis.

The principle of PTS management revolves around lowering venous pressure. This is accomplished by elevating the affected limb and giving external limb support, such as elastic support stockings. The patient has to understand that successful care can only be achieved through individual effort, so keeping the affected limb elevated and wearing the elastic stockings should become part of their lives. However, in patients with suspected peripheral arterial disease, an ankle–brachial index (ABI) exam is indicated. An elastic stocking is relatively contraindicated in an individual with an ABI <0.6. While the benefit of an elastic stocking may still outweigh its risk in these patients, the decision of whether to use this therapy should be individualized.

Therapeutic considerations for valvular insufficiency may be indicated on the basis of the site and severity of valvular reflux. For example, a patient with severe valvular reflux in the superficial system without involvement of the deep system may be adequately treated with either sclerotherapy, surgical vein stripping, or endovascular ablation; patients with deep vein reflux would be better served with surgical deep venous reconstruction. The VNUS Closure device (VNUS Medical Technologies, Sunnyvale, CA, USA) is a percutaneous catheter-based system that delivers radiofrequency current and causes permanent obliteration of the long saphenous vein [59–63]. When compared with surgical stripping for treating varicosity of the long saphenous vein, this technique may provide a shorter recovery period and may be more cost-effective [62]. Patients with perforator vein incompetency near the site of a venous ulcer may be best treated by interruption of these veins via sclerotherapy or endovascular therapy.

References

1. Anderson FA Jr, Wheeler HB, Goldberg RJ, et al. A population-based perspective of the hospital incidence and case-fatality rates of deep vein thrombosis and pulmonary embolism. The Worcester DVT Study. *Arch Intern Med* 1991;151:933–8.

2. Silverstein MD, Heit JA, Mohr DN, et al. Trends in the incidence of deep vein thrombosis and pulmonary embolism: a 25-year population-based study. *Arch Intern Med* 1998;158:585–93.

3. Goldhaber SZ. Pulmonary embolism. *N Engl J Med* 1998;339:93–104.

4. Goldhaber SZ, Visani L, De Rosa M. Acute pulmonary embolism: clinical outcomes in the International Cooperative Pulmonary Embolism Registry (ICOPER). *Lancet* 1999;353:1386–9.

5. Heit JA, Mohr DN, Silverstein MD, et al. Predictors of recurrence after deep vein thrombosis and pulmonary embolism: a population-based cohort study. *Arch Intern Med* 2000;160:761–8.

6. Mustafa S, Stein PD, Patel KC, et al. Upper extremity deep venous thrombosis. *Chest* 2003;123:1953–6.

7. Seligsohn U, Lubetsky A. Genetic susceptibility to venous thrombosis. *N Engl J Med* 2001;344:1222–31.

8. Weinmann EE, Salzman EW. Deep-vein thrombosis. *N Engl J Med* 1994;331:1630–41.

9. Rosendaal FR. Risk factors for venous thrombotic disease. *Thromb Haemost* 1999;82:610–9.

10. Deitcher SR, Gomes MP. Hypercoagulable state testing and malignancy screening following venous thromboembolic events. *Vasc Med* 2003;8:33–46.

11. Deitcher SR, Caiola E, Jaffer A. Demystifying two common genetic predispositions to venous thrombosis. *Cleve Clin J Med* 2000;67:825–6, 829, 833–6.

12. Anderson FA Jr, Spencer FA. Risk factors for venous thromboembolism. *Circulation* 2003;107(23 Suppl. 1):I9–16.

13. Emmerich J, Rosendaal FR, Cattaneo M, et al. Combined effect of factor V Leiden and prothrombin 20210A on the risk of venous thromboembolism – pooled analysis of 8 case-control studies including 2310 cases and 3204 controls. Study Group for Pooled-Analysis in Venous Thromboembolism. *Thromb Haemost* 2001;86:809–16.

14. den Heijer M, Koster T, Blom HJ, et al. Hyperhomocysteinemia as a risk factor for deep-vein thrombosis. *N Engl J Med* 1996;334:759–62.

15. Ridker PM, Goldhaber SZ, Danielson E, et al. Long-term, low-intensity warfarin therapy for the prevention of recurrent venous thromboembolism. *N Engl J Med* 2003;348:1425–34.

16. Kearon C, Ginsberg JS, Kovacs MJ, et al. Comparison of low-intensity warfarin therapy with conventional-intensity warfarin therapy for long-term prevention of recurrent venous thromboembolism. *N Engl J Med* 2003;349:631–9.

17. Francis CW, Berkowitz SD, Comp PC, et al. Comparison of ximelagatran with warfarin for the prevention of venous thromboembolism after total knee replacement. *N Engl J Med* 2003;349:1703–12.

18. Lee AY, Levine MN, Baker RI, et al. Low-molecular-weight heparin versus a coumarin for the prevention of recurrent venous thromboembolism in patients with cancer. *N Engl J Med* 2003;349:146–53.

19. Neuerburg JM, Handt S, Beckert K, et al. Percutaneous retrieval of the Tulip vena cava filter: feasibility, short- and long-term changes – an experimental study in dogs. *Cardiovasc Intervent Radiol* 2001;24:418–23.

20. Millward SF, Bhargava A, Aquino J Jr, et al. Gunther Tulip filter: preliminary clinical experience with retrieval. *J Vasc Interv Radiol* 2000;11:75–82.

21. Millward SF, Oliva VL, Bell SD, et al. Gunther Tulip Retrievable Vena Cava Filter: results from the Registry of the Canadian Interventional Radiology Association. *J Vasc Interv Radiol* 2001;12:1053–8.

22. Decousus H, Leizorovicz A, Parent F, et al. A clinical trial of vena caval filters in the prevention of pulmonary embolism in patients with proximal deep-vein thrombosis. Prevention du Risque d'Embolie Pulmonaire par Interruption Cave Study Group. *N Engl J Med* 1998;338:409–16.

23. Mewissen MW, Seabrook GR, Meissner MH, et al. Catheter-directed thrombolysis for lower extremity deep venous thrombosis: report of a national multicenter registry. *Radiology* 1999;211:39–49.

24. Fedullo PF, Tapson VF. Clinical practice. The evaluation of suspected pulmonary embolism. *N Engl J Med* 2003;349:1247–56.

25. Wells PS, Anderson DR, Rodger M, et al. Evaluation of D-dimer in the diagnosis of suspected deep-vein thrombosis. *N Engl J Med* 2003;349:1227–35.

26. Stein PD, Athanasoulis C, Alavi A, et al. Complications and validity of pulmonary angiography in acute pulmonary embolism. *Circulation* 1992;85:462–8.

27. Buller HR, Davidson BL, Decousus H, et al. Subcutaneous fondaparinux versus intravenous unfractionated heparin in the initial treatment of pulmonary embolism. *N Engl J Med* 2003;349:1695–702.

28. Kucher N, Wallmann D, Carone A, et al. Incremental prognostic value of troponin I and echocardiography in patients with acute pulmonary embolism. *Eur Heart J* 2003;24:1651–6.

29. Horlander KT, Leeper KV. Troponin levels as a guide to treatment of pulmonary embolism. *Curr Opin Pulm Med* 2003;9:374–7.

30. Mehta NJ, Jani K, Khan IA. Clinical usefulness and prognostic value of elevated cardiac troponin I levels in acute pulmonary embolism. *Am Heart J* 2003;145:821–5.
31. Konstantinides S, Geibel A, Olschewski M, et al. Importance of cardiac troponins I and T in risk stratification of patients with acute pulmonary embolism. *Circulation* 2002;106:1263–8.
32. ten Wolde M, Tulevski II, Mulder JW, et al. Brain natriuretic peptide as a predictor of adverse outcome in patients with pulmonary embolism. *Circulation* 2003;107:2082–4.
33. Nagaya N, Ando M, Oya H, et al. Plasma brain natriuretic peptide as a noninvasive marker for efficacy of pulmonary thromboendarterectomy. *Ann Thorac Surg* 2002;74:180–4; discussion 184.
34. Tulevski II, Mulder BJ, van Veldhuisen DJ. Utility of a BNP as a marker for RV dysfunction in acute pulmonary embolism. *J Am Coll Cardiol* 2002;39:2080.
35. Ly B, Arnesen H, Eie H, et al. A controlled clinical trial of streptokinase and heparin in the treatment of major pulmonary embolism. *Acta Med Scand* 1978;203:465–70.
36. Verstraete M, Miller GA, Bounameaux H, et al. Intravenous and intrapulmonary recombinant tissue-type plasminogen activator in the treatment of acute massive pulmonary embolism. *Circulation* 1988;77:353–60.
37. Molina JE, Hunter DW, Yedlicka JW, et al. Thrombolytic therapy for postoperative pulmonary embolism. *Am J Surg* 1992;163:375–80; discussion 380–1.
38. Diehl JL, Meyer G, Igual J, et al. Effectiveness and safety of bolus administration of alteplase in massive pulmonary embolism. *Am J Cardiol* 1992;70:1477–80.
39. Gonzalez-Juanatey JR, Valdes L, Amaro A, et al. Treatment of massive pulmonary thromboembolism with low intrapulmonary dosages of urokinase. Short-term angiographic and hemodynamic evolution. *Chest* 1992;102:341–6.
40. Vujic I, Young JW, Gobien RP, et al. Massive pulmonary embolism: treatment with full heparinization and topical low-dose streptokinase. *Radiology* 1983;148:671–5.
41. Goldhaber SZ, Vaughan DE, Markis JE, et al. Acute pulmonary embolism treated with tissue plasminogen activator. *Lancet* 1986;2:886–9.
42. Goldhaber SZ, Kessler CM, Heit J, et al. Randomised controlled trial of recombinant tissue plasminogen activator versus urokinase in the treatment of acute pulmonary embolism. *Lancet* 1988;2:293–8.
43. Levine M, Hirsh J, Weitz J, et al. A randomized trial of a single bolus dosage regimen of recombinant tissue plasminogen activator in patients with acute pulmonary embolism. *Chest* 1990;98:1473–9.
44. Goldhaber SZ, Haire WD, Feldstein ML, et al. Alteplase versus heparin in acute pulmonary embolism: randomised trial assessing right-ventricular function and pulmonary perfusion. *Lancet* 1993;341:507–11.
45. Jerjes-Sanchez C, Ramirez-Rivera A, de Lourdes Garcia M, et al. Streptokinase and heparin versus heparin alone in massive pulmonary embolism: a randomized controlled trial. *J Thromb Thrombolysis* 1995;2:227–9.
46. Konstantinides S, Tiede N, Geibel A, et al. Comparison of alteplase versus heparin for resolution of major pulmonary embolism. *Am J Cardiol* 1998;82:966–70.
47. Goldhaber SZ. Integration of catheter thrombectomy into our armamentarium to treat acute pulmonary embolism. *Chest* 1998;114:1237–8.
48. De Gregorio MA, Gimeno MJ, Mainar A, et al. Mechanical and enzymatic thrombolysis for massive pulmonary embolism. *J Vasc Interv Radiol* 2002;13:163–9.
49. Konstantinides S, Geibel A, Heusel G, et al. Heparin plus alteplase compared with heparin alone in patients with submassive pulmonary embolism. *N Engl J Med* 2002;347:1143–50.
50. Goldhaber SZ, Agnelli G, Levine MN. Reduced dose bolus alteplase vs conventional alteplase infusion for pulmonary embolism thrombolysis. An international multicenter randomized trial. The Bolus Alteplase Pulmonary Embolism Group. *Chest* 1994;106:718–24.
51. Ellis DA, Neville E, Hall RJ. Subacute massive pulmonary embolism treated with plasminogen and streptokinase. *Thorax* 1983;38:903–7.
52. Goldhabert SZ, Kessler CM, Heit JA, et al. Recombinant tissue-type plasminogen activator versus a novel dosing regimen of urokinase in acute pulmonary embolism: a randomized controlled multicenter trial. *J Am Coll Cardiol* 1992;20:24–30.
53. Goldhaber SZ. A contemporary approach to thrombolytic therapy for pulmonary embolism. *Vasc Med* 2000;5:115–23.
54. Daniels LB, Parker JA, Patel SR, et al. Relation of duration of symptoms with response to thrombolytic therapy in pulmonary embolism. *Am J Cardiol* 1997;80:184–8.
55. Fava M, Loyola S, Flores P, et al. Mechanical fragmentation and pharmacologic thrombolysis in massive pulmonary embolism. *J Vasc Interv Radiol* 1997;8:261–6.
56. Fava M, Loyola S, Huete I. Massive pulmonary embolism: treatment with the hydrolyser thrombectomy catheter. *J Vasc Interv Radiol* 2000;11:1159–64.
57. DiFelice GS, Paletta GA Jr, Phillips BB, et al. Effort thrombosis in the elite throwing athlete. *Am J Sports Med* 2002;30:708–12.
58. Chan AW, Bhatt DL, Wilkoff BL, et al. Percutaneous treatment for pacemaker-associated superior vena cava syndrome. *Pacing Clin Electrophysiol* 2002;25:1628–33.

59. Sybrandy JE, Wittens CH. Initial experiences in endovenous treatment of saphenous vein reflux. *J Vasc Surg* 2002;36:1207–12.
60. Fassiadis N, Kianifard B, Holdstock JM, et al. A novel approach to the treatment of recurrent varicose veins. *Int Angiol* 2002;21:275–6.
61. Fassiadis N, Kianifard B, Holdstock JM, et al. Ultrasound changes at the saphenofemoral junction and in the long saphenous vein during the first year after VNUS closure. *Int Angiol* 2002;21:272–4.
62. Rautio T, Ohinmaa A, Perala J, et al. Endovenous obliteration versus conventional stripping operation in the treatment of primary varicose veins: a randomized controlled trial with comparison of the costs. *J Vasc Surg* 2002;35:958–65.
63. Chandler JG, Pichot O, Sessa C, et al. Defining the role of extended saphenofemoral junction ligation: a prospective comparative study. *J Vasc Surg* 2000;32:941–53.

Abbreviations

4S	Scandinavian Simvastatin Survival Study
AAA	abdominal aortic aneurysm
ABC	airway–breathing–circulation
ABI	ankle–brachial index
ACA	anterior cerebral artery
ACAS	Asymptomatic Carotid Atherosclerosis Study
ACE	angiotensin-converting enzyme
ACEI	angiotensin-converting enzyme inhibitor
ACS	acute coronary syndromes
ACT	activated clotting time
ADP	adenosine diphosphate
AHA	American Heart Association
AICA	anterior inferior cerebellar artery
APC-R	activated protein C resistance
ATLANTIS	Alteplase Thrombolysis for Acute Noninterventional Therapy in Ischemic Stroke
AV	arteriovenous
AVM	arteriovenous malformation
BA	basilar artery
BOA	Bypass Oral Anticoagulants or Aspirin
CAMPER	Clopidogrel and Aspirin in the Management of Peripheral Endovascular Revascularization
CAPRIE	Clopidogrel versus Aspirin in Patients at Risk of Ischemic Events
CASPAR	Clopidogrel and Acetylsalicylic Acid in Bypass Surgery for Peripheral Arterial Disease
CAVATAS	Carotid and Vertebral Artery Transluminal Angioplasty Study
CBF	cerebral blood flow
CCA	common carotid artery
CEA	carotid endarterectomy
CFA	common femoral artery
CHARISMA	Clopidogrel for High Atherothrombotic Risk and Ischemic Stabilization, Management, and Avoidance
CI	confidence interval
CRS	captopril renal scanning
CT	computed tomography
DFA	deep femoral artery
DSA	digital subtraction angiography
DSB	detachable silicone balloon
DVT	deep venous thrombosis
ECA	external carotid artery
ECASS	European Cooperative Acute Stroke Study
EPD	emboli protection devices
ESRD	end-stage renal disease
EVAR	endovascular abdominal aortic aneurysm repair

FDA	Food and Drug Administration
FMD	fibromuscular dysplasia
GDC	Guglielmi detachable coil
GP	glycoprotein
HOPE	Heart Outcomes Prevention Evaluation
HPS	Heart Protection Study
IA	intra-arterial
ICA	internal carotid artery
ICH	intracranial hemorrhage
Ig	immunoglobulin
IMA	inferior mesenteric artery
INR	international normalization ratio
IS	ischemic stroke
IV	intravenous
IVC	inferior vena cava
IVT	Interventional Therapeutics
IVUS	intravascular ultrasound
JR	Judkins right
LAO	left anterior oblique
LIMA	left internal mammary artery
LMWH	low molecular weight heparin
MAP	mean arterial pressure
MCA	middle cerebral artery
MRA	magnetic resonance angiography
MRI	magnetic resonance imaging
NASCET	North American Symptomatic Carotid Endarterectomy Trial
NBCA	n-butyl cyanoacrylate
NINDS	National Institutes of Neurological Disorders and Stroke
OCP	oral contraceptive pill
PA	posteroanterior
PCA	posterior cerebral artery
PCI	percutaneous coronary intervention
PE	pulmonary embolism
PEI	percutaneous endovascular intervention
PICA	posterior inferior cerebellar artery
PICC	percutaneous inserted central catheter
PIOPED	Prospective Investigation of Pulmonary Embolism Diagnosis trial
PO	by mouth (Latin: per os)
PROACT	Prolyse in Acute Cerebral Thromboembolism
PROMPT	Platelet Receptor Antibodies in Order to Manage Peripheral Artery Thrombosis
PT	prothrombin
PTA	percutaneous transluminal angioplasty
PTCA	percutaneous transluminal coronary angioplasty

PTFE	polytetrafluoroethylene
PTS	postthrombotic syndrome
PVA	polyvinyl alcohol
PVD	peripheral vascular disease
PVR	pulse volume recording
RAO	right anterior oblique
RAS	renal artery stenosis
RDC	renal double curve
r-pro-UK	recombinant pro-urokinase
rt-PA	recombinant tissue plasminogen activator
SAH	subarachnoid hemorrhage
SAPPHIRE	Stenting and Angioplasty with Protection in Patients at High Risk for Endarterectomy
SCA	superior cerebellar artery
SCVIR	Society of Cardiovascular and Interventional Radiology
SFA	superficial femoral artery
SIROCCO	Sirolimus-coated Cordis SMART Nitinol Self-expanding Stent for the Treatment of Obstructive Superficial Femoral Artery Study
SMA	superior mesenteric artery
SPECT	single positron emission computed tomography
STAR	SCVIR Transluminal Angioplasty and Revascularization
SVC	superior vena cava
SVS	Society for Vascular Surgery
TAA	thoracic aortic aneurysm
TASC	Transatlantic Inter-Society Consensus
TBO	test balloon occlusion
TCD	transcranial Doppler ultrasound
TIA	transient ischemic attack
TIMI	Thrombolysis in Myocardial Infarction
TOF	time-of-flight
TOS	thoracic outlet syndrome
TPN	total parenteral nutrition
UFH	unfractionated heparin
USRDS	United States Renal Data System
VA	vertebral artery
VB	vertebrobasilar
VTE	venous thromboembolism
WASID	Warfarin–Aspirin Symptomatic Intracranial Disease

Index

Page numbers in **bold** refer to figures.
Page numbers in *italics* refer to tables.

A

M

N

O

P

T